Health, disease and society in Europe 1500–1800

Health, disease and society in Europe 1500–1800

A source book

edited by
Peter Elmer and Ole Peter Grell

Manchester University Press
Published in association with

The Open University

Published by Manchester University Press
Altrincham Street, Manchester M1 7JA, UK
www.manchesteruniversitypress.co.uk

British Library Cataloguing-in-Publication Data
A catalogue record for this book is available from the British Library

Library of Congress Cataloging-in-Publication Data applied for

978 0 7190 6737 2 paperback

First published 2004

First reprinted 2007

This publication forms part of an Open University course: A218 *Medicine and Society in
Europe, 1500–1930*. Details of this and other Open University courses can be obtained
from the Course Information and Advice Centre, PO Box 724, The Open University, Milton
Keynes MK7 6ZS, United Kingdom: tel. +44 (0)1908 653231, e-mail general-enquiries@open.
ac.uk. Alternatively, you may visit the Open University website at http://www.open.ac.uk
where you can learn more about the wide range of courses and packs offered at all levels
by The Open University.

Printed by Bell and Bain Ltd, Glasgow

Contents

Contents

Acknowledgements

The editors and publisher would like to thank the following for help in preparing this anthology: Rod Boroughs, Laurence Brockliss, Mark Jenner, Sachiko Kusukawa, Elizabeth Rabone, Silvia de Renzi and Andrew Wear.

The editors and publisher would also like to thank the following for permission to publish the enclosed documents: Galen, *Selected Works*, ed. P. N. Singer (Oxford, Oxford University Press, 1997), reprinted by permission of Oxford University Press. Dean Putnam Lockwood, *Ugo Benzi: Medieval Philosopher and Physician 1376–1439* (Chicago, University of Chicago Press, 1951), reprinted by permission of University of Chicago Press. Guy de Chauliac, *Great Surgery*, from *The Portable Medieval Reader*, by James Bruce Ross and Mary Martin McLaughlin, copyright 1949 by Viking Penguin, Inc. Copyright renewed © 1976 by James Bruce Ross and Mary Martin McLaughlin. Used by permission of Viking Penguin, a division of Penguin Group (USA). Jon Arrizabalaga, John Henderson and Roger French, *The Great Pox: The French Disease in Renaissance Europe* (New Haven & London, Yale University Press, 1997), reprinted by permission of Yale University Press. Doreen Evenden Nagy, *Popular Medicine in Seventeenth-Century England* © 1988. Reprinted by permission of The University of Wisconsin Press. Margaret Pelling, 'Appearance and Reality: Barber-Surgeons, the Body and Disease' in A. L. Beier and R. Finlay (eds), *London 1500–1700: The Making of the Metropolis* (London & New York, Longman, 1986), reprinted by permission of author. Nancy Siraisi, *Medicine and the Italian Universities 1250–1600* (Leiden, Boston and Cologne, Brill, 2001), reprinted by permission of Brill. Vivian Nutton, 'The Rise of Medical Humanism: Ferrara, 1464–1555', *Renaissance Studies*, 11 (1997), reprinted by permission of Blackwell Publishing. Nancy G. Siraisi, *Medieval and Early Renaissance Medicine: An Introduction to Knowledge and Practice* (Chicago & London, University of Chicago Press, 1990), reprinted by permission of University of Chicago Press. Andrew Cunningham, *The Anatomical Renaissance: The Resurrection of the Anatomical Projects of the Ancients* (Aldershot, Scolar Press, 1997), reprinted by permission of Ashgate Publishing Limited. Andreas Vesalius, *On the Fabric of the Human Body*, trans. W. F. Richardson with J. B. Carman (2 vols, San Francisco, Norman Publishing, 1999), reprinted by permission of Norman Publishing. Andrew Cunningham, 'Fabricius and the "Aristotle Project" at Padua' in A. Wear, R. K. French and I. M. Lonie (eds), *The Medical Renaissance of the Sixteenth Century* (Cambridge, Cambridge University Press, 1985), reproduced with permission of Cambridge University Press and the author. Paracelsus, *Four Treatises of Theophrastus Von Hohenheim Called Paracelsus* © 1941, H. E. Sigerist. Reprinted with permission of The Johns Hopkins University Press. Charles Webster, 'Paracelsus: Medicine as Popular Protest' in Ole Peter Grell and Andrew Cunningham (eds), *Medicine and the Reformation* (London & New York, Routledge, 1993), reprinted with permission from Routledge. Ole Peter Grell, 'The Protestant Imperative of Christian Care and Neighbourly Love' in Ole Peter Grell and Andrew Cunningham (eds), *Health Care and Poor Relief in Protestant Europe 1500–1700* (London & New York, Routledge, 1997), reprinted with permission from Routledge. Hugh Trevor-Roper, 'The Court Physician and Paracelsianism' in Vivian Nutton (ed.), *Medicine at the Courts of Europe, 1500–1837* (London & New York, Routledge, 1990), reprinted with permission from Routledge. Allen G. Debus, *The French Paracelsians: The Chemical Challenge to Medical and Scientific Tradition in Early Modern France* (Cambridge, Cambridge University Press, 1991), reproduced with permission of Cambridge University Press Publishing and the author. Carlo M. Cipolla, *Fighting the Plague in Seventeenth-Century Italy* (Madison, Wisconsin & London, University of Wisconsin Press 1981), reprinted by permission of The University of Wisconsin Press. Paul Slack, *The Impact of Plague in Tudor and Stuart England* (London, Routledge & Kegan Paul, 1985), reprinted with permission from Routledge. Katherine Park, 'Healing the Poor: Hospitals and Medical Assistance in Renaissance Florence' in Jonathan Barry and Colin Jones (eds), *Medicine and Charity Before the Welfare State* (London, Routledge, 1991), reprinted with permission from Routledge. 'An Account of the Establishment of the County Hospital at Winchester' in John Woodward, *To Do the Sick No Harm: A Study of the British Voluntary Hospital System to 1875* (London & Boston, Routledge & Kegan Paul, 1974), reprinted with permission from Routledge. *Mending Bodies, Saving Souls: A History of Hospitals* by Guenter B. Risse © 1999 by Oxford University Press, Inc. Used by permission of Oxford University Press, Inc. Andrew Cunningham, 'William Harvey: the Discovery of the Circulation of the Blood' in Roy Porter (ed.), *Man Masters Nature: 25 Centuries of Science*, reproduced with the permission of BBC Worldwide Limited. Copyright © 1987. *Treatise of Man* by René Descartes, edited and translated by Thomas Steele Hall, Cambride, Mass.: Harvard University Press, copyright © 1972 by the President and Fellows of Harvard College. Howard B. Adelmann, *Marcello Malpighi and the Evolution of Embryology* (Vols I–V). Copyright © 1966 Cornell University Press. Used by permission of the publisher, Cornell University Press. *The Letters of Dr. George Cheyne to the Countess of Huntingdon*, ed. Charles Mullett (San Marino, California, Huntington Library, 1940), reprinted with the permission of the Henry E. Huntington Library. Nicholas D. Jewson, 'Medical Knowledge and the Patronage System in 18th Century England', *Soci-*

ology 8 (1974), reprinted by permission of Sage Publications Ltd (© BSA Publications Limited, 1974). Laurence Sterne, *The Life and Opinions of Tristram Shandy, Gentleman*, ed. Ian Campbell Ross (Oxford, Clarendon Press, 1983), reprinted by permission of Oxford University Press. *The Woman Beneath the Skin: A Doctor's Patients in Eighteenth-Century Germany*, by Barbara Duden, translated by Thomas Dunlap (Cambridge, Mass.: Harvard University Press) copyright © 1991 by the President and Fellows of Harvard College. Also reprinted with permission from Klett-Cotta, publisher of the original German edition. Angus McLaren, 'The Pleasures of Procreation: Traditional and Biomedical Theories of Conception' in W. F. Bynum and R. Porter (eds), *William Hunter and the Eighteenth-Century Medical World* (Cambridge, Cambridge University Press, 1985), reprinted with the permission of the author and publisher. Doreen Evenden, 'Mothers and their Midwives in Seventeenth-Century London' in Hilary Marland (ed.), *The Art of Midwifery. Early Modern Midwives in Europe* (London, Routledge, 1993), reprinted with permission from Routledge. Adrian Wilson, *The Making of Man-Midwifery: Childbirth in England 1660–1770* (London, UCL Press, 1995), reprinted with permission from Taylor and Francis Books Ltd (UCL Press). Michael MacDonald, *Mystical Bedlam: Madness, Anxiety, and Healing in Seventeenth-Century England* (Cambridge, Cambridge University Press, 1981), reproduced with permission of Cambridge University Press Publishing and the author. Excerpts from H. C. Erik Midelfort, *A History of Madness in Sixteenth-Century Germany*. Copyright © 1999 by the Board of Trustees of the Leland Stanford Jr. University. Used with the permission of Stanford University Press, www.sup.org. *The Apologie and Treatise of Ambroise Paré containing the Voyages made into divers Places with many of His Writings upon Surgery*, ed. Geoffrey Keynes (New York, Dover Publications, 1968), reprinted with permission from the publisher. Christopher Lloyd (ed.), *The Health of Seamen: Selections from the Works of Dr. James Lind, Sir Gilbert Blane and Dr. Thomas Trotter* (London, Navy Records Society, 1965), reprinted with the permission of the Navy Records Society. Laurence Brockliss and Colin Jones, *The Medical World of Early Modern France* (Oxford, Clarendon Press, 1997), reprinted by permission of Oxford University Press. Margo Todd, *The Culture of Protestantism in Early Modern Scotland* (New Haven & London, Yale University Press, 2001), reprinted with the permission of Yale University Press. Michel Foucault, *Power/Knowledge: Selected Interviews and Other Writings 1972–1977*, ed. Colin Gordon (Brighton, The Harvester Press, 1980), reprinted by permission of Pearson Education Limited. Andrea A. Rusnock, 'The Weight of Evidence and the Burden of Authority: Case Histories, Medical Statistics and Smallpox Inoculation' in Roy Porter (ed.), *Medicine in the Enlightenment* (Amsterdam & Atlanta, Georgia, Rodopi, 1995), reprinted by permission of the publisher. Voltaire, *Letters concerning the English Nation*, ed. Nicholas Cronk (Oxford & New York, Oxford University Press, 1994), reprinted by permission of Oxford University Press. *A System of Complete Medical Police: Selections from Johann Peter Frank*, ed. Erna Lesky (Baltimore, Maryland, John Hopkins

University Press, 1976), reprinted with permission from the Israel Program for Scientific Translations, Keter Publishing House, Jerusalem. Ludmilla Jordanova, 'Earth Science and Environmental Medicine: the Synthesis of the late Enlightenment' in L. J. Jordanova and Roy Porter (eds), *Images of the Earth: Essays of the Environmental Sciences* (Chalfont St Giles, 1979), reprinted with permission from The British Society for the History of Science. Alfred W. Crosby, *Ecological Imperialism. The Biological Expansion of Europe, 900–1900* (Cambridge, Cambridge University Press, 1986), reproduced with permission of Cambridge University Press Publishing and the author. Karen Ordahl Kupperman, 'Fear of Hot Climates in the Anglo-American Colonial Experience', *William and Mary Quarterly* 41 (1984), reprinted with permission from the Omohundro Institute of Early American History and Culture. Reprinted by permission of The University of Tennessee Press, extract by Guenter B. Risse from chapter 'Medicine in New Spain' from *Medicine in the New World: New Spain, New France, and New England* edited by Ronald L. Numbers. Copyright © 1987 by The University of Tennessee Press. Excerpts from Simon Varey (editor), *The Mexican Treasury. The Writings of Dr. Francisco Hernández*. Copyright © 2000 by the Regents of the University of California. Used with the permission of Stanford University Press, www.sup.org. Andrew Wear, 'The Early Modern Debate about Foreign Drugs: Localism versus Universalism in Medicine', reprinted with permission from Elsevier (*The Lancet*, 1999, 354, pp. 149–51). Richard B. Sheridan, *Doctors and Slaves: A Medical and Demographic History of Slavery in the British West Indies, 1680–1834* (Cambridge, Cambridge University Press, 1985), reprinted with the permission of the publisher. From *Working Cures: Healing, Health, and Power on Southern Slave Plantations* by Sharla M. Fett. Copyright © 2002 by the University of North Carolina Press. Used by permission of the publisher. Sir George Clark, *A History of the Royal College of Physicians of London* (2 vols, Oxford, Clarendon Press, 1964–6), reprinted with permission from the Royal College of Physicians of London. 'Letter of Georg Spangenberg to the Collegium Medicum of Braunschweig (May 1747)', Lindemann, Mary. *Health and Healing in Eighteenth-Century Germany*, pp. 3–6. © 1996 The Johns Hopkins University Press. Reprinted with permission of The Johns Hopkins University Press. Pinel, Philippe. *The Clinical Training of Doctors. An Essay of 1793*, pp. 77–9, 85–93. © 1980 Dora B. Wiener. Reprinted with permission of The Johns Hopkins University Press.

Introduction

This volume of primary and secondary sources deals with health, disease and society in Europe between 1500 and 1800. As such it is representative of its subject – the social history of medicine – which has developed rapidly within the last thirty years. Accordingly, it provides examples of the role and importance of early modern medicine not only within its broader social and political framework, but also within its cultural and religious contexts. However, it should appeal not only to students of the social history of medicine, but also to history students and that illusive character, the interested general reader, who are looking for historical examples to illustrate new approaches and trends in social and cultural history in general, and the social history of medicine in particular. Thus, the volume provides insight into medical treatment as seen from the patient's point of view, the significance of gender, the influence of religion on medicine, the importance of popular as well as learned medicine, and new attitudes to madness, just to mention a few of the areas covered in this volume. This collection of secondary and primary sources is a first of its kind; in fact, to our knowledge no attempt has so far been made to produce a volume of sources for early modern social history of medicine. This volume therefore meets an important need for the growing number of students studying the discipline.

In our selection of examples we have sought to provide as comprehensive an European cover as possible, but the fact that much of the research in this field until fairly recently has remained the prerogative of Anglo-Saxon scholars working on British history, has dictated that a somewhat stronger focus on Britain has been unavoidable. For reasons of space alone no source-collection for a topic as wide-ranging as medicine and society in Europe between 1500 and 1800 can be fully comprehensive. Accordingly, this volume seeks to exemplify areas within this field which we, and, for that matter, a considerable number of scholars working within it, have considered the most central and rewarding to study. As such this volume should provide an up-to-date reflection of the most recent scholarly concerns within the discipline. It also includes much original material – some of it translated for the first time – which has hitherto been neglected by scholars and students because of its inaccessibility.

This book is an integral part of the Open University course *Medicine and Society in Europe, 1500–1930* (A218). As such the readings offered here have been chosen to illustrate and problematise key aspects of the course which are discussed more fully in the companion volume of essays entitled: *The Healing Arts: Health, Disease and Society in Europe, 1500–1800* (Manchester University Press in association with The Open University 2003). The latter in particular provides detailed help in reading and analysing these texts, and in promoting their use as aids to understanding the social history of medicine. Alternatively, they are designed in such a way as to be accessible to historians and others with a specific interest in this period, as well as the interested general reader. It can, however, be used or studied separately by anyone interested in the social history of European medicine from 1500 to 1800. The volume is divided into thirteen parts, to complement the thirteen chapters in the teaching book, each containing from four to fourteen source-extracts of different length.

Part one provides extracts that illustrate the state and nature of medical knowledge in Western Europe around 1500. It demonstrates how this knowledge remained rooted in Greek medical theory, emphasising the significance of the medical learning coming from the universities and the role and significance of learned doctors and surgeons for the Christian societies in which they worked. It offers among other things examples of Galen's approach to health and disease, the role and significance of the Hippocratic oath, and reactions of classically trained physicians to new diseases such as the pox or French disease at the Papal court.

Part two deals with the sick and their healers. It exemplifies how the sick in early modern society did not rely exclusively on learned physicians for their medical advice, but drew on a variety of medical practitioners, ranging from free assistance from family and friends, via paid treatment from uneducated quacks and empirics, to the more expensive treatment provided by trained surgeons and physicians. It provides, for instance, examples of how women who offered medical treatment and advice were perceived by early modern physicians, how barber surgeons provided a range of services which improved the bodily appearance of their customers, and popular and learned critiques of Renaissance medicine.

Part three is concerned with the medical renaissance. Focusing on the famous sixteenth-century anatomist Andreas Vesalius, and especially his approach to blood-letting, it shows the role and variety of medical humanism and how Vesalius' approach to anatomy was conditioned by contemporary social and religious concerns. Among other things it offers insight into the emergence of medical humanism in Ferrara from the late fifteenth century till the mid-sixteenth century, an eye-witness account of Andreas Vesalius' first public anatomy in Bologna in 1540, and extracts from Vesalius' *On the Fabric of the Human Body* demonstrating the various ways he sought to legitimate his new approach to anatomy.

Part four examines the connections between medicine and religion in the sixteenth century. It emphasises the continued demand for sacred and miraculous healing in sixteenth-century Europe even in those areas which, as a consequence of the Reformation, became Protestant. It also illustrates the significance of the Reformation, and later the Counter-Reformation, for the changes in health care and poor relief which were instituted across Europe in the sixteenth century. Likewise, it points up the importance of the Reformation for the emergence in the sixteenth century of a new, specifically Christian medicine, known as Paracelsianism. It provides examples of Luther's views of physicians and medicine, the healing of living saints in Italy, Paracelsus' view of the medical benefits of travel, the role and obligations of the Christian physician in times of plague as seen by the Bremen physician Johan Ewich, and a translation of the rules for the Order of the Ministers of the Sick who looked after the patients in the Maggiore Hospital in Milan in 1616.

Part five covers the legacy of Paracelsian medicine, and how it challenged the Galenic status quo, in particular on the continent, but also in England. It then traces the transformation of Paracelsianism into chemical medicine and Helmontianism; and exemplifies how in this latter form it made a concerted effort to challenge the powers of the College of Physicians in London in the years immediately after the Restoration (1660). It offers an extract from the works of the English sixteenth-century follower of Paracelsus, Richard Bostocke, insight into the revival of a sanitised type of Paracelsianism within some of the courts of late sixteenth-century Europe, the role of Helmontianism in the medical reforms of Cromwellian England as seen from the writings of Noah Biggs, and finally examples from the public debate which raged in Restoration England between advocates of alchemical medicine, such as George Thomson, and defenders of the Galenic status quo, such as William Johnson, who spoke on behalf of the London College of Physicians.

Part six shows how contagious diseases were understood by early modern communities. It discusses examples of how these societies tried to contain and prevent the plague, the major epidemic disease in the sixteenth and most of the seventeenth centuries, and how plague increasingly became associated with poverty. It deals with health policies in Stuart England and the related issue of social control, and looks at similar policies in eighteenth-century continental Europe where the health of the national populations were increasingly seen as an important goal for rulers who wanted to expand their influence and power. Furthermore, the section also illustrates how hospitals treated diseases and how medical experts in the course of this period came to exert greater influence on health issues. It offers examples of how the magistrates of Pistoia in Tuscany sought to protect their community against the plague which had struck the region in 1631, and how outbreaks of plague increasingly came to be linked with poverty in early modern England. It also provides a number of examples of how the poor and sick were treated in hospitals from Florence in Italy, via London and Winchester in England, to Edinburgh in Scotland in the eighteenth century.

Part seven exemplifies the new models of the body, which emerged between 1600 and 1800, from the mechanical, over the mathematical, to the sensible body. Based on pioneering anatomical investigations and physiological experiments the map of the body became increasingly detailed, so that the human body studied by medical students towards the end of the eighteenth century became fundamentally different from that which had been studied by their counterparts a hundred and fifty years earlier. Despite these changes, which were closely related to the general social and cultural developments of the period, the new models of the body had little or no influence on popular perceptions of the body and illness, which continued to rely on the traditional holistic view, and consequently left medical practice largely unchanged. This section provides insight into Harvey's discovery of the circulation of the blood, Descartes' discovery of the mechanical body, as expressed in his *Treatise of Man*, the Newtonian medicine of the physician George Cheyne, and finally an exploration of the relationship between medical theories and patronage and its influence on medical practice in eighteenth-century England.

Part eight provides extracts illustrating the role of women within early modern medicine. It raises a series of questions linked to gender: how was the female body viewed in the period, how was it seen to differ from its male counterpart, and how much did these perceptions change over time? Likewise, views of the role of the female body in generation are offered to illustrate the contemporary debate over conception and pregnancy. This section also deals with the role of women practitioners of the period, especially midwives and the implications of the arrival and growing influence of man-midwifery by the end of the seventeenth century. Extracts on specific female complaints such as the flux are included, as is a discussion of popular and learned theories of conception in early modern England. Finally, this section also includes three extracts illustrating the role of midwifery in early modern Europe, including the emergence of the man-midwife in Georgian England

Part nine is concerned with the experience and treatment of mental illness in early modern Europe. It shows how some of the mad came to be treated in specialised hospitals such as Bethlem by the eighteenth century, even if the majority remained at home. It also emphasises the role of new ideas about madness, especially those associated with the development of nervous theory, while underlining that much in terms of treatment had changed little since the seventeenth century. By the eighteenth century, most physicians were still reliant on a traditional regime of evacuation, bleeding and vomiting, as practised in the previous century by doctors such as Richard Napier. Extracts which provide evidence of the demography of madness in early modern England, showing the role of gender, age, and marital and social status, are included, alongside an account of a growing phenomenon in early modern medical circles – the disease of melancholy – by the sixteenth-century English physician, Philip Barrough. Similarly, examples of how the insane were treated in a German Protestant hospital (Haina) and in a Catholic Counter-Reformation hospital (Würzburg) respectively are provided.

Part ten deals with war and medicine in early modern Europe. It seeks to demonstrate how and why surgery and medicine developed as a consequence of the so-called military revolution. It underlines the particular, often experimental environment, in which medical practitioners in the field (usually surgeons) operated. It also illustrates how military surgeons and physicians became increasingly preoccupied with hygiene, the environment and epidemic disease in the eighteenth century. Finally, it provides examples of the significance and rationale behind the growing number of medicalised, military hospitals in the eighteenth century. A number of extracts from the writings of the famous French sixteenth-century surgeon Ambroise Paré are included, illustrating among other things his approaches to surgery, burns and amputations. Likewise extracts from James Lind's *A Treatise of the scurvy* describes the origins of Lind's pioneering diagnosis and treatment of scurvy, while an extract from Sir John Pringle, *Observations on the Diseases of the Army,* offers Pringle's view on the causes of hospital or jail fever. Finally, an extract deals with the rise of the French military hospitals from the late seventeenth century.

Part eleven exemplifies the relationship between health, environment and population in Europe from 1500 to 1800. It shows how air and health were linked in early modern thinking, and emphasises the role of healing wells and springs after the Reformation, not to mention the role and significance of spas in the eighteenth century. It touches upon new approaches to the understanding of disease as expressed by Thomas Sydenham. It discusses the meaning and interpretation in the eighteenth century of the increasingly used term: medical police. It also offers insight into the growing understanding and focus on smallpox in the eighteenth century and the move towards inoculation, not to forget measures for improved cleanliness and ventilation in institutions, especially hospitals. Among the extracts in this section is one from a tract by Du Laurens dealing with the significance of air as part of the Hippocratic six non-naturals. Other extracts include a section from Johann Peter Frank, *A System of Complete Medical Police,* and a section on the use and benefit of artificial ventilators in hospitals taken from the writings of Stephen Hales.

Part twelve deals with European medicine and health and its encounter with the New World, which was largely colonised during the seventeenth and eighteenth centuries. It illustrates the disastrous consequences of contact with Europeans for the indigenous people of the Americas following their exposure to new illnesses against which they carried no resistance. Likewise, it exemplifies how the settlers in North America combined their perceptions of health with their new environment and how Western medicine was introduced into the Spanish colonies of central and South America. It also deals with the Europeanisation of native American drugs, not to mention examples of how Western medicine was imposed on the African slaves brought to America to work on the new settlers' plantations. Among the extracts here is the Elizabethan Thomas Hariot's attempt to promote the colonisation of Virginia on grounds of health, and examples of how native American drugs were 'Europeanised' through the writings of the Spanish physician Francisco Hernández.

Finally, part thirteen incorporates examples of the changes that took place in medical training, organisation, and the medical marketplace in the Age of Enlightenment. It focuses on challenges to traditional licensing practices, and the changes medical education underwent, especially the convergence of the training of physicians and surgeons. Furthermore, it shows how the divisions between licensed and unlicensed medical practitioners were breaking down during the eighteenth century, and how trained medical practitioners competed with quacks in a single medical marketplace. This section includes extracts from the famous case against the London apothecary William Rose (1704), brought by the College of Physicians, and an example of the difficulties faced by an eighteenth-century state-physician in Germany. It also incorporates an extract from the new medical curriculum taught in Toulouse in the 1770s and the French physician Philippe Pinel's experiences of clinical education in the late eighteenth century, not to mention examples of alternative treatments in Georgian England.

The secondary sources that we have selected for this volume are mainly reproduced here without the scholarly annotations of their original authors. Elsewhere, footnotes have been kept to a minimum. We have adopted this approach in order to make the extracts as accessible as possible, both for the general reader as well as undergraduates for whom time is of the essence. Those who want to see the full texts in their annotated form should consult the sources from which our readings have been taken. For those who have not yet engaged with the full Open University course for which this volume is produced, we hope that this volume may serve to encourage them to do so.

Finally, the editors would like to thank the whole course team of *Medicine and Society in Europe, 1500–1930* (A218) for their assistance in the preparation of this source book.

Peter Elmer

Ole Peter Grell

Part one

Medical practice and theory: the classical and medieval heritage

---

1.1

Galen's approach to health and disease: *The Art of Medicine*

Galen, *The Art of Medicine* in Galen, *Selected Works*,
ed. P. N. Singer (Oxford and New York, Oxford University Press,
1997), pp. 345–8, 374–6.

Galen (129–c. 210) was born in Pergamum in a Greek-speaking enclave of the Roman Empire. After completing his medical studies, he travelled to Rome, where he became established as one of the foremost physicians in the city, numbering among his clientele the emperor, Marcus Aurelius. His voluminous medical writings betray a broad range of interests, both philosophical and medical, and were widely read in the Middle Ages and the Renaissance. His greatest achievement, however, was to produce a vast synthesis of earlier medical thinking, centred on the importance of a humoral understanding of the function of the human body. In this extract, taken from his treatise, *The Art of Medicine*, Galen expounds on what constitutes a healthy body, and how this might be maintained through close observation of the six *non-naturals*.

Medicine is the knowledge of what is healthy, what is morbid, and what is neither. It makes no difference if one uses the term 'diseased' instead of 'morbid'. The term 'knowledge' is to be understood in its common, not its technical, sense.

[. . .]

There is, further, an ambiguity in the definition as a whole. For when one says that medicine is the knowledge of what is healthy, what is morbid, and what is neither, this can mean the knowledge of *all* individual things which are healthy, morbid, or neither; the knowledge of *what kind of* things are healthy, morbid, or neither; or the knowledge of *some* things which are healthy, morbid, or neither. But the knowledge of all would be indefinable and impossible; the knowledge of some would be deficient and unscientific. The knowledge of what kind of things fall into each category is both scientific and sufficient for all the individual parts of the art, and so we say that this is what is contained in the definition of medicine. Let us, then, begin first with bodies, and consider of what kind are the healthy, the morbid, and those which are neither. We shall then turn to consideration of signs and of causes.

A body is healthy in the general sense when it has from birth a good mixture of the simple, primary parts, and good proportion in the organs which are composed of these. A body is healthy with application to the present when it enjoys this state for the time being. Such a body will also be (for the duration of its healthy state) of good mixture and proportion; but it will not be possessed of the best type of mixture and proportion, rather of that suitable to itself. Of generally healthy bodies, the 'always' healthy is the one with the best mixture and proportion, while 'for the most part' is that which falls short of the best state by only a little.

A body is morbid in the general sense when it has from birth a bad mixture in the homogeneous parts, or a bad proportion in the organic ones, or both. A body is morbid with application to the present when it is suffering from a disease at the time when this term is used of it. Clearly such a body too – for the duration of its morbid state – will be subject to bad mixture in the homogeneous parts, or to bad proportion in the organic, or to both. And the 'always' morbid is that body which from birth is of a very poor mixture in all its simple, primary parts, or in some of them, or in the most important; or, equally, of extremely poor proportion in the organic parts – here similarly, in all, in some, or in the most important. A body is morbid 'for the most part' when it is in a less bad state than this last one, but still not situated in the mean position.

Now, the 'neither' body has three subdivisions (that which has no share in either of the extremes, that which shares in both of them, and that which shares sometimes in one, sometimes in the other).

2

[. . .]

The causes of change in the body are divided into the 'necessary' and the 'not necessary'. By 'necessary' I mean those which it is impossible for a body not to encounter; by 'not necessary', all others. Constant contact with the ambient air is necessary, as are eating and drinking, waking and sleeping; contact with swords and wild beasts is not. The art concerned with the body is thus performed by means of the former, not of the latter. And if we make a classification of all the necessary factors which alter the body, to each of these will correspond a specific type of healthy cause. One category is contact with the ambient air; another is motion and rest of the body as a whole or of its individual parts. The third is sleep and waking; the fourth, substances taken; the fifth, substances voided or retained; the sixth, what happens to the soul.

The body cannot but stand in some relationship or other to all these. By the effects of the ambient air it will be heated, cooled, dried, or moistened, or will undergo some combination of these, or even a total change of its substance. By the effects of motion or rest, similarly – if either of these is more than normal – it will be heated, dried, cooled, or moistened, or will undergo some combination of these. As a result of sleep and waking, too, it must be affected in some way. So too as a result of substances taken, voided, or retained. All these cause change in the body (some directly, some by the action of other, intermediate causes), and loss of health. . . .

Now, all these categories of healthy causes which we are now discussing are *materials*: the correct employment renders them causative of preservation and healthy, while errors with regard to their proper balance render them morbid. From which it is clear that it is wrong to set up a different category apart from these phenomena for the substances of health as opposed to those of disease; it is the same substances which, according to context, are either healthy or morbid. When, for example, the body is in need of motion, exercise is healthy and rest morbid; when it is in need of a break, rest is healthy and exercise morbid. The same applies to food, drink, and so on. Any of these is healthy when the right sort is given in the right quantity to a body which is in need of it; when given to a body which does not need it, or given in the wrong measure, it is morbid. Quantity and quality of what is offered are the two variables to be borne in mind generally in matters of the healthy and morbid. . . .

Now the consideration of these variables applies equally in the case of the healthy causes previously listed and in the case of the type which we are considering now; let us return to these healthy causes.

3

When the constitution of the body is optimal, and the ambient air of a good mixture, then a perfect balance of all those elements mentioned above – rest and motion, sleep and waking, substances taken and voided – will be suitable. When it is not of a good mixture, the balance of these elements must be altered in accordance with that defect. The points to be borne in mind are: that the ambient air should cause neither shivering nor sweating; that exercise should cease as soon as the body begins to suffer; that food should be properly digested, and excretions preserve a good balance in both quality and quantity. In such persons appetite will be well attuned to digestion, so that they will need no supervision in order to get the right amount of each substance taken. The best natures only desire as much as they are able to digest well. The amount of sleep, too, is naturally regulated in cases of optimal constitution: they will finish sleeping when their bodies no longer require sleep. And if their lifestyle follows this pattern, then their excretions will also be free of disturbance – those of the stomach, urine, and all others.

The latter features are rendered healthy by a balanced diet; when we come to the transpiration of breath throughout the whole body, this is affected by the employment of exercise. Obviously one must refrain from excess of all affections of the soul: anger, grief, pride, fear, envy, and worry; for these will change the natural composition of the body. As for sex, Epicurus' view[1] was that no indulgence in it is healthy; the truth is that it should be practiced at sufficient intervals of time that there is no sensation of loss of strength during the act, and that one gains the impression of becoming lighter and in better breath. The correct time for sexual activity is when the body is in a precisely medial state with respect to all external influences: neither overfilled nor empty, neither excessively heated nor cooled, dried nor moistened. And if there is any error in these respects it must be a small one; and it is better to err on the side of hot rather than cold, of full rather than empty, and of wet rather than dry when performing the sexual act.

The exact nature of each of these elements must also be chosen in relation to the best constitution. Exercise will be such that each part of the body moves in proportion, none being worked either too hard or not hard enough. Food and drink will be of the best-balanced varieties, these being most appropriate to the best-balanced natures. And the same goes for all the other factors.

---

[1] Epicurus (341–270 BC) was an ancient Greek philosopher who advocated an austere doctrine of temperance in all matters relating to the body. His basic principle – that pleasure was the goal of existence – was widely misconstrued in the Renaissance. Pleasure, for Epicurus, consisted of the avoidance of pain and bodily disturbance, including excessive indulgence in material pleasures.

1.2

A medieval *consilium*: Ugo Benzi (1376–1439)

Dean Putnam Lockwood, *Ugo Benzi: Medieval Philosopher and Physician 1376–1439* (Chicago, University of Chicago Press, 1951), pp. 54–6.

Ugo Benzi (1376–1439) was a physician and scholar, who produced numerous commentaries on the works of Galen and the Arab physicians. Born at Siena, he taught at the university there in the medical faculty, as well as at Bologna and Parma. He later became physician to the king of France. As a practising physician, he was frequently asked his judgement in difficult cases, which he gave in the form of written *consilia*, literally 'letters of advice'. In the example here, he follows a typical formula in which the particular needs of the individual patient are attended to by following a detailed regimen and diet.

The case

The distinguished and noble gentleman, Messer Mariscoto of Nullano (?), about sixty years of age, of a complexion naturally tending to hot and moist, suffers from gout in his whole body and likewise at times from arthritis, whose matter is mixed, although at present, as usual, phlegm predominates. And at intervals he is so free from discomfort that he can easily walk or ride horseback, although in some of his joints a certain degree of stiffness persists. And I will give him here a brief regimen, supported by medical treatment, to the end that his health be preserved as well as possible.

Regimen

First, then, let him occupy a good chamber between two roof-terraces or balconies. The chamber should be warmed in cold weather by a fire of dry wood. And in general he should be amply protected against the cold by clothes, shoes, and other appropriate means.

And let him sleep seven or eight hours per night, and when that is not sufficient, let him sleep in the morning before tierce,[2] with his head well elevated and his body well covered.

---

[2] Nine o'clock in the morning; the third hour of the canonical day.

And let him be sure that he has a movement every day, and if nature does not respond, let him use a clyster.[3]

And for his exercise let him walk or ride horseback every day before eating, but not if it gives him much pain; and after eating let him refrain from effort.

And let him forego sexual intercourse as much as possible.

In regard to his food, he should always incline to moderation, making it a rule to leave the table before his appetite is completely satisfied. Similarly in regard to drink. And let him secure a vessel of seventeen ounces and fill it half full of water of honey, and fill the remaining half with wine, and let him not consume more than the contents of this vessel at lunch or at dinner. His wine should be red, clear, and of moderate strength.

For food let him eat the meat of chicken, partridges, pheasants, larks, and other small birds; also squab,[4] doves, and quail; and similarly kid, veal, and the flesh of young sucklings and of castrated animals; also young rabbits, and young deer. He should refrain from waterfowl, domestic pork, lamb, and beef; also from dried meats and all other forms of the flesh of the above-mentioned animals.

Let him use bread made of good flour, well cooked and well leavened; and let him avoid cheese. Fresh eggs, however, are good, i.e., the yolks lightly cooked, in the shell or poached or otherwise dished up, or in a tender omelet fried in sweet oil, or prepared in other ways, provided they be not overdone nor mixed with cheese. Farinaceous foods, such as pancakes, rolls, and so forth he should forego.

As for vegetables, none are good, but he can make a dish of spelt,[5] barley, panic,[6] millet, spinach, blite,[7] borage, bugloss,[8] balm, fennel, anise, parsley, marjoram, and savory herbs, such as sage and thyme, along with bread crumbs and eggs – singly or jointly.

And he should eat but little fish; the less harmful sort are those which are small and scaly, living in clear water and of good odor. Crayfish, however, are not good.

And of fruits the following are suitable: raisins, figs either fresh or dried, almonds, pine-nuts, filberts. And for dessert he can have pears stewed with wine and anise and fennel; but from other moist fruits he had better refrain, such as apples and cherries and peaches and so

---

[3] An enema or suppository.
[4] A newly-hatched or very young bird.
[5] A wheat-related grain grown in southern Europe.
[6] A variety of Italian millet.
[7] Wild spinach.
[8] A variety of borage.

forth, save that a small quantity, e.g., of melons or plums, may be taken before a meal in summer.

And as for condiments, he must forego vinegar, but he may use verjuice[9] and cinnamon and pepper and good spices. And he shall not use raw herbs.

So much for his regimen.

Medicinal treatment

Coming now to medicinal treatment, at the middle of February or a little earlier he should start taking the following syrup:

[in the following proportions] of compound syrup without vinegar, [4 troy ounces][10]

of oxymel of squills,[11] [2 troy ounces]

of sage-water, parsley-water, fennel-water and marjoram-water, each, [3 troy ounces]

Strain and flavour with ginger and muscat nut.

This will be sufficient for four doses. To be taken hot at dawn.

Item, [in the following proportions] of fetid pills and of greater hermodactyl[12] (?), each [half a drachm].

To be divided into seven doses. To be taken two hours before sunrise and after the syrup.

And on this day he should use great precaution against cold and not eat before the eighteenth hour. And on the following morning let him use a cleansing clyster, and take [2 drachms] of theriac with [2 troy ounces] of honey-water seven hours before lunch. And a similar purge should be made at the beginning of October. During the intervening periods he should be purged without supervision at least once a month, taking [1 drachm] of the following pills at midnight or thereabouts:

[in the following proportions] of pills of the eightfold antidote, [half a drachm]

of larch fungus, [half a drachm]

of sal-gem, [half a scruple]

Make into pills with sage-water, and they are for one dose only, but he may have them prepared in advance for many doses.

---

[9] The juice of sour fruits.

[10] In apothecaries' weights, one pound was the equivalent of 12 troy ounces, 96 drachms, and 288 scruples.

[11] Honeyed syrup concocted from the bulb of the sea onion, or *scilla*.

[12] Cholchium, a herbal remedy used for gout.

Item, in winter once a week he should take [2 drachms] of mithridate five hours before eating.

Item, in cold weather he should wear on his feet at night little bags of ground salt.

And often in the morning before breakfast he should wash his legs and feet and knees with the the following water:

of sage, camomile, and laurel, each, [2 minims][13]

of water, [20 pounds]

of salt, [5 pounds]

To be boiled over a fire, until the salt dissolves, and used frequently as a hot footbath.

1.3

The history of surgery:
Guy de Chauliac (1298–1368)

Guy de Chauliac, *Great Surgery* in James B. Ross and
Mary M. McLaughlin (eds), *The Portable Medieval Reader*
(Harmondsworth, Penguin Books, 1977), pp. 640–9.

Guy de Chauliac (1298–1368) was one of the most eminent surgeons of the Middle Ages. His *Chirurgia Magna* or *Great Surgery* (1363) was a standard text for surgeons until well into the seventeenth century. Having taken holy orders, Guy proceeded to study at the universities of Toulouse, Montpellier, Paris and Bologna. He spent most of his life, however, at Avignon, where he served as surgeon to three popes. In this extract, he attempts to create a noble lineage for the art and practice of surgery and to place the work of the surgeon on a par with the learned physician.

The workers in this art [i.e. surgery], from whom I have had knowledge and theory, and from whom you will find observations and maxims in this work, in order that you may know which has spoken better than the other, should be arranged in a certain order.

The first of all was Hippocrates who (as one reads in the *Introduction to Medicine*) surpassed all the others, and first among the Greeks

[13] A minim was the smallest fluid measure, a drop, or more accurately the sixtieth part of a fluid drachm.

led medicine to perfect enlightenment. For according to Macrobius and Isidore, in the fourth book of the *Etymologies* . . . medicine had been silent for the space of five hundred years before Hippocrates, since the time of Apollo and Aesculapius, who were its first discoverers.[14] He lived ninety-five years, and wrote many books on surgery, as it appears from the fourth of the *Therapeutics* and many other passages of Galen. But I believe that on account of the good arrangement of the books of Galen the books of Hippocrates and of many others have been neglected.

Galen followed him, and what Hippocrates sowed, as a good labourer he cultivated and increased. He wrote many books, indeed, in which he included much about surgery, and especially the *Book on Tumors Contrary to Nature*, written in summary; and the six first *Books on Therapeutics*, containing wounds and ulcers, and the last two concerning boils and many other maladies which require manual operation. In addition, seven books which he arranged, *Cuturyeni* (that is, about the composition of medicaments according to kinds), of which we have only a summary. Now he was a master in demonstrative science in the time of the Emperor Antoninus [Marcus Aurelius], after Jesus Christ about one hundred and fifty years. He lived eighty years, as is told in *The Book of the Life and Customs of the Philosophers*. Between Hippocrates and Galen there was a very long time, as Avicenna says in the fourth of the *Fractures*, three hundred and twenty-five years, as they gloss it there, but in truth there were five hundred and eighty-six years.[15]

After Galen we find Paul [of Aegina][16] who . . . did many things in surgery; however, I have found only the sixth book of his *Surgery*.

Going on we find Rhazes, Albucasis and Alcaran,[17] who (whether they were all one and the same, or several) did very well, especially in

[14] Ambrosius Theodosius Macrobius (fl. c. 400 AD) was a Roman scholar and philosopher. He was the author, among other works, of an etymology, *On the differences and similarities between Greek and Latin words*. St Isidore of Seville (b. c. 560–636) was a theologian and the author of an important encyclopaedia of the ancient world, containing the remains of much ancient wisdom, entitled *Etymologies*. It remained a popular work of reference throughout the Middle Ages. The Greek God, Apollo, was the father of Aesculapius or Asclepius and was worshipped for his gift of healing.

[15] The Persian scholar Avicenna, or Abu Ali Ibn Sina (980–c. 1036), was the author of the *Canon of medicine*, one of the most important compilations of medical knowledge in the Middle Ages. In this work, Avicenna subordinated the medical principles of Galen to the natural philosophy of Aristotle. Its influence on Western medical thinking was vast and the *Canon* was regularly invoked in medical treatises and university courses as late as the seventeenth century.

[16] Paul of Aegina was a seventh-century writer on medicine.

[17] Rhazes or Rhasis (Abu Bakr Muhammad ibn Zakariyya Al-Razi, c. 825–c. 924) was an Arab physician, philosopher and poet.

the *Books for Almansor* and in the *Divisions*, and in the *Surgery* called Albucasis. In these as Haly Abbas says, he put all his particulars, and in all the *Continens* (which is called *Helham* in Arabic) he repeated the same things, and he collected all the sayings of the ancients, his predecessors; but because he did not select and is long and without conclusion, he has been less prized.

Haly Abbas[18] was a great master, and besides what he sowed in the books on *The Royal Disposition*, he arranged on surgery the ninth part of his *Second Sermon*.

Avicenna, illustrious prince, followed him, and in very good order (as in other things) treated surgery in his fourth book.

And we find that up to him all were both physicians and surgeons, but since then, either through refinement or because of too great occupation with cures, surgery was separated and left in the hands of *mechanics*. Of these the first were Roger [of Salerno], Roland [of Parma], and the Four Masters, who wrote separate books on surgery, and put in them much that was empirical. Then we find Jamerius who did some rude surgery in which he included a lot of nonsense; however, in many things he followed Roger. Later, we find Bruno [of Longoburgo],[19] who, prudently enough, made a summary of the findings of Galen and Avicenna, and of the operations of Albucasis; however, he did not have all the translation of the books of Galen and entirely omitted anatomy. . . .

[. . .]

And I, Guy of Chauliac, surgeon and master in medicine, from the borders of Auvergne, diocese of Mende, doctor and personal chaplain to our lord the pope, I have seen many operations and many of the writings of the masters mentioned, principally of Galen; for as many books of his as are found in the two translations, I have seen and studied with as much diligence as possible, and for a long time I have operated in many places. And at present I am in Avignon, in the year of our Lord 1363, the first year of the pontificate of Urban V. In which year, from the teachings of the above named, and from my experiences, with the aid of my companions, I have compiled this work, as God has willed.

[. . .]

Let us return to our theme, and put down the conditions which are req-

[18] Haly Abbas or Majusi (fl. late tenth century) was a Persian physician and the author of *The complete medical art*, which was translated into Latin twice in the late eleventh and early twelfth centuries.

[19] Guy lists here a number of medieval authorities on surgery who were writing during the twelfth and thirteenth centuries.

uisite to every surgeon, who wishes by art to exercise on the human body the aforesaid manner and form of operating, which conditions Hippocrates, who guides us well in everything, concludes with a certain subtle implication, in the first of the *Aphorisms*: life is short, and art prolix, time and chance sharp or sudden, experience fallacious and dangerous, judgment difficult. But not only the doctor must busy himself in doing his duty but also the sick person and the attendants, and he must also put in order external things.

[. . .]

The conditions required of a surgeon are four: the first is that he be educated; the second, that he be skilled; the third, that he be ingenious; the fourth, that he be well behaved. It is then required in the first place that the surgeon be educated, not only in the principles of surgery, but also of medicine, both in theory and practice.

In theory he must know things natural, non-natural and unnatural. And first, he must understand natural things, principally anatomy, for without it nothing can be done in surgery, as will appear below. He must also understand temperament, for according to the diversity of the nature of bodies it is necessary to diversify the medicament. . . . This is shown by the virtue and strength of the patient. He must also know the things which are not natural, such as air, meat, drink, etc., for these are the causes of all sickness and health. He must also know the things which are contrary to nature, that is sickness, for from this rightly comes the curative purpose. Let him not be ignorant in any way of the cause, for if he cures without the knowledge of that, the cure will not be by his abilities but by chance. Let him not forget or scorn accidents; for sometimes they override their cause, and deceive or divert, and pervert the whole cure. . . .

In practice, he must know how to put in order the way of living and the medicaments; for without this surgery, which is the third instrument of medicine, is not perfect. Of which Galen speaks in the *Introduction*; as pharmacy has need of regimen and of surgery, so surgery has need of regimen and pharmacy.

Thus it appears that the surgeon working in his art should know the principles of medicine. And with this, it is very fitting that he know something of the other arts. That is what Galen says in the first of his *Therapeutics* against Thessales, that if the doctors have nothing to do with geometry, or astronomy, or dialectics,[20] or any other good discipline, soon the leather workers, carpenters, smiths, and others, leaving

---

[20] Logic.

their occupations, will run to medicine and make themselves into doctors.

In the second place, I have said he must be skilled and have seen others operate; I add the maxim of the sage Avenzoar,[21] that every doctor must have knowledge first of all, and after that he must have practice and experience. To the same testify Rhazes, in the fourth *Book for Almansor*, and Haly Abbas on the testimony of Hippocrates, in the first of his *Theory*.

Thirdly, he must be ingenious, and of good judgment and good memory. That is what Haly Rodan[22] says in the third of his *Techni*; the doctor must have good memory, good judgment, good motives, good presence, and sound understanding, and that he be well formed, for example, that he have slender fingers, hands steady and not trembling, clear eyes, etc.

Fourth, I have said, he should be well mannered. Let him be bold in safe things, fearful in dangers, let him flee false cures or practices. Let him be gracious to the sick, benevolent to his companions, wise in his predictions. Let him be chaste, sober, compassionate, and merciful; not covetous, or extortionate, so that he may reasonably receive a salary in proportion to his work, the ability of his patient to pay, the nature of the outcome, and his own dignity.

1.4
The Hippocratic oath

The Hippocratic oath in Owsei Temkin and C. Lilian Temkin (eds), *Ancient Medicine: Selected Papers of Ludwig Edelstein* (Baltimore, Johns Hopkins Press, 1967), p. 6.

The Hippocratic oath, attributed to the ancient Greek physician, Hippocrates, was adapted worldwide as a guide to medical ethics and continues in use in many medical schools on graduation. In its original

---

[21] Avenzoar or Ibn Zuhr (d. 1162) was a pupil and friend of the great Arab scholar Averroes at Cordoba in Moslem Spain, who showed a willingness in his medical writings to criticise Galen.

[22] Haly Eben Rodan or Ridwan (fl. eleventh century) wrote a commentary on Gerard of Cremona's translation of Galen's *Ars parva*, in which he showed a preference for practice over theory.

form, it binds both teacher and student to follow certain prescribed obligations and duties, as well as pledging all trained doctors to a specific series of ethical commitments which they are sworn to uphold in their day-to-day practice.

I swear by Apollo Physician and Asclepius and Hygieia and Panaceia[23] and all the gods and goddesses, making them my witnesses, that I will fulfil according to my ability and judgment this oath and this covenant:

To hold him who has taught me this art as equal to my parents and to live my life in partnership with him, and if he is in need of money to give him a share of mine, and to regard his offspring as equal to my brothers in male lineage and to teach them this art – if they desire to learn it – without fee and covenant; to give a share of precepts and oral instruction and all the other learning to my sons and to the sons of him who has instructed me and to pupils who have signed the covenant and have taken an oath according to the medical law, but to no one else.

I will apply dietetic measures for the benefit of the sick according to my ability and judgment; I will keep them from harm and injustice.

I will neither give a deadly drug to anybody if asked for it, nor will I make a suggestion to this effect. Similarly I will not give to a woman an abortive remedy. In purity and holiness I will guard my life and my art.

I will not use the knife, not even on sufferers from stone, but will withdraw in favor of such men as are engaged in this work.

Whatever houses I may visit, I will come for the benefit of the sick, remaining free of all intentional injustice, of all mischief and in particular of sexual relations with both female and male persons, be they free or slaves.

What I may see or hear in the course of the treatment or even outside of the treatment in regard to the life of men, which on no account one must spread abroad, I will keep to myself holding such things shameful to be spoken about.

If I fulfil this oath and do not violate it, may it be granted to me to enjoy life and art, being honored with fame among all men for all time to come; if I trangress it and swear falsely, may the opposite of all this be my lot.

[23] Asclepius (or Aesculapius), the son of Apollo, was taught the art of medicine by Chiron, guardian of the underworld. Hygieia (hence the word, hygiene) and Panaceia were the daughters of Asclepius, who inherited his healing powers.

1.5
Reactions to the 'French Disease' at the papal court

Jon Arrizabalaga, John Henderson and Roger French, *The Great Pox: The French Disease in Renaissance Europe* (New Haven and London, Yale University Press, 1997), pp. 113–19, 131–42.

Syphilis or the pox, frequently styled the 'French Disease' (*Morbus Gallicus*), first appeared in Europe shortly after the discovery of the New World in the late 1490s. The appearance of this dreadful disease, which caused acute pain and disfigurement in those who contracted it, provoked widespread debate in medical circles. In particular, it challenged accepted medical thinking and drew a variety of responses from experts in the field who sought to integrate an understanding of the disease and its cure into contemporary frameworks of medical theory and practice. In the extract cited here, the authors focus on the reactions of two papal physicians, Gaspar Torrella (c. 1452–c. 1520) and Pere Pintor (c. 1423/24–1503), who, from slightly different perspectives, both published learned tomes on the disease.

It was the time of Alexander VI, pope from 1492 to 1503, who had been born Rodrigo Borjia (henceforth Borgia) in Játiva, Valencia, in 1431. He comes into our story only indirectly, as the centre of the court, for he did not contract the disease himself. But many at the papal court did. Several members of the papal *familia* were early affected . . . [including] Rodrigo's own son Cesare, cardinal of Valencia. . . . Alexander VI and his *familia* had seven physicians in their retinue; we are concerned with the two Spaniards, Gaspar Torrella (c. 1452–c. 1520) and Pere Pintor (c. 1423/4–1503), who published on the French Disease.

Torrella and Pintor shared to an extreme degree the problems of all physicians facing *Morbus Gallicus*. The disease was apparently new, or at least had no ancient name by which it could be understood within learned medicine. It was very widespread and was known to be a particularly intractable disease. But the problem was not primarily that the doctors were unsuccessful in curing it, and were therefore forfeiting the confidence of the public. . . . The main problem was that the disease was seen as divine punishment or as having been generated by conjunctions of the planets, and that therefore the scope for any human endeavour to alleviate it was seen as very limited. The physicians' prob-

lems were more professional. The learned, university-trained physicians were under great pressure to act – to bring relief to the suffering,
to prevent the spread of the disease and to give advice. There was pressure not only from their patients, but also from civil authorities who
were concerned with the health of populations. Lastly they were under
pressure to preserve the professional status quo, for inaction or admitted failure would give an opportunity to unlicensed practitioners to
take the initiative. That is, because the disease did not have an ancient
name, it could not be handled by the theoretical apparatus of learned
and rational medicine, on which the reputation and advantages of the
university-trained physician rested. He was in no better position than
the empirical practitioner who claimed to have a specific, that is, a
remedy proven by experience rather than reason (and probably kept
secret).

These pressures must have been more extreme in the papal court
than in very many other situations. Clearly the publications of Torrella
and Pintor were strategies towards a solution. Much of what we see at
the papal court can be recognised as actions prompted by the pressures
generated by this new and disastrous scourge. We shall look mainly at
two areas where the papal physicians were active. We shall examine
first their resources, whether intellectual or material, and second the
strategies they adopted. We shall see that part of the story is the competition between different classes of practitioner, from the unlicensed
empiric to the university doctor, and also between different types of
university doctor, especially between Torrella and Pintor.

It is clear that to maintain his position and to solve the problem of the
pox, the learned and rational doctor had to bring it into the medical
system. It had to be identified with something that the medical literature contained, for only then could he talk of causes, remedies and prevention and in this way be learned and rational about it. It was his
knowledge of the medical literature that quickened his eye when looking at poxed patients and what his fellows had written about them.
What was significant in the disease was what was in the literature, and
therefore in this sense the learned physician constructed a picture of
the pox.

It is not surprising that two learned medical men should see rather
different things as significant. Partly this had to do with their training.
Torrella and Pintor both came from Valencia, the home too of Alexander VI, who perhaps showed them special favour on that account. Both
men belonged to families of Jews who had converted to Christianity,
and who later suffered persecution by the Inquisition in Valencia.
Pintor's family was destroyed and he found protection with the cardi-

nal, Rodrigo Borgia. Of Torrella, as of many other fellow countrymen who decided to stay in Italy after completing their university studies there, we can only presume that his choice of Rome as a place to settle was related to the situation created by the Inquisition in Valencia. The social climate resulting from the inquisitorial offensive in Valencia was unfavourable to the return of those who had reached elsewhere some professional level and where they could enjoy a greater degree of intellectual and religious freedom. It was therefore natural that both of them should settle in Italy. But there were differences as well as similarities between the two men. Torrella was a priest and had studied medicine in Siena and Pisa; Pintor, a generation older, did not leave Spain for his medical training and studied the subject in Lérida, the *studium generale* of the Crown of Aragon.

The differences between Torrella and Pintor derive mostly from their different universities. While both accepted the Avicennan Galenism that was the common property of the learned physicians as a group, Torrella shows evident traces of the Italian intellectual world of his time. He was at his Tuscan universities at the time – the 1470s – when the Neoplatonist circle of Marsilio Ficino[24] was active in Florence, and one of his teachers, Pierleone da Spoleto, was an outstanding member of the circle. Torrella adopted some humanist values from Italy, although we should not . . . regard him strictly as a humanist. In all this he was different from Pintor, who was thirty years older and without an Italian training. It is clear from what they wrote that there was an intense rivalry between them. Perhaps it was intellectual, the result of their different training, or perhaps it was because they had to compete for the favour of the same patron; at all events their rivalry is not only revealed in their work on the French Disease but was a factor in encouraging them to write.

Publication indeed was one of the main resources available for these two physicians when faced with the general problem of the pox and with the problems of their own personal situation. But publication now meant something different: the printing press had not existed when Pintor was born, and not all medical men were sure that it was a good thing. To us the press means an invariant text, more copies and a consequent more rapid spread of knowledge. . . . The close connection of

---

[24] Marsilio Ficino (1433–99) was one of the leading scholars of his day and the central figure in an important and influential coterie of intellectuals that met in Florence under the patronage of the Medici. His major achievement was the rediscovery and publication of the works of the Greek philosopher, Plato, as well as those early Christian Neoplatonists, who sought to reconcile Christianity with Platonism.

the two men with the pope and Torrella's personal position as physician to Alexander's son Cesare must have ensured them a wide audience, demonstrating the power of the press as a resource. No wonder that Torrella decided to resort to the press for the first time two years before Pintor. Books formed a related resource. Torrella was appointed librarian of the Vatican library by Alexander in May 1498. He was there for two years at least, and he probably took advantage of the manuscripts and printed works in producing his own written material.

Pintor's education was also a resource for him. His training in medicine in Lérida began in the late 1430s and he was practising medicine by 1445. He was much more a practical physician than Torrella, whose medical degree was secured only with the help of Alexander VI, some years after Torrella had finished his studies. Pintor was the city's examiner of physicians in Valencia four times between 1445 and 1481, and lectured in the Valencia school of surgery for periods between 1468 and 1485. Indeed, he was instrumental in setting up the school in 1462 and in reorganising it in 1480; it was the core of the new medical faculty when the *university* of Valencia was established in 1499. Clearly the surgical component of medicine was important for Pintor, which must have been significant when he came to write on the pox, which was often seen as a skin condition and therefore surgical. He had, moreover, been practising medicine for about forty years when he ran up against the Inquisition and left Valencia by 1484 to become personal physician to Rodrigo Borgia in Rome.

Given that the two men had very different backgrounds and different resources on which to draw, it is not surprising that they differed in their reactions to the pox and its problems. There is a strong sense in which they were both successful. That is not to say that either found a cure or a preventive regimen, but that both were perceived to be successful. That is, the strategies they developed from their resources worked. Both remained as papal physicians and Torrella survived the purge of the Borgias instituted by Julius II, Alexander's successor.[25] . . . Julius suffered from the French Disease and he chose to keep Torrella in his position as papal physician, despite his connection with the Borgias. Clearly Torrella's strategies had worked, and he had a reputation as a pox-doctor. Both popes showered him with benefices.[26]

The writings of both men enable one to examine their strategies at work. Of Torrella's output, five medical works and an astrological pre-

[25] Giuliano della Rovere (1443–1513) was elected pope, as Julius II, in 1503. He immediately set about purging the papal court of all earlier Borgia influence.

[26] Clerical positions.

17

diction survive from the period 1497–1506. The prediction was actually a letter addressed to Cesare Borgia in 1502 and was published in 1506 at the request of the apostolic *datarius*, Giovanni Gozzadini, who was interested in the astrological effects of a comet that appeared over Rome in that year.[27] It is interesting that even if at this time astrology was beginning to come under attack, both Torrella and Pintor used it, albeit in rather different ways.

Torrella's more strictly medical works are mostly directed at infectious diseases. His *Consilium* on the pestilence known as 'modorrilla', which broke out in the Castilian fleet at Flanders and spread over the Iberian kingdoms, was published twice, in Rome and Salamanca, in 1505. Another *Consilium* was directed against a pestilence that occurred in Rome in 1504. Then there was his *Regimen Sanitatis* [*Rule of Health*], a preventive regimen presented as a dialogue addressed to Julius II in 1506. All these followed his *Tractatus cum Consiliis* [*Treatise with Letter of Advice*] on the pox of 1497 (republished in about 1498) and his *Dialogus* on the same subject in 1500. Clearly Torrella saw publishing on infectious diseases, both pestilential and not, as a strategy to deal with the problems that faced him.

The same can be said of Pintor, although only two of his works are known, on pestilence and pox, published respectively in 1499 and 1500. He addressed them to his patron – Alexander VI which, as in all patron-client relationships, had advantages to both parties. The patron was flattered and furthered his reputation, and the client strengthened his security of employment. Like Torrella, Pintor found that to publish on infectious diseases during the first years of a disastrous new scourge was to become an authority. A further similarity is that both men found a proper medical name for the pox. Torrella called it *pudendagra*, because often it first appeared in the genital organs, *pudenda* (*-agra* was a common ending for a disease name, as *podagra* was 'disease of the feet'). After searching the literature, Pintor came up with the term *aluhumata*.

That Torrella should invent a neologism and Pintor should find a term from the medical literature is characteristic of the two men. Pintor's long medical practice, his greater age, his Spanish training all made him want to find a solution from within available sources. His first work, on pestilence, reveals the same tendencies. He called it an *Agregator Sentenciarum*, a collection of opinions of the learned. This was a medieval technique, even a genre of literature, and renaissance authors some-

---

[27] The *datarius*, or datary, was an officer of the papal court responsible for registering and dating all documents issued by the pope.

times looked down their noses at it. Pintor collected summaries of opinions of people like Pietro d'Abano.[28] The surgeon Guy de Chauliac[29] had expressed the principle of 'aggregation' as the cumulative addition of works by means of which knowledge grows and the art progresses. Guy was doubtless one of Pintor's major intellectual mentors, particularly since, unlike Torrella's, Pintor's medicine included a large and practical interest in surgery.

These then are some of the differences between the two physicians who were facing the problem of the pox at the Roman court. Their first step towards a solution was the epistemological one of identifying the disease. . . . [S]ome doctors, like the Bolognese teacher Natale Montesauro,[30] accounted for the apparent newness and strangeness of the disease by assuming that it was a compound entity, combining features of more than a single disease. But Torrella and Pintor followed the simpler course of taking it as a single disease. It had then a single cause for the pains and the sores which made their task in explaining the nature of the disease much more straightforward.

It is necessary to underline here their difficulty in dealing with a very real phenomenon that had only a vernacular name. It was partly that the professional knowledge of the learned physician was so structured that it could not deal with an unnamed disease. It was also partly that it was a common medieval belief that names *meant* something about the essence of the things they signified. The laboured etymologies of the middle ages from Isidore onwards were expressions of this. But this system worked only in Latin and, in an age when Latin was the language of medicine and philosophy, for something to have only a vernacular name was to devalue it.

Thus, in seeking a Latin name for the new disease, Torrella and Pintor had to grasp its essential nature. This meant also discovering how it had arisen. This was more than discovering historically whether or not it was indeed a new disease, and meant learning about its nature from the causes that produced it. Torrella held that the disease had originated in the French Auvergne in 1493 and had subsequently spread by contagion to the rest of Europe and indeed the world. He was expressing the devalued worth of a vernacular name when he said in 1500 that the French Disease was first seen among the French troops in Naples, and

---

[28] Pietro d'Abano (1257–c. 1315) taught medicine at Padua and was the author of the influential treatise, *Conciliator*, in which he argued for the importance of philosophy in the education of the learned physician.

[29] For Guy de Chauliac, see extract 1.3 above.

[30] Natale Montesauro (fl. 1490s) was strongly influenced by the Arab medical tradition and was one of the first to write on the French disease.

that the Italians thought that it was 'connate to the French people'; correspondingly, when Charles took his diseased troops back to France, the French thought that the pox had originated in Naples and gave it an appropriate name, the 'Neapolitan disease'. The variety of vernacular names also lessened their authority. Torrella reports that the French also called it the *grosse vérole*,[31] the Valencians, Catalans and Aragonese the *mal de siment*,[32] and the Castilians the 'curial disease' because it 'followed the court'. Pintor agreed that the disease was commonly known as the French Disease, *Morbus Gallicus*, and, like Torrella, felt the difficulty of the range of vernacular names (but he does not particularise).

Another reason why vernacular names devalued medical things was that they were used by vernacular people. The unlicensed, the empiric, the apothecary and the common surgeon would not have used Latin, and it was for professional reasons that the physicians insisted on Latin. They identified the use of the vernacular with groups of practitioners with whom they were in competition. The French Disease had to have a Latin name so that the physicians could draw it into the apparatus that distinguished them from other groups and justified their claims to superiority.

Part of this apparatus was that diseases fell into categories. There were *kinds* of disease, species within genera. They made a point of entry for the pox. If it could be shown that the disease resembled another then it might be a new species of some genus. Torrella, for example, was prepared to accept that the French Disease was a nameless species of a kind of disease called *scabies* in the Latin version of Avicenna. He could not allow it a vernacular name, of course, and in inventing a name for it he was extending the subdivision in Avicenna's classicifaction of disease.

Pintor was in a similar position. As a learned and rational doctor he saw that to allow the disease to be new, with only a vernacular name, was to allow competing medical groups a double advantage. He too made it partly new, so to speak, by claiming that it was to be identified with a third and obscure species of the *variola* kind of disease, a species which he found in Avicenna and Rhazes, called *aluhumata*. So his strategy, to pick up and expand an obscure part of the learned apparatus, differed from Torrella's, which was to insert a new subcategory into the apparatus. The 'part newness' of the disease according to

---

[31] 'Great pox'.

[32] In earlier editions of his work on syphilis, Torrella says that it was described as 'mal de San Sement' or 'morbus Sancti Sementi'.

Pintor was also due to the fact that it had an astrological cause. Such things of their nature were infrequent, and the pox was, says Pintor, unknown before its recent irruption. Both authors are giving their topic a history, in two senses. First . . . to enquire into the causes of the disease, whether or not astrological, was to learn about its essence. Secondly, in general terms, to give a new thing a history was to give it the dignity and authority of age. To show that some new scheme of things had been perhaps adumbrated but not systematised by the ancients made it more credible. Torrella and Pintor were achieving that credibility by fitting the pox into the apparatus of the ancients and the Arabs.

Pintor thought that he had been particularly successful in this strategy, and while ignoring what had been published by others he made great claims for his own intellectual understanding of *aluhumata* – systematised from Avicenna and Rhazes – and for his ability to treat it. Pintor too was rewarded by his patron, and his strategy was in that sense successful. The essential thing about a strategy was that it had to be intelligible and convincing to the patient or patron. The specialist knowledge of the doctor was of the same kind as that of most learned men and was simply more extensive in a way that they recognised. So in returning to his resources, the medical literature, and modifying it by accommodating the French Disease, Pintor looked as though he was refining medical knowledge.

[. . .]

It was consistent with their standing as university-trained rational and learned physicians that both Torrella and Pintor claimed to use for the pox a treatment that was 'rational', 'regular' and 'canonical'. Not to have done so would have been to rely solely on experience. The learned doctor did not indeed deny experience and valued it as something that could be made more meaningful than mere empiricism by the use of reason. But within this formula, as we would expect, Torrella and Pintor, with their different notions on the identity and cause of the pox, differed considerably in their practical treatment of the disease.

The most striking feature of Torrella's view of *Morbus Gallicus* was his optimistic opinion that it was both known and curable. He claimed that he had treated successfully seventeen cases in just the two months of September and October 1497. To emphasise the point in his earliest work (of the same year) he included the medical reports – *consilia* – of five of his allegedly cured patients, which also allowed him to illustrate several species of the disease. *Consilia* constituted a well-known form of medical literature in the middle ages, but Torrella was the only one of the early physicians writing on the pox to use the form. He probably did so as part of his confident, even aggressive rhetoric of success. Clearly, one strategy open to a man at the top of his profession, who had by now fitted an apparently new disease into the extant medical apparatus, was the bold one of announcing his mastery of it. Since it was seen as a new disease, there were no common expectations about its durability or curability. Torrella seems to have decided to fill that space with the help of the printing press, with claims about his own insights into the disease and his practical ability to cure it. He accordingly seized on the differences between his own claims and those of others who saw the disease as unknown and incurable. Whether these others were merely straw-men, Torrella used this pessimistic approach as a rhetorical mirror to reflect his own views:

> M[any] modern people have believed that this disease arose from an upper cause, so that it missed no region or time and did not respect the age, sex or complexion [of its victims] and did not follow a regular sequence of invasion, by reason of the diversity of its peccant matter. . . . Thus they did not give attention to its cure and decided to do nothing but wait until nature had eliminated it, because some of their attempted cures of people ill with the disease did more harm than good. For this reason they claimed that the disease corresponded to no specific and adequate category [of the medical apparatus] and was irregular and incurable.

Torrella attacked such passive pessimism with a charge of impiety. Medieval physicians not uncommonly used, to justify their profession, an argument taken from Ecclesiasticus: God created medicine and He is the only one able to cure us; but He has not forgotten to teach God-fearing people the art of curing.[33] Torrella used the argument too, claiming that it would be a sin not to intervene as a physician in these cases of pox. He accordingly advised 'everyone to remember that they are mortal and sinners, and first of all to praise God's help as is proper, and afterwards to consult physicians, since God Himself . . . allows both physicians to understand this disease and medicines to act according to the properties given to them by Him.' In other words, here is a university-trained, rational and learned physician claiming for his kind no less than a uniquely God-given ability to *understand* the disease, that is, to fit it into his professional learning and rationality. It is also a personal claim for Torrella because not all university physicians were so optimistic about the disease: they had not adopted Torrella's strategy. Torrella added this personal claim to the evidence provided by the *consilia* for the value of the medical 'product' he was offering, in order to emphasise his own professional worth. In addition, in dedicating the

---

[33] Ecclesiasticus 38:1–15.

Tractatus to Cesare Borgia and claiming to have cured him of the pox, Torrella is also using his patron's name as authority for his own virtues:

> No one can question the degree to which humanity is indebted to you [Cesare Borgia] since in your time and because of you we now know not only the essence of the disease, which everyone considered incurable, but also the method of cure. It is thanks to precisely this knowledge that those infected will be optimistic and confident. . . . [T]his confidence will enable them to regain and maintain their health. . . . From this it is obvious that your most Reverend Lordship has cured the infected and kept others healthy as the result of their expectation of health.

So what was there in Torrella's treatment of the pox to justify this optimism? The starting point of his cure was the standard regimen, based on manipulating the six non-naturals, with an eye on the individuality of the patient, and with the view of digesting and evacuating the peccant matter. In other words it was just the same as Pintor's preventive regimen and hundreds of others. Torrella's difference lies in the emphasis he gave to the sixth non-natural, the 'accidents of the soul', that is, the mutual effects of the soul and the body. He treats it first and devotes a large amount of space in the *Tractatus* to it. . . . [I]ts message is that confidence itself in the treatment and the cure is the most important therapeutic device available to Torrella. He linked the patient's confidence to his faculty of imagination, *virtus imaginativa*. This was not simply the patient's 'imagination' in our sense, but was more literally the power to conjure *images*, whether directly from the sense or indirectly from the memory. It was part of the medieval apparatus that linked the internal senses with the external. These links made it possible for Torrella to discuss the matter theoretically, and so to justify it in practice. They also provided him with the avenues of approach to the patient in whom he in practical terms wanted to generate confidence. Torrella used the same linkages to provide an apparatus for (to 'understand') other therapeutic devices like exorcism and charms. What is notable in this side of Torrella's medical thought is the extent of his Platonism, which he may have been cultivating since his days as a medical student and which was always in line with the tastes of contemporary courtly culture, including Borgia's Roman court.

Next Torrella turned to some standard pharmaceutical practice. The purpose of giving medicine to the patient was ultimately to remove the morbific matter of the *pudendagra*. The physician's objective in many diseases was the removal of morbific matter or peccant humours, and there were a number of ways of doing it, often called 'intentions'. Torrella's three intentions were evacuation, resolution and desiccation, and consumption (or destruction). His first 'intention' was to let blood when he thought that this humour partook in the morbific matter. This too was standard practice . . . With other morbific matter, Torrella first used 'digestive' or 'alterative' medicines that prepared the matter for evacuation, perhaps by changing its nature, and secondly purges to eliminate it. When he considered that enough of the morbific matter had been evacuated Torrella employed his second intention, which was to move the largely vaporous remainder of the peccant matter from its interior location to the skin, whence it could be expelled. This needed resolutive techniques to break down and mobilise the matter and drying techniques to draw it to the skin. In practical terms this meant making the patient sweat by fumigations, baths and especially the 'dry stove', a device big enough to contain the patient wholly.

Torella's third 'intention' followed, to remove the skin lesions. These were generally taken to be the appearance and actions of the morbific matter at the skin, and so their appearance during treatment could be taken as a sign that the first two intentions had been successful in drawing the matter to the skin. It was also the point at which the arguments and learning of the university doctor in his traditional practice of internal medicine met the practical, external and experiential learning and practice of the surgeon. Torrella, like most university physicians of the time, then used ointments, liniments and lotions. Like the surgeons too he used a range of corrosive and abrasive substances: mercury; yellow litharge, sulphur, ceruse, watered calx, ammonia and verdigris. By 1500 he was also using 'live' calx, alum, rock salt, tartar emetic, ink, vitriol and aqua fortis. To these minerals he added vegetable substances like turpentine, mastic, incense, myrrh, galbanum and *opopanax*. The most notorious of them was mercury, and we shall later meet the troubles it caused to our two courtly physicians (and their different explanations of them).

[. . .]

Pintor's practice in the case of the pox was formed by the same kind of constraints as Torrella's. Like Torrella, he had related the apparently new disease to another well known in the medical apparatus, so that he was bound to be partly guided by the therapeutic indications offered by the apparatus (which was the point of so relating the disease to it in the first place). The details of Pintor's recommended course of action were somewhat different to Torrella's because he had chosen a different part of the apparatus in which to 'understand' the pox. It was still a question of attacking the morbific matter, changing or digesting it and expelling it, whether by phlebotomy or purges or by encouraging it to come to the skin. It was still a matter of the learned and rational physician's personal skill to decide on the timing of these measures in view of the success of the intentions, the severity of the symptoms and the individual characteristics of each patient.

In other words, most of Pintor's practice derived from the fact that he had made the pox, his *aluhumata*, a kind of *variola*. But Pintor had made pain the distinguishing feature of the pox, which distinguished it from other kinds of *variolae*. It was pain that could itself kill the patient, and was therefore more than a symptom or sign. One means of attacking the pain was the usual technique of applying alterative and evacuative remedies to the matter that caused it, but Pintor was unusual in believing that because it was so important to limit the pain it was permissible to use narcotic or sedative remedies. While such things were always harmful, the localised and minor damage they caused was justified by their control of the dangerous pain. In practice all of these remedies were ointments containing mercury, generally in what we would call chemical combination. Pintor, like Torrella and others, had techniques which he believed would modify the known danger of mercury without limiting its effectiveness. When he says it was to be 'extinguished with the saliva of a fasting person' he seems to have had in mind some combustive process upon metallic mercury. He also used medical simples for the same purpose, to lessen the danger but not the effect of mercury. He drew authority not so much from the great classical authors as from the Arabs and medieval Westerners, including Rhazes, Avicenna, Bernard de Gordon[34] and Guy de Chauliac, all of whom had used ointments of this kind to treat disease like *scabies*, *malum mortuum*, *impetigo*, *serpigo* and *pruritum*, most of them skin diseases, like the sores of the pox.

[. . .]

The practice of making the patient sweat was well known to Galenist physicians, and they used sudorific medicines for the purpose. . . . Another strategy was the use of mercury, and here too our two authors differed. Mercury had been a resource in the treatment of skin disorders, including *scabies* and lice (*pediculi*), since the time of Avicenna and Rhazes. Although as an external and practical treatment it fell within the province of surgery, these Arabic authors gave the method respectability in the physicians' eyes. . . .

The treatment of the pox with ointments or lotions containing mercury lasted from five to thirty days or more. During this period the

---

[34] Bernard de Gordon (b. 1258) taught and practised medicine at Montpellier for over thirty years.

mercury would be applied at least once a day and in a closed room near a fire, as in the stove, to help the patient sweat.[35] University physicians believed that this evacuated the moisture of the morbid matter and so relieved the pain and reduced the pustules. When the patient relapsed, the treatment was repeated. Torrella commonly used the method for a period of three to six days, Pintor for about eight. Pintor made a point of anointing the parts where the pain was most severe twice a day, making sure that, as in Torrella's treatment with the stove, the patient had not eaten before the treatment. The hand that applied the ointment – presumably Pintor's own – was first warmed before the fire, to ensure that the warmed ointment entered the pores of the flesh more easily; Pintor believed that it reached the membranes surrounding the bones and nerves. He claimed that the pustules disappeared after four to six days of the treatment, while the pains, although at first growing stronger, vanished by the eighth day.

There were two principal disadvantages with mercurial applications used by university-trained physicians. First, they caused serious side effects. Second, they were tainted by a history among the surgeons and unqualified practitioners ... For professional reasons it was essential that the rational and learned physician should draw mercury into *his* realm and show that its correct use belonged to his kind of doctor. One of the ways in which he did this was by claiming that the side effects of mercury treatment were the result of its wrong use at the hands of the *unqualified* practitioner, a strategy which also served for the specific and empirical remedy for pox, guaiac wood. Another way of drawing mercury into learned medicine was to argue that although administered externally as an ointment its effect was internal and thus part of the physician's business.

We can see these forces at play in Pintor's long discussion of mercury-containing 'narcotic' medicines, which takes up as much as a tenth of the whole work. He was clearly concerned about their use in treating the pains and sores of the *aluhumata* and like Torrella had to balance their effectiveness against their side effects. His conclusion was that the advantages outweighed the disadvantages *only if used* by a physician who was 'rational', 'learned' and 'very prudent', especially in relation to those taken by the mouth. Then, he claimed, a complete cure would be effected (provided that the amount of morbid matter was not large) by the help that was given to the native heat in dissolving the matter. We can see the force of his words, for these were mercury com-

---

[35] In some cases, patients were placed in 'dry stoves' to encourage sweating as part of their treatment.

pounds and very poisonous. The prudence he advised consisted in deciding the dose, the moment of taking the medicine, the duration of treatment, the nature of the patient and the prognosis. These were parts of a learned practice that the university physician jealously guarded and for which there were rules in the learned literature. Indeed, the prescription of internal medicines was claimed by the university physicians as their monopoly; it was no accident when Pintor said that internal application of narcotics was a final resort, after the failure of the partly surgical ointments, and when the patient began to weaken. This by implication is when the learned and rational physician is most needed, for he understands the body, disease and how medicines have their effects.

Pintor expressly contrasts the practice of the 'rational, learned and prudent' physicians with the 'inexperienced and ignorant' people who recklessly applied narcotic ointments, anointing not only the painful parts but the groin and armpits, which, the learned doctor believed, gave direct access to the vital parts of the body. The result of this, claimed Pintor, was that the patients suffered pustules and sores, even in the windpipe and lungs, threatening 'the greatest constriction and suffocation' of the throat, 'which is a pernicious thing increasing the danger of death'. But these undesirable side effects, he says elsewhere, are almost exactly the same as the common symptoms of *aluhumata*. Clearly, the difference between a side effect and a symptom depended on the position from which it was viewed.

For the benefit of university physicians and educated people, Pintor discusses seven narcotic ointments, all containing mercury 'extinguished with the saliva of a fasting person'. . . . He advised against one of them, which he believed had caused the death of a cardinal. . . . One other ointment was for use in certain cases only, but the remaining five, less harmful, were recommended by him for patients of different complexions. He was, therefore, claiming for his own type of practitioner and its patrons the most effective type of medicine, that which was accommodated to the individual. It is another opportunity to pour scorn on the 'vulgar and inexperienced' who were producing an increasing number and variety of what he saw as very dangerous remedies. He directs his peers to places in the learned literature where they can find remedies that will enable them to outshine the vulgar and inexperienced practitioners.

[. . .]

The same factors governed Torrella's choice of remedies as Pintor's. In the first place he believed that he was prescribing the most effective medicine for the pox. But it had also to be seen to be better than the prescriptions of the unqualified practitioners and so had to have some learned and rational authority. He was also in competition with other learned and rational physicians, most notably Pintor, and his remedies had to be distinctive if he was going to enhance his reputation as a pox doctor. It was probably for this reason that he recommended none of the ointments prescribed by Pintor. Moreover, in 1500 he singled out for condemnation four 'pernicious ointments', all containing quicksilver, and urged that people should 'flee from these ointments as from the plague'. Two of them were the two that Pintor had also warned against, and in this case we see Torrella and Pintor as learned physicians attacking those who were unqualified. But two of them had been recommended by Pintor; and when Torrella called upon the *protomedici*[36] to take action against 'the ignorant, the impostors and swindlers', who made a great deal of money from and did much damage with such remedies, it was a charge not only against the quacks outside his own professional group but almost certainly against Pintor.

In other words, one of the reasons why Torrella abandoned the use of metallic mercury was because Pintor persisted with it. In his tract on the pox Pintor revealed that he had been attacked by 'someone' – almost certainly Torrella – for his use of quicksilver in remedies. His answer was . . . that it was better to use even a dangerous remedy than allow the pain to kill the patient by overcoming his vital powers. Both Torrella and Pintor knew how dangerous mercury could be, and that mercury was implicated in the death of the cardinal of Segorbe.[37] It was important then that its use was tightly disciplined. Pintor clearly thought such discipline could be achieved, Torrella evidently thought not. Containing the danger and exercising discipline were areas which gave opportunity for medicalising and empirical remedy so that it could be seen to be used in an elaborate and rational way. For the rational doctor mercury was given in doses that were calculated, not empirical.

How much mercury was to be given depended on where it stood on the scale of degrees of the qualities. . . . The qualititative nature of mercury was much discussed in the sixteenth century, largely because of

---

[36] A form of medical police or bureaucracy found throughout Spain and Italy, which performed numerous functions including the issue of licences to practitioners, collection of fees, regulation of medical publications and the oversight of measures directed against contagious diseases such as plague.

[37] Bertomeu Marti was a close friend and possibly a relation of Rodrigo Borgia. On moving to Rome he became a bishop and head of Rodrigo's palace household before the latter's elevation to the pontificate. He was made a cardinal by Borgia, now Pope Alexander VI, in 1496, but died of the pox four years later.

the therapeutic implications for the pox, and Pintor's is a very early discussion. Was it true, he asked, that mercury was hot and humid in the fourth degree? Or cold and humid in the second degree? He did not want it to be cold, for then it would not seem capable of expelling the morbid matter. He pushed the argument in the direction he wanted, as medieval scholars so often did, by making a *distinctio*, that is, by drawing two different meanings out of a term and using one preferentially. Pintor 'distinguished' between natural or mineral quicksilver – that found in mines – and 'artificial' quicksilver, formed by burning mercury ore. He could then maintain that mineral quicksilver was cold in the second degree, but that the artificial sort was hot (because it had been burned) in the fourth degree. The same kind of reasoning might also lie behind his claim that mercury sublimate, having been sublimed, was hotter still. This was an argument against his opponent, whom we have with some caution identified as Torrella. Certainly Torrella was using the sublimate, which Pintor now argued, from Avicenna, was often fatal.

Part two

The sick body and its healers, 1500–1700

2.1

Medicine: trade or profession?

Margaret Pelling, 'Trade or Profession? Medical Practice in Early Modern England' in M. Pelling (ed.), *The Common Lot: Sickness, Medical Occupation and the Urban Poor in Early Modern England* (London and New York, Longman, 1998), pp. 240–5.

Margaret Pelling has written extensively on issues relating to the practice of medicine in early modern England. In this extract, which is taken from a revised version of an earlier essay published in 1987, she explores the question of whether or not it is possible to talk about a medical profession at this time given the large numbers of people engaged in the various forms of medical practice, and the tendency for many of these to pursue more than one occupation or career.

There are major features of medicine in the early modern period which seem to point to the value of shifting the emphasis away from the conventional definition of a profession as a full-time, autonomous activity, and towards other crafts, trades and occupations. [T]he tendency in the past has been to take the claims of certain minorities at their own valuation. Raach's approach had the merit of looking beyond London institutions to reveal the high incidence of academically qualified physicians even in small rural centres.[1] This is confirmed by . . . the finding that more than half of sixteenth-century medical graduates of Cambridge, and a larger proportion of the licentiates and unlicensed practitioners

[1] J. H. Raach, *A Directory of English Country Physicians 1603–1643* (London, Dawsons, 1962).

30

from the university, settled in the provinces. However, it is not clear that this is definitive of professional activity when many such graduates may have practised only sporadically. Much has been gained historically by taking Raach's quantitative approach further, to make an assessment of the occupation of medicine as a whole. This has involved both the adoption of a generic category of 'medical practitioner' in place of the conventional tripartite distinctions, and the inclusion in this category of any individuals recognised by their contemporaries as involved in the care of the sick. Behind this approach lies the assumption that 'any balanced view of medicine in the early modern period, or in non-western societies, must take into account all practitioners involved in dispensing medical care'. The inclusive view is also warranted on the grounds of the lack of historical justification for most criteria of selection:

> the difficulties involved in framing consistent and historically fruitful criteria for isolating responsible medical practitioners from empirics and quacks have often not been fully appreciated. Terms such as empiric tend to be used without consistency or sound historical justification. Adoption of technical criteria for the isolation of empirics based on the legal code, professional attachments, or educational attainment is practicable, but it tends to generate a trivial and unrealistically narrow conception of legitimate medical practice. Reference to more meaningful criteria related to professional efficiency, reliability and responsibility, or the ideal of service rather than pecuniary gain, is difficult to operate because of lack of evidence, but if applied objectively it is likely to reinforce the use of a broader rather than narrower conception of responsible medical practice.[2]

Even if fairly strict criteria are adopted, a high ratio of practitioners to population emerges. An estimate for London in the late sixteenth century, which is consistent with estimates of later date, leads to a ratio to population of at least 1:400. This body of *c.* 500 practitioners comprised: 50 fellows, candidates and licentiates of the Physicians' College; 100 members of the Barber-Surgeons' Company, including those prosecuted by the College; 100 apothecaries, some of them also the subject of prosecutions; and 250 practitioners (of all descriptions but excluding midwives and nurses) lying outside the London institutions except for (in some instances) the possession of licences. At the parish level, where occupational realities are often best reflected, a single London parish at the same period contained a barber-surgeon of some repute; a grocer free of the Barber-Surgeons' Company; two unlicensed practi-

---

[2] M. Pelling and C. Webster, 'Medical Practitioners', in C. Webster (ed.), *Health, Medicine and Mortality in the Sixteenth Century* (Cambridge, Cambridge University Press, 1979), p. 166. The previous quote is from the same source, p. 186.

tioners and one immigrant practitioner; 'a professor of physic and other curious arts', and a poor man who also professed physic; and a woman described as a 'counterfeit' physician and surgeon. A similar quantitative approach applied to Norwich over the period 1550–1640 revealed a group of 150 physicians, barber-surgeons, surgeons, lithotomists[3] and bonesetters, all of whom had some formal connection with the barber-surgeons' company of the city; and an additional group of 120, apparently lacking any such connection, which included physicians, women practitioners, immigrant practitioners, midwives, clerical practitioners, practising schoolmasters, and keepers of lazarhouses (male and female) who practised medicine. Even though the apothecaries were excluded, this more exhaustive assessment produced an even higher ratio of practitioners to population. That the present estimates are minimal rather than over-high is indicated by the fact that many of the practitioners have been identified by their being prosecuted for unlicensed practice, by the College or by the ecclesiastical authorities. Other evidence suggests strongly that prosecution by either authority was far from exhaustive. These estimates have led to the conclusion that medicine was a much more significant occupation in the early modern period, both economically and culturally, than previous analysis had suggested.

What was there for so many practitioners to do? There seem to be a variety of answers to this question. Perhaps most importantly, all the evidence suggests that the 'patient' in the early modern period was extremely 'active', being critical, sceptical and well-informed to a degree not anticipated in analysis of the professions, except in the extremely limited context of the pre-professional patronage relationship. This latter phenomenon is . . . assumed to go with low demand. However, it seems clear that the critical consumer of the early modern period absorbed enormous quantities of medical care, of all kinds, and that this consumption probably increased at crisis periods such as the later sixteenth and early seventeenth centuries, just as the consumption of similar consolations such as alcohol also increased. Poverty did not inhibit the consumption of certain forms of medicine at least; in periods of economic difficulty, loss of health or mobility was more threatening than ever. Not only was a scale of payment generally adopted, from pennies and payment in kind to high fees; there is some evidence to suggest that high fees failed to deter many patients, and that municipalities and parishes regarded medical expenses as being as legitimate an object of charity as losses by fire, or shipwreck. Poverty could also be seen by

---

[3] A lithotomist specialised in cutting out stones in the kidneys.

authority and the poor alike as a justification for practising medicine, especially in the case of women, and this suggests there were grounds for confidence that poverty could be alleviated by such means. . . . One example was Adrian Colman, the widow of a practitioner of physic, who was licensed at Whitehall in 1596 to practise on women and children in Norfolk, because she had no other means of support. Clerics also pleaded poverty as an excuse for practising medicine. Poverty could thus increase both supply and demand. At the same time, by 1600 medical care was already an aspect of the consumption of services in towns like Norwich and York, which early became centres for professional and social life. Holmes attributes the 'rise of the doctor' in the early eighteenth century to increased middle-class prosperity, along with a generalised tendency for towns to become service centres.[4] This argument was previously applied to the nineteenth century, along with the assumption of a shift from patronage to commodity relations associated with industrialisation. . . . [W]ith respect to medical personnel this interpretation has not been precisely articulated in historical terms, and tends to be based on minorities, rather than on the whole occupational group. Here it should be stressed that prosperity was not the only engine either of consumption or of the proliferation of medical practice.

This phenomenon of high but fluctuating consumption is complemented by a characteristic which increasingly is being shown to apply to a wide range of other occupational groups, and which may not be irrelevant to later periods when the professions seem firmly established. Both formally and informally, a great many medical practitioners either practised medicine part-time, or combined it with a range of associated activities. This was a feature of urban as well as of rural life, where it is more familiar. Barber-surgeons traditionally diversified into tallowchandling, knitting, netmaking and wigmaking; in towns dominated by the textile trades they also engaged in these in a minor level. Particularly strong and widespread was their involvement in music, which was one aspect of the social and public context represented by the shops of barbers and barber-surgeons. The latter offered a range of personal services which, in sophisticated urban environments, led to a natural intermingling with other tradesmen concerned with dress and ornament, such as dyers and perfumers. As well as continuing their traditional diversifications, medical practitioners showed themselves highly responsive to new economic opportunities. Among these, in the

---

[4] G. Holmes, *Augustan England: Professions, State and Society, 1680–1730* (London, George Allen & Unwin, 1982), pp. 11–18.

seventeenth century if not earlier, were the manufacture of small consumer goods relating primarily to dress and accessories, the selling of
tobacco, and distilling. An enterprising surgeon of the early seventeenth century was William White of Midhurst, Sussex, a small centre
near Chichester. White possessed a range of surgical instruments but
also barber's gear, distilling equipment, apothecary drugs, a considerable library of books, a stock of wine, and tobacco. The alertness of the
apothecaries to new botanical discoveries, and the growth in imported
drugs are both well-established developments. ... Barber-surgeons and
physicians as well as apothecaries were involved in distilling of various
kinds. Such flexibility could be formal: a citizen waxchandler around
1660 could accept an apprentice in 'the several arts of chirurgery and
distillation'. When distilling reached the level of an industrial process,
thus prompting attempts to monopolise it under the sponsorship of the
crown, objections were heard from the barber-surgeons as well as from
the apothecaries and the vintners. Distilling related to the production of
new drugs as well as of strong liquors. . . .

Practitioners of physic diversified as well as surgeons and barber-surgeons. At one extreme there is the 'professor' of physic of London . . .
who also practised 'other curious arts'; at the other is the well-known
tendency of schoolmasters and clerics also to be physicians. Scriveners
and physicians enjoyed close relations, and were sometimes (as with
surgeons) combined in one person, possibly because of the congruence
of skills and occasions. The latter could include attendance at the time
of will-making, if not the actual death-bed. . . . Also striking as a characteristic response to economic opportunities is the involvement of
practitioners in the Muscovy Company, which was founded in an
attempt to dominate trade with Russia in the mid-sixteenth century.
Physicians as well as surgeons and midwives formed part of the diplo-
matic commerce between England and Russia, which tended to focus
on the person of the monarch, and many of these took the opportunity
to engage in trade, one leading example being Arthur Dee, the son of the
astrologer John Dee.

Taken as a whole, medical practice in early modern England was neither well organised nor firmly controlled. No system of surveillance had
more than a partial application. The tripartite structure more strictly
adopted in continental Europe remained the aim of minority groups.
This intermittent kind of regulation is compatible with the occupational
flexibility just described, which seems entirely at odds with the full-
time, self-sufficient, life-long commitment characteristic of the professional as usually defined.

2.2

Women practitioners: the prescriptions of Lady Grace Mildmay

Linda Pollock, *With Faith and Physic: The Life of a Tudor Gentlewoman Lady Grace Mildmay 1552–1620* (London, Collins & Brown, 1993), pp. 123–4.

Lady Grace Mildmay (1552–1620) was a Northamptonshire gentle-woman who devoted much of her time to providing medicine for the poor and sick of the neighbourhood. Well read and conversant with much of the medical literature of her day, her papers include hundreds of recipes for the preparation of drugs and copious notes of her medical practice, with descriptions of the symptoms and outcomes of her patients' illnesses. Her papers have allowed historians to begin to reconstruct the activities of female healers in the early modern period. In the following extract, one can see how she understood and treated headache.

Of the headache

It is distinguished into 3 kinds. The first is cephalgia which is a pain new begun in the head. The second is called cephalia which is an inveterate pain in the whole head. And the third is himecrania which is a pain in half the head.

In the headache first consider if the pain be within the skull or without. If within, it will extend to the roots of the eyes. If without, the patient cannot endure the outside of the head to be touched.

If it come of accidental heat as long being in the sun, much exercise, hot baths, much anger, hot diseases, or hot savours, or watching, or fasting; then their head will feel hot, the skin drier, eyes red. And avoid no excrement at the nose and unapt to sleep and cool things outwardly do give ease. If the pain be occasioned by accidental cold and long tarrying in the cold air of extreme cold things applied to the head and idleness, the face will be full and pale and the eyes swollen and swart,[5] avoid much excrements at their nose, sleep much. If of blood and plenitude of humours caused of nourishing meats and drinks plentifully taking, neglect of natural and artificial evacuations; the face and eyes

---

[5] Dark, swarthy or baleful in appearance.

will be red, the veins swollen and those of the temples beat, the pulse great and vehement and a heaviness will accompany the pain. If of choler caused of meats that engender that humour, the signs are like those proceeding of accidental heat, saving that the pain will be more pricking and the face pale and wan. If it arise from phlegm, the signs will be like those proceeding of accidental cold. If it arise from wind, the signs are distension in the head without heaviness and beatings (which signified inflammation) and noise in the ears.

The increase of this kind cometh to the vertigo, to the falling sickness[6] and apoplexy. And when it comes to the vertigo it is occasioned either of gross humours in the brain itself, out of which by heat a vaporous wind is resolved or from vapours arising to the brain, from the abundance of corrupt humours in the stomach. Which vapours, from whence soever coming, turns about the animal spirits contained in the brain.

The signs of the first cause are as before said in the headache. And the signs of the second are as the signs of the headache from consent of other parts which followeth. If the headache arise from consent of other parts as from the stomach, caused by the vapours of sharp humours in the mouth thereof; the signs are the pain will be a gnawing and biting pain and the patient will have a desire to vomit. And the more they fast the more vehement is the pain and the more the malice of the humour increaseth.

For remedy of the headache of what kind soever it be, according to the signs of the offending humour, apply cordials or coolers inward or outward. And if it be from consent of other parts which of both have recourse for remedies to mitigate the humour where it is, and to draw it to the natural sewers, to the chapters of the greater diseases in the head and to the chapters of opening the passages from thence to the several places of evacuations.

Now followeth several courses of physic practised by the advice of several physicians upon several patients for the headache.

If giddiness or other grief in the head have been occasioned by staying corrupt fluxes, then must rectifying with opening things be given.

[6] Epilepsy.

2.3

The place of women in learned medicine:
James Primrose's *Popular Errours* (1651)

James Primrose, *Popular Errours. Or the Errours of the People*
in Physick, First Written in Latine . . . Translated into English
by Robert Wittie Doctor in Physick (London, W. Wilson,
1651), pp. 19–21.

James Primrose (d. 1659) practised medicine in Kingston-upon-Hull. A
Huguenot emigré, he settled in the north of England and published
numerous works on a variety of medical subjects, including the debate
over the circulation of the blood in which he appears as a conservative
opponent of William Harvey. *Popular Errours* was originally published in Latin in 1638 and was translated by his colleague, Robert
Wittie, a puritan physician who practised in Yorkshire in this period.
The work itself is a typical defence by the physician of his learned art
from the encroachments of a whole range of medical interlopers,
including women.

Having taken upon me to point out some Errours of the people, or at
least the common Errours of many, I have willingly favoured Churchmen (as much as I could possibly) so I resolve also concerning Women.
For it is not a thing of such consequence, nor ought any Physician of
note, or Surgeon to think worse of Women, which are borne for the care
and service of men, if they doe their whole endeavour for the good of
Mankinde; for they know how to make a bed well, boyle pottage, cul-
lices[7], barley broth, make Almond milke, and they know many remedies
for sundry diseases. But they especially are busied about Surgery, and
that part chiefly which concernes the cure of Tumours and Ulcers:
Notwithstanding the cure of Ulcers and Wounds doth require very much
art; at first all their differences must bee known, to wit, whether it be a
simple Wound, or corroding, contused, with putrefaction of the bone,
corrupt, cancrous, fistulous, &c. Then the variety of remedies and circumstances in curing, makes the art to be fallacious, uncertaine and
conjecturall. All which things, seeing they cannot be known but by a
skilfull Physician, women ought not so rashly and adventurously to
intermeddle with them. Againe, they usually take their remedies out of

---

[7] Strong broths made of meat.

English bookes, or else make use of such as are communicated to them by others; and then they think they have rare remedies for all diseases. But *Galen* in his bookes of *Method*, teaches that remedies are to bee altered according to the person, place, part affected, and other circumstances; for in some a deterging Medicine[8] will draw unto suppuration, as Frankincense; in others the same remedy will generate flesh, and *Galen* gives an example of a Surgeon, who in an Ulcer where hee saw great putrefaction, did daily apply a strong deterger, *viz*. Verdigrease,[9] and the oftner he did so, by so much the more did the putrefaction encrease, because the remedy was stronger than the disease. The same Ulcer in the Legge doth require a different remedy from that in the breast, or another part, because of the diverse nature of the parts. If therefore they understand well all the differences and causes of ulcers, as also a right method, and a right use of suppurating, deterging, flesh-generating, and cicatrizing[10] medicines, and the reason of varying them according to the nature of the parts, ages, temperaments, and other circumstances, I will easily believe that they may be able to exercise this Art. But seeing that these things cannot bee attained unto without much labour and study, I can scarce be brought to believe that they are able to understand, or performe what they promise. But because a Physician ought to be but little solicitous, who, and how many they be that practise Physick, we will say no more of Women, it sufficeth that wee have manifested their errours to the people.

2.4

Lay and learned medicine in early modern England

Doreen Evenden Nagy, *Popular Medicine in Seventeenth-Century England* (Bowling Green, Ohio, Bowling Green State University Press, 1988), pp. 43–8, 53.

In this extract, Evenden Nagy demonstrates the extent to which the boundary between 'popular' medicine, usually depicted by historians as superstitious and rooted in folk lore, and learned medicine, the

---

[8] A cleansing medicine.
[9] Verdigris or acetate of copper.
[10] Cures that leave a scar.

domain of university-educated professionals, was largely a myth. Two examples of the intermingling of lay, amateur medicine with the practice of learned professionals are discussed here: firstly, the extent to which many of the latter depended upon, and utilised, herbs and other concoctions that formed part of popular medicine; and secondly, the emergence of a vernacular medical literature in mid-seventeenth-century England, which was aimed at the popular market.

Although the medical profession laid claim to a corpus of medical knowledge which it deemed inaccessible to those lacking the formal education in the classics and humanities offered by the universities, or, in the case of surgeons, the expertise derived from a lengthy apprenticeship, evidence points to the fact that in reality there was no clearly defined separation between the methods used by authorized practitioners and those used by lay or popular practitioners in the treatment of illness. Doctors' records from the period illustrate the striking similarity between their treatments and those used by lay practitioners, including those which were drawn from an oral tradition and handed down from generation to generation.

[. . .]

Dr. John Hall[11] was a university-trained physician who used the treatments commonly associated with Galenic medicine: laxatives, enemas, emetics and bleeding, although he appeared to use phlebotomy or bleeding much less frequently than other forms of removing unhealthy 'humours' from his suffering patients. Hall's prescriptions were commonly concoctions of readily available herbs, roots and spices. When Mr. Drayton, a poet,[12] was suffering from a Tertian ague,[13] Hall gave him an 'emetick infusion mixed with syrup of violets' which, Hall noted, worked 'very well both upwards and downwards.' He treated Mrs. Chandler, who was ill with child-bed fever, with a mixture of hartshorn, spring water, syrup of lemons, rosewater, sugar and syrup of red poppies, which he claimed cured her. The young son of a minister who Hall diagnosed as suffering from 'Falling sickness,' was treated by having 'round pieces' of peony root hung about his neck, as well as a sponge soaked in vinegar and rue, applied to his nostrils. The medieval practice of hanging peony root around children's necks as a preventive measure against convulsions . . . was recommended in medical literature as late

---

[11] Hall, who practised in Stratford-upon-Avon, was the son-in-law of William Shakespeare.
[12] Michael Drayton (1563–1631), poet and celebrated author of *Poly-olbion*.
[13] A fever characterised by convulsions every third day.

as 1739, and may have originated with Dioscorides[14] who advised hanging the peony plant 'about one' to avoid poisons, bewitchings, fears and devils as well as fevers and agues.

Hall gave a fifty-year old woman who was bleeding from the mouth a mixture which contained syrup of poppies, rosewater, conserve of roses, bloodstone and sealed earth. To treat a man who had not voided for three days, Hall prescribed a mixture of winter cherry berries, parsley seed, milk, syrup of marshmallows and Holland powder followed by local applications of hot onion and garlic fried in butter and vinegar; the latter treatment 'procured urine within an hour, with some stone and gravel.' An 'electuary' made of finely chopped dates mixed with purified honey cured Mrs. Harvey, five weeks post-partum, of excessive vaginal discharge, pain and weakness in her back. Although Hall has been credited with combining 'medical procedures and herbal decoctions with an enlightened cure for scurvy', his prescriptions for scurvy which contained scurvy-grass, water cress and brook-lime were basically the same as or inferior to those used by lay practitioners, many of which also contained oranges and lemons. For example, Lady Sedley's receipt book contained five prescriptions for scurvy: one of these was credited to the renowned anatomist, Richard Lower.[15] But one recipe containing lemons, and one from a layman containing orange juice, were far superior to Dr. Lower's, as well as to Dr. Hall's receipts. Susanna Avery's receipt book (inscribed 1688), contained 'A Drinke for the Scurvy' which called for oranges, among other ingredients. In his treatise on diseases of the eye, Richard Banister[16] mentioned a woman who was 'famous for curing the Scorby'. She administered a drink made from brook-lime and water cresses, 'nine times daily'. This unknown woman, then, was using a herbal treatment (which is now known to be high in the content of Vitamin 'C' and specific for the treatment of scurvy) many years before Hall's records were published.

John Symcotts was another university-trained and fully qualified practitioner whose treatments combined elements of folk medicine, superstition, and Galenic tradition. In 1648 he treated the youngest son

[14] Dioscorides (c. 40–c. 90 AD) was a Greek surgeon in Nero's army and the author of *De materia medica*, a compilation of plants and their curative qualities.

[15] Richard Lower (1631–91) studied medicine at Oxford and was an associate of Robert Boyle and other early members of the Royal Society. In his treatise on the heart, *Tractatus de corde*, published in 1669, he famously suggested that it was the 'nitrous' property of the air in the lungs that imparted life-sustaining qualities to the arterial blood.

[16] Richard Banister (d. 1626), of Stamford, was a celebrated eye specialist who was responsible for the publication of the translation of Jacques Guillemeau's *A treatise of on hundred and thirteene diseases of the eye and eye-lidds* (London, 1622).

of the Earl of Bridgewater who had apparently suffered a stroke. A partial list of his efforts to save the unconscious young man's life included blowing tobacco up his nostrils (as well as sneezing powder), warm applications to his head, striking his hands and feet 'mightily', inserting mustard and vinegar in his mouth, enemas, suppositories, cupping, scarification, applying plasters and dead pigeons to his feet, holding a hot frying pan close to his head and applying leeches to his rectum. Despite (or more probably because of) Symcott's efforts, the young man died. Among Symcott's recipes were two which Symcotts acknowledged as receipts from lay people; one was a prescription for a salve for a 'spleen plaster,' the other a list of ingredients for a remedy against the plague or the ague which Symcotts ascribed to 'Mrs. Rolt of Pertenhall.' The latter contained no less than twenty roots, plants or herbs in a base of white wine. When this recipe used by Dr Symcotts is compared with a recipe found in a seventeenth-century manuscript from the Dorset region which was based on orally-transmitted traditions, the Dorset recipe known as 'Mrs. Hodges cordiall Water, useful for agues or any infectious diseases,' duplicates Symcotts' (or Mrs. Rolt's) recipe almost ingredient for ingredient. Further research is needed to establish firmly the debt which seventeenth-century physicians owed to lay practitioners of earlier generations, but again, the generalization can be made that licensed practitioners could offer no guarantee of cures which were the exclusive property of the professionals.

Symcotts' records offer a further illustration of the blurring of the line between popular and 'learned' medicine. In 1635 when Dr. Symcotts was suffering from gout, his brother, a London merchant, wrote to suggest that his brother try the treatment by which he had cured himself the previous year; this 'cure' consisted of a paste made from yeast, egg white and alum which was spread on brown paper and bound about the foot. . . . [As such] it is an excellent example of how contemporary lay people perceived the limited capacity of the medical profession, even to the extent of their inability to treat themselves effectively.

[. . .]

The analysis of 83 medical treatises which were published between 1640 and 1660, reveals that while 39 were ostensibly intended for use by the professionals, only 9 were written in Greek or Latin, thus placing them out of the reach of all but the formally educated. A further 10 publications were directed to lay as well as professional use. Thus, of the literature for licensed physicians and surgeons, some 40 treatises offered 'cures' which could be easily duplicated by lay persons (indeed in some cases, cures or treatments were ascribed to lay practitioners). The remaining 30 odd treatises were clearly intended for lay use.

Ralph Williams, 'practitioner in Physick and Chyrurgerie,'[17] stated that he wrote for the professions; he described treatments for plague, tertian fevers and gout, all based on herbs, roots, bark or other readily available ingredients. Williams included Galen's cure for gout: old cheese soaked in the broth of a gammon of bacon and made into a plaster for local application. Robert Bayfield of Norwich also wrote for the professions, especially 'to help young and greene students in Physick and Chyrurgery.'[18] His prescription for various cordials to treat the plague are made up of readily available materials such as root of angelica, wormwood vine, conserve of roses, treacle and mithridate.[19] For inflammation of the breast, Bayfield prescribed the same concoction as for stomach ache with vomiting: syrup of roses, syrup of rhubarb and senna.

Three Fellows of the College of Physicians in London published a scholarly work in 1650: *A Treatise of the Rickets Being a Disease Common to Children.* The authors, headed by the highly respected Francis Glisson,[20] left no doubt that their work . . . was intended for the benefit of professional practitioners. The treatment of rickets which they outlined, however, offered nothing new or original that lay beyond the compass of traditional or popular medicine. Their research undoubtedly assisted lay practitioners in the diagnosis of rickets, while the treatments which they recommended were customarily non-specific, described by the doctors as simples and compounds *'readily available* in shops such as rue, spica roots, Fernbrake, betony, Fennell, caraway, dill.' The regimen, typically Galenical, included an initial preparation of the passages with enemas, vomits and purges, and finally, external applications of camomile, marigold and earthworms, as well as ointments made of herbs, butter and nutmeg. Glisson and his colleagues failed to make any connection between their clinical dis-

---

[17] Williams was the author of *Physical rarities, containing the most choice receipts of physick, and chyrurgerie, for the cure of all diseases incident to mans body* (London, J. M., 1651).

[18] Robert Bayfield, *Enchiridion medicum: containing the causes, signs, and cures of all those diseases that do chiefly affect the body of man* (London, E. Tyler, 1655).

[19] An antidote for poisons and infectious diseases, usually composed from the plant, candy tuft.

[20] Francis Glisson (1597–1677) was Regius Professor of Medicine at Cambridge and a celebrated physician and anatomist, who also wrote original works on the liver and the relationship between the soul and the body. His work on rickets – a collaborative project with two other physicians, George Bate and Ahaseurus Regemorter – was originally published in Latin in 1650. The first pirated English translation appeared in 1651.

coveries, which related to diagnosis and description, and their treatment of the disease; in the case of rickets, it was pointless to seek the help of licensed physicians. Indeed, in one medical compendium published by a lay person for non-professionals, a receipt which contained the specific treatment for rickets appeared in 1655.

[. . .]

Aside from the books whose authors were clearly identified with the medical profession in one way or another, other compendia were published for the benefit of the lay practitioner or to give directions for self-treatment. The most ambitious of these was published in 1655 under the pseudonym 'Philiatros' and purported to contain one thousand seven hundred and twenty 'Receipts fitted for the cure of all sorts of Infirmities whether Internal or External, Acute or Chronical that are incident to the body of Man.' The 'receipts' were contributed or approved by a variety of persons and provide an interesting commentary not only on the minimal control exercised by the universities and the doctors in the dissemination of medical knowledge, but also on the way that a prescription from a lay person was perceived as having as much merit as one from a licensed practitioner. Contributors include 22 doctors, 41 males from either the aristocracy or gentry, 13 women with the title of Countess or lady, 32 women with the designation 'Mrs.', one good wife and two women without any designation; the heaviest contributor was a Mrs. Downing, with 16 prescriptions. In this publication, then, the contributions of lay practitioners outnumbered those by doctors by four to one.

In the same year [1655], W.M., who claimed to have been a former servant of the Queen,[21] published *The Queen's Closet opened*, a book which proved so popular, subsequent editions appeared in 1671, 1674, 1683 and 1698. One possible reason for the book's popularity was the author's claim that the queen had actually used many of the prescriptions. Listed among the contributors of receipts to the 'Queen's Closet' were 29 physicians and surgeons, 15 men with titles or from the gentry, 16 countesses and ladies, 1 bishop and only 3 from what could be considered the lower classes.

Moreover, there appears to be no distinction between the illnesses for which the physician offered receipts and those for which lay persons offered their favoured cures. Philiatros published two cures for the gout which were attributed to Mr. Peacock and Mr. John Cornwallis, as well as five or six treatments by unnamed contributors. Of the

---

[21] Queen Henrietta Maria, the widow of Charles I, who had been executed in 1649.

latter, one was designated, the 'best' cure for gout; it contained black soap and the yolks of raw eggs bound to the afflicted part by a plaster of egg whites and flour. W.M.'s treatise offered 'Dr. Stevens' cure for gout,' made up of his famous 'water', plus sheep's suet, boar's grease, wax and 'neet's foot oyl';[22] a prescription for gout by a lay person contained sheep's suet and wax, as well as herbs while another unnamed contributor included the 'neet's foot oil' favoured by Dr. Stevens. Lady Oxford's 'Oyl of Excester' was described as a cure for gout and sciatica. It contained olive oil plus seventeen herbs, plants and flowers. Mr. Peacock's cure, while more modest in content, also contained flowers and leaves. It can be seen, therefore, that there was no great distinction between the ingredients used by professionals and lay practitioners.

[. . .]

In conclusion, any sharp distinction between 'popular' and professional medical practice and treatment in Stuart England appears to be untenable. The concepts of a unique corpus of established, academic knowledge on the one hand, and of a backward, simple folk medicine on the other, are equally misleading. Within the published literature as well as available physicians' and lay records, the two merged together into a largely amorphous whole. The recognition of this fact is vital in assessing the nature and position of popular medicine in this period. In essence, it was neither 'fringe' nor 'alternative' health care, but an integral part of an unconscious, interdependent 'system.' Evaluated in these terms, the continued vitality of popular medicine throughout the century was reasonable and, in the main, noncontentious.

---

[22] An oil made from the foot of an ox.

2.5

Physical appearance and the role of the barber surgeon in early modern London

Margaret Pelling, 'Appearance and Reality: Barber-Surgeons, the Body and Disease' in A. L. Beier and R. Finlay (eds), *London 1500–1700: The Making of the Metropolis* (London and New York, Longman, 1986), pp. 89–95.

In this extract, Pelling demonstrates the importance of bodily appearance, and the need to disguise physical imperfections, in the broader cultural worldview of early modern men and women. Integral to the process of caring for the body's appearance was the barber surgeon, who provided a range of services that were designed both to promote the health of his clients, as well as offering various physical pleasures and other stimulants.

In any period before antibiotics, scarring, and more importantly, chronic failure to heal, must greatly have prejudiced the individual's chances of appearing clear and unspotted before the world. It could be argued that the individual's response to this situation has varied little, being consistently negative, while the terms in which responses were cast, on the other hand, have varied greatly according to the beliefs of the society in which they were produced. An appearance of indifference can be given, in that scars and deformities, like such features as unusual height and hair colour, could provide important means of identifying individuals and even establishing credentials. In European folklore, however, the idealized protagonist typically combined a person entirely free of deformity with an identifying mark or feature which was small and hidden. In periods before the present day, medical practitioners and the laity alike placed great stress on disfiguring conditions, especially those affecting the face; modern medicine concentrates more exclusively on life-threatening conditions, although there is little evidence that the laity shares this comparative indifference.

It is notable that, while northern Renaissance portraiture shows a fascination with extremes of ugliness, it signally fails to depict the more minor defects which are so plentifully recorded in such sources as popular medical literature, satire, and private correspondence. . . .

Such attitudes seem not to have been confined to any class or classes in society, whether rural or urban. Urban life, however, added new

45

dimensions to attitudes to the body as the city became the main arena for competition among social aspirants. The pre-eminence of London was sealed by the increasing presence there of courts which were famous for their stress on personal good looks and accomplishments. Society still expected the individual to summarize his estate in his own person; now a new flamboyance and even fastidiousness was required. It would be surprising if a climate of acute social competition were to foster indifference to personal appearance, death or decay. Early modern London produced infinite variations on the theme of false appearances; but this evidence of sophistication should be seen as based on relatively stable attitudes to physical life. It was still customary to seek the mind's construction in the face (and hands), even though one might, like Shakespeare's Duncan, despair of the attempt, or alternatively, look to more and more subtle means (physiognomy, chiromancy) of achieving the truth.[23]

[. . .]

The preoccupation with disguise obviously had a humorous and even positive side, just as the London playwrights and others were also prepared to make ribald or cynical use of every detail of physical frailty collected by the satirists. In the concealments and revelations which occur so often in plays of the period, enormous and significant stress is placed on clothing and accessories and their power to determine, in the eye of the beholder, the personality, occupation, rank, and sex of the wearer. Inventories and wills which carefully identified and disposed of single garments, show clearly the high capital cost of outer clothing, its status as a durable, and the significance vested in it by the wearer. Protests against the rapidly changing fashions and frivolous assumption of styles of dress, which were typical of the urban setting and above all of London, had considerable social and economic justification. At the same time, London fashion was acting as an engine of economic growth and change.

Elizabethan and Jacobean clothing, although strong in outline and attractive in surface, played an important role in concealing the body from public view. Very little of the surface of the body was allowed to appear. Refinements introduced into the town dress of the wealthier classes pointed to the same desire to combine ostentation with concealment. It seems reasonable to connect this with a high incidence of, and even increased sensitivity to, defect or deformity caused by disease

---

[23] W. Shakespeare, *Macbeth* 1.4.12–13. Physiognomy was the art of judging character from the features and lines of the face. Chiromancy was the ancient art of palmistry.

in the context of a crowded society. Beggars offended by baring their limbs and sores in public, as well as by breathing on passers-by. The few areas of the body normally left uncovered by clothing acquired, for the more prosperous, accessories which attempted to make a virtue of necessity. Decorative gloves were an important item and permanently perfumed gloves were especially prized. The pre-eminence of the face was stressed by many styles of the period, notably ruffs. Small looking-glasses were attached to the costume like fobs. It is not surprising to find that masks were also worn from about mid-century by both sexes, and that face-patches were adopted during the 1590s. Cosmetics were also applied, particularly those calculated to improve the appearance of the skin. For most of the Elizabethan period, the hair of men was generally kept short, and women's hair was mostly covered; by a similar characteristic tension between desire and fulfilment, men's hair became longer and women's hair more visible just when it seemed that the likelihood of hair loss by disease was at its greatest. Wigs rapidly evolved to fill the gap. This expedient also solved the perennial problem of infestation by lice and other parasites, with its ugly *sequelae* caused by scratching and infection.

Clothing at this time had other functions which were important for all classes, in both town and country. Parts of the body which were uncovered were also unprotected, a belief which has considerable justification in temperate climates and at a time when minor injuries could lead by unchecked infection to major disaster. This again points to the special sensitivity of the face and hands. . . . [I]t would not be an exaggeration to suggest that, at this period, covering the body was thought to be necessary for survival. However, change, or 'shifting' of clothing was also essential, even for the poorest.

It is usually assumed, on the basis of scanty evidence, that the Tudor and Stuart periods, coming after the communal and ritual bathing of the medieval period, and before the allegedly superior regard for cleanliness adopted by fashionable society in the eighteenth century, were distinguished by their dirtiness. The question deserves much greater attention, but enough has been said to suggest that, at the least, there was no lack of sensitivity on matters relating to the body and its state of health. Stray comments by contemporaries on dirty habits are usually taken as incriminating, without also being considered as evidence of a kind of fastidiousness. It is also worth stressing that there are more ways than one of being clean. Even in the present day, in Western society, many people make a strong distinction between their persons and their surroundings with respect to cleanliness. Ritual bathing apart, regular and prolonged immersion of the whole body is, for good and obvious reasons, a very recent habit, and even now is probably more partially adopted than bathroom furniture might suggest.

Similarly, it is only recently that it was thought acceptable for any major area of the outer clothing to be in contact with the skin. The main burden of absorbing dirt and vermin from the body, and protecting the outer garments which were often worn daily for long periods, fell on the intervening layers or underclothing. Very few items survive from the period under discussion, pointing to great wear and tear followed by the use of the material for other purposes, and it is not even certain what was worn. It seems reasonable, however, to suggest that the layer next to the skin has been under, rather than overestimated. It is difficult otherwise to imagine (for instance) what work was carried out by the numerous washerwomen of the time. Washing has received little attention as an occupation yet, to take one example, it was the single most common occupation of poor women in Norwich in the 1570s if the textile-related occupations are left out of account, and was also commonly adopted as a second-string occupation. Clothing was also cleaned by mechanical means, including brushing and beating, the latter being particularly important against vermin such as lice. Both the capital value of clothing and its relation to health and disease are further underlined by the frequent reference to clothes acting as fomites, or carriers of infection, with respect to contagious diseases like plague, or the French pox.

Although total immersion seems to have been rare, washing of the all-important face and hands, and even the whole head, may have been a regular and even daily occurrence. The persistently high incidence of death by drowning was in some cases at least due not to suicide, or the role of water in transport and industry, but (with the almost universal inability to swim) to the use of rivers and ditches for washing, either of clothes or bodies. Self-medication was a universal habit in which forms of washing or bathing could play a vital and little-considered part. Like substances now commonly regarded merely as foods, water itself very often had a potent or medicinal role and there was widespread contemporary awareness of the properties of different waters. In addition a very broad range of health-giving, curative, or merely soothing procedures involved bathing part or even all of the body in waters imbued with herbs and other substances. Causing the body to sweat was also a very common and related procedure. Thus [William] Bullein[24] recommended fennel, balm and bay for washing-water and 'barbers' baths', and fennel with endive as 'very good to wash one's feet to bedward'.

[24] William Bullein (d. 1576) was a Galenic physician, who practised in Durham and Northampton, and wrote a number of popular treatises on medicine.

Perfumed waters, although liable to perversion by 'light wanton people', had similar virtues; 'what is pleasanter in sweet water, to wash hands, head and beard, and good in apparel, and may be rightly used', was a gift of God. The potency of soap was not underestimated; it was used as an active ingredient combined with others (including heavy metals) to combat tetters,[25] black morphew,[26] ringworms, spots, melancholy infecting the skin, scalding, stinking scabs, and itch'. Although Bullein's prescriptions were not for the poor, it may be concluded that lack of personal hygiene in the modern sense (in which water is given a neutral role) was partly compensated for by the universal tendency to domestic self-help with respect to health. In the present context what is relevant is that the most important locality outside the home for washing, grooming, and every function relevant to hygiene and the presentation of the body to the outside world, was the barber-surgeon's shop.

The short hair and constantly changing beardstyles of earlier Elizabethan men obviously required regular attention. Beards were dyed as well as shaped; later, not surprisingly, barber-surgeons became involved in wig-making as well as the shaving of heads so that wigs could be worn. However, there seem to have been few limits to the personal services offered by barber-surgeons. Among these, bloodletting and toothdrawing are well-known; but barber-surgeons also cleaned teeth by scraping them, pared nails, picked or syringed ears (which could involve the removal of worms or 'small beasts'), plucked with tweezers, and had a special role in the removal and mitigation of marks and blemishes. Soapballs were used for washing, and perfumes were applied with casting-bottles. Even if the customer failed to follow the example of centuries, and did not confide in his attendant, the barber-surgeon was in an excellent position to acquire knowledge of state of health from skin, breath, odour, and even the state of the hair. In using such signs barber-surgeons could justifiably argue that they were following the best traditions of Hippocratic medicine. Even if he did not often practise the more extreme forms of surgery, the barber-surgeon was in a better position even than the tailor to know both the appearance and the reality of his clients. He was responsible for the crucial exposed areas of head and hands, but also dealt in what was hidden.

Barber-surgeons' shops in towns and cities emerge as places of resort for men, offering music, drink, gaming, conversation, and news, as well as the services already mentioned. After 1600 many added to their attractions by selling tobacco, a contemporary obsession which first

---

[25] Generic name for any pustular, herpes-like eruptions of the skin.
[26] Leprous or scurfy condition of the skin.

earned credit for curing diseases, including venereal disease. Direct evidence is hard to find, but it seems plausible to propose that the barbershop also served as the first port of call for advice on sexual matters, being, unlike the brothel itself, primarily a male preserve. The later history of the barbershop suggests continuity in this as in other respects. It should be stressed that for the first half of the seventeenth century at least there was a 'marked surplus' of men – particularly younger men – in London's population. It is unlikely that every barber-surgeon in London offered the full spectrum of attractions mentioned here, if only because of the number of competing outlets for such items as drink. Nonetheless, the range is sufficient to explain both the large numbers of this occupation in London, and the evennesses and concentrations of their distribution in the capital.

2.6

Renaissance critiques of medicine: Pico and Agrippa

Nancy Siraisi, *Medicine and the Italian Universities 1250–1600* (Leiden, Boston and Cologne, Brill, 2001), pp. 187–200.

The following extract is taken from chapter 9 of Siraisi's book on academic medicine in late medieval and Renaissance Italy entitled 'Renaissance Critiques of Medicine, Physiology, and Anatomy'. It focuses on the criticisms of two leading controversialists in early sixteenth-century Europe, Gianfrancesco Pico della Mirandola and Henricus Cornelius Agrippa. Pico (1469–1533) was the nephew of the even more celebrated intellectual, Giovanni Pico della Mirandola, one of the central figures in the Italian Renaissance and the revival of neoplatonism. The younger Pico was a profound critic of contemporary learning and its claims to certainty. In his *Examen vanitatis doctrinae gentium et veritatis christianae disciplinae* (*An examination of the futility of pagan learning and of the truth of Christian teaching*) of 1520, cited here, he claimed that all the sciences, including medicine, were essentially erroneous as they relied exclusively on the evidence of the faulty and corrupt senses.

Pico's critique of Renaissance medicine was largely academic in tone and content, aimed at demonstrating the inconsistencies and illogical claims of university-educated physicians. Agrippa (1486–1535), on the other hand, adopted a more vitriolic and populist approach in his critique of the medical profession, in particular focusing on the failure of physicians to heal their patients. His comments are contained in a work first published in 1530 entitled *De incertitudine et vanitate scientiarum declamatio invectiva* (*An invective declamation concerning the uncertainty and vanity of the sciences*), in which Agrippa employed a wide range of humanist rhetorical strategies, including invective, irony and humour, in order to get his message across.

[W]hen Pico focused his critique on the issue of the certitude of physiological and pathological knowledge, he was not introducing a consideration hitherto absent in medieval and Renaissance medical discourse. Rather, his analysis gained in effectiveness precisely because it used skeptical criteria as the basis of a fresh evaluation of two of the most central and frequently discussed problems in the Latin academic medical literature of the thirteenth to the fifteenth century: the kind and level of knowledge afforded by medicine, or the several parts of medicine, and the differences over physiology between 'the philosophers and the physicians'. Furthermore, physiology was precisely the branch of medical knowledge for which the status of a science offering certitude was most likely to be seriously claimed by medical writers in the Latin scholastic tradition.

Chapter 16 of Book I of the *Examen vanitatis*, on the subject of the 'remarkable dissension that seems to have flourished among the philosophers and even the physicians of the nations about the formation, conditions, and properties of the human body' is a rhetorical tour de force. In it, Pico followed the human body from conception, through sexual differentiation, normal or abnormal embryonic development, birth, growth, nourishment, disease and aging to natural death, while simultaneously pointing out that two thousand years of argument had not led to agreement as to how any of these physiological processes actually operate. His presentation laid particular emphasis upon the diversity and multifarious nature of ancient opinion among both philosophers and physicians; for each of the physiological events discussed he listed the views of an array of ancient authorities, including not only Aristotle, Plato, the Stoics, Hippocrates, Celsus[27] and Galen,

---

[27] Celsus (fl. c. 30 AD) was not a physician by training or profession, but the author of one of the most important compendia of ancient Greek and Roman medicine.

but also various Presocratics and early medical figures known chiefly by report. For the supposed physiological opinions of ancients in the two last categories, Pico relied in part upon the collection of ancient views about conception and embryology put together by Censorinus, and on other similar doxographical sources.[28] He also made use of the reports, or polemics, about their predecessors contributed by Aristotle and Galen, especially Aristotle. In the physiological chapter, as in the *Examen vanitatis* as a whole, a major goal was to show that Aristotle represented only one strand of ancient teaching and was internally inconsistent into the bargain.

One example of the way Pico handled particular physiological topics must suffice. On the subject of semen, Pico addressed two questions: how and where it is produced in the body, and whether it is produced by both men and women. In the first, the main emphasis is on Aristotle's treatment of the subject. Pico used Aristotle's attack on pangenesis[29] in *De generatione animalium* [*On the generation of animals*] . . . to point out the difference of opinion between Aristotle and other ancient authorities. And he also drew attention to the apparent inconsistency between Aristotle's own teaching in *De generatione animalium* . . . that semen is the final residue of aliment, and the statement in *Problemata* . . . that it comes down from the brain, which is why 'castrated cattle do not grow horns and children do not go bald.' Pico characterized this second supposed opinion of Aristotle's as 'against Alcmaeon', evidently an allusion to Aristotle's report in *Historia animalium* (*The history of animals*) . . . that the fifth-century physician Alcmaeon of Croton associated the growth of hair [that is, pubic hair] with the production of semen.

On the second question, Pico reviewed opinions ascribed to Pythagoras, Democritus, Hippocrates, Epicurus, Aristotle . . . Galen, Averroes, and Zeno.[30] Once again, rhetorical effectiveness depends on the suggestion that there are not just one or two but a multiplicity of 'authorities' with irreconcilable views. But the most substantial ancient discussions of the respective contributions of male and female to conception were in fact those by Aristotle and Galen, whose differing opin-

[28] A doxographer was someone who collected the opinions of the ancient Greek philosophers. Censorinus' *De die natali* was composed some time around 238 AD. It was primarily concerned with chronology, calendars, and the various periods of life, and drew widely on earlier authorities.

[29] Pangenesis refers to the belief that both the man and the woman contribute to the process of conception. Aristotle rejected this approach, asserting that only the male contributed to generation through the production of sperm.

[30] Zeno of Citium (fl. fourth to third century BC) was the founder of the ancient school of Stoicism.

ions on the subject were of course well known, and much debated among scholastic physicians. As Pico said, 'almost all the later crowd of *medici* [physicians] used to fight at some time over this, and to this day they are clearly still fighting.' In this instance, in short, Pico deliberately chose a topic that was a scholastic cliché, a standard *quaestio* in thirteenth- to fifteenth-century Latin medical works, in order to provide the most effective illustration possible of the absence of certain knowledge about even the most frequently discussed issues in physiology.

But academically trained medical writers of the thirteenth to fifteenth centuries were in fact well aware of ambiguities and conflicts in the status ascribed to medical knowledge by Hippocrates, Galen, Avicenna and Averroes, and of irreconcilable elements in the discipline as they themselves encountered it. In numerous discussions (often in the form of an introductory *quaestio* at the beginning of general medical works) physicians took up the question of whether medicine should properly be defined as *scientia*, *ars*, or some combination of the two. *Scientia* for physicians trained in Aristotelian logic and epistemology implied certain knowledge, based on accepted principles, arrived at by syllogistic demonstrations, and enunciating universally valid truths. *Ars* involved the orderly and rational transmission of knowledge, but did not necessarily yield certitude about general truths. Evidently, the multifarious and unsystematic particulars of practical or operative medicine were difficult to fit into the definition of *scientia*, and even in some respects into that of *ars*. On the other hand, the theoretical part of the university medical curriculum, in which disputation about physiology was a principal component, which made use of Aristotelian scholastic methodology, and which overlapped in subject matter with Aristotelian natural philosophy, appeared to have a better claim to *scientia* in the Aristotelian sense. As a result, scholastic writers often ended up by asserting that medicine was somehow both *scientia* and *ars*, but that theoretical medicine (and hence physiology) partook of the nature of *scientia* more fully than did the rest of medicine.

[. . .]

Unlike Pico, who treated physiology from a standpoint on the boundaries of natural philosophy and medicine, Agrippa was primarily concerned with medicine as a therapeutic system. His chapter 'On medicine in general,' dealing with the nature of medical knowledge and with physiology, occupied only about one-sixth of the space he devoted to medicine as a whole; most of the rest is taken up by a lengthy chapter 'On operative medicine.' These chapters are as filled with invective, exaggeration, and anecdote as the rest of *De incertitudine*, so that

Agrippa's intentions in respect of medicine are just as hard to discern as his overall objectives in composing the *declamatio*. Elements of irony and satire are clearly present in his handling of his medical subject matter, as is a display of rhetorical skill in invective, involving the assembly of all possible arguments attacking a given target, but these features do not of themselves exclude the possibility of serious intention. It remains a problem to delineate the direction of such intention and the areas in which it operates. . . .

Agrippa's chapters on medicine appear to convey a double message. The first part of this message is a repudiation just as thorough-going as Pico's of traditional physiological theories and of the possibility of arriving at a systematic physiological knowledge, accompanied in Agrippa's case by a denial of the value of any such knowledge – even if it could be obtained – in medical practice. The second part is a scathing criticism, biting, rhetorical and humorous, of current medical practice and practitioners, which, however, by no means repudiates the possibility of valid medical practice, and includes elements of a call for reform.

[. . .]

[Agrippa's main concern was] the critique of medical practice. His chapter on 'operative medicine' first cites various admissions by Hippocrates, Galen, and Avicenna about the difficulty of cure, and the role of the patient's confidence and of chance in procuring it, and then dwells at length upon the vices of the medical profession. The whole is richly seasoned with invective and sprinkled with a fine array of allusions, drawn partly from Pliny,[31] to ancient authorities who denounced medicine and ancient peoples who lived without it. A number of items in Agrippa's list of medical vices were very well-worn *topoi* in twelfth- to fifteenth-century critiques of medicine. The disgusting preoccupation of physicians with excrement, which is responsible for their unhealthy pallor, is familiar to us from Petrarch; their avarice was a medieval commonplace.[32] And despite his supposed medical studies or associations in Italy at a time when interest in anatomy was beginning to expand in advanced medical circles there, Agrippa denounced anatomical dissection in terms reminiscent of, but much harsher than,

---

[31] Pliny the elder (c. 23–79) was the author of a great compendium of classical science entitled *Historia naturalis* (*A natural history*).

[32] Petrarch, *Invectiva contra medicum*. One of the leading figures in the early Italian Renaissance, it was Petrarch who famously said that 'I have never believed in doctors nor ever will'.

Salutati.[33] According to Agrippa, the cruelty of surgery is only exceeded by that of anatomy:

> a form of public execution in which at one time they used to cut up condemned criminals, still alive and breathing, with savage tortures. Today, on account of reverence for the Christian religion, they are made a little milder, and the man is first killed. Then with their own hand or that of the lecturer in the cadaver they proceed with these crimes, and tearing the human body in pieces they seek out and pry into the site, order, size, functions, nature, and hidden things of all the members. [They do this] in order to learn how and in what places [the body] should be cured by means of this cruel diligence and spectacle as impious as it is abhorrent and abominable.[34]

Indeed, the main difference between Agrippa's accusations against practitioners and those made by many previous authors often seems to be chiefly that Agrippa's are more extreme and violently expressed. Thus, for example, Matteo Villani,[35] writing soon after the Black Death, had remarked, reasonably enough, that the deaths of physicians during the plague showed that their claim to be able to cure disease was feigned. And although Salutati said medicine tortured more people than law, he also recounted a joke the point of which was merely the mild and doubtless justified comment that the physicians claimed to cure illnesses that were actually self-limiting.[36] But Agrippa said that medical practitioners deliberately prolonged and exacerbated disease in order to magnify their own profits and reputation, and actually caused their patients' deaths by ignorantly or carelessly prescribing poisonous mixtures.

The novelty of Agrippa's approach lies in the way he combined this amplification and intensification of themes found in earlier hostile external evaluations of medicine with a reformist program emanating from within self-consciously progressive academic medical circles of his own day, namely the call for a pharmacology that was to be both philologically and physically purged of adulteration and based on accurate first-hand botanical knowledge. These ideas had been given promi-

---

[33] Coluccio Salutati (1331–1406), the humanist chancellor of Florence, was the author of *De nobilitate legum et medicinae* (*On the nobility of law and medicine*) in which he stressed the horror and grief inspired by the sight of a dissected cadaver.

[34] Agrippa, *De incertitudine*, ch. 86.

[35] Matteo Villani, author of *Cronica*, from which above is taken [book 2].

[36] Siraisi refers here to an anecdote found in Salutati's *De nobilitate* in which he refers to a patient hiding the medicines prescribed by a physician who, when congratulated by the latter on his recovery, proceeded to show him his unused and redundant remedies.

nence in the writings of Leoniceno and Manardo,[37] and by the 1530s were providing the motivation for activities of medical botanists in both Italy and Germany.

Yet Agrippa turned this theme too against the medical profession, in this case by reversing a *topos*. Scholastic learned physicians . . . were accustomed to contrast the merely empirical practice of the *vetula*, the ignorant old woman, with their own true science. In the course of denouncing polypharmacy and exotic *materia medica*,[38] and asserting that Nature provided locally grown remedies for the diseases of each region, Agrippa contrasted favorably the true knowledge an old peasant woman has of the virtues, colors, shapes, tastes and smells of the plants in her own garden with the guesswork with which uselessly learned physicians compound and prescribe medicines.

2.7

Cardano's description of the death of a patient

Girolamo Cardano, *Opera omnia* (Lyons, 1663) translated by
Nancy G. Siraisi, *The Clock and the Mirror: Girolamo Cardano
and Renaissance Medicine* (Princeton, Princeton University
Press, 1997), p. 210.

Girolamo Cardano (1501–76) was born in Pavia and studied medicine at Padua, where he obtained his M.D. in 1526. Following a brief period of medical practice near Padua, he was repeatedly refused admission to the College of Physicians in Milan on account of his illegitimacy. Eventually, however, he was admitted in 1539, and in 1543 he began lecturing as professor of medicine in the University of Pavia. His interests, however, extended beyond medicine. He was the author of various astrological and mathematical treatises, and in 1550 he published a compendium of natural philosophy entitled *De subtilitate*. A second volume, *De varietate rerum*, followed in 1557. He travelled widely in Europe and eventually acquired a position on the prestigious medical

[37] Nicolò Leoniceno (1428–1524) and Giovanni Manardo or Manardi (1462–1536) were academic physicians who taught at the University of Ferrara. Both were committed to the humanist goal of ridding ancient medical texts of their errors, Leoniceno, most famously, in his work of 1492 entitled *On the errors of Pliny*.

[38] Literally, 'the matter of medicine', i.e. the constituent parts of plants, herbs and other natural products, that were used in the composition of medicines.

faculty at Bologna (1562–70). He finally moved to Rome in 1570, following an accusation of heresy, and continued to practise medicine until his death in 1576.

Vicenzo Cospo of Bologna, a senator and a friend of mine, fifty years old, of tall stature, thick body, thin thighs, bad color, excessively timid, carrying a *fons*[39] in his arm already for many years, exerting himself a lot, and afterwards resting; he devoured many different coarse, bad foods, such as chestnuts, *itria*,[40] vegetables, and cheese, with other things too, at one meal. This year he used to eat three or four watermelons in one day. On October 21 1569, he was seized by a double tertian fever; but there was rigor on Friday, and with it vomiting and dark feces; he was not sweating: the fever was ending. Having been called the fifth day, around evening, I knew of no other symptoms. In the morning he seemed to be more or less all right: but he had already taken food, bread cooked with liquid; however, he also drank water for the accession [of fever] was threatening. In the evening when I came back, I noticed his pulse was weak. He was cheerful, lying on his left side so that he could receive (I believe) visitors. Where I kept on trying to feel the pulse, I did not find it, and I was wondering if this happened because of me, that is, on account of my stupidity. I undertook to touch him again; I noticed I had not been deceived, for indeed I found the pulse, but it was very languid, small, not very fast but rather frequent. Certain therefore about his condition and having warned the other physician, I prescribed him a little bit of diluted wine for supper, along with a dish of egg yolk. The following morning we gave him theriac[41] and fomented his belly with absinth and even anointed the heart. Fever followed, without vomiting or defecation. A sufficiently robust pulse, and as usual, large, rapid, and frequent. Copious sweating followed, since he had also sweated the previous night. When the seventh day had gone past, we were afraid of the circuit [of critical days]; the remedies of the previous day were applied. When I came about the sixteenth hour (but he had already taken food), I found him feverish, since the accession had not yet supervened (but it was exacerbated on even days and took place later). When the accession [of fever] and a little rigor came, his forces collapsed but he defecated a little, as on the sixth day, and he vomited nothing. Before sunset, he died.

---

[39] A point on the body used for bloodletting or the release of other humours.

[40] Unidentified by the translator.

[41] Theriac was the name for a general tonic in this period, but in its earliest form in the ancient world it was specifically an antidote for snakebites.

Part three

The medical renaissance of the sixteenth century: Vesalius, medical humanism and bloodletting

3.1
Leoniceno and medical humanism at Ferrara

Vivian Nutton, 'The Rise of Medical Humanism: Ferrara, 1464–1555', *Renaissance Studies* 11 (1997), pp. 2–8.

During the late fifteenth and early sixteenth centuries, the University of Ferrara in Italy (founded in 1391) was a major centre for humanist studies. Its medical faculty was fortunate in securing the services of some of the leading medical humanists of the day, including Nicolò Leoniceno (1428–1524), whose career is reassessed in this article by Vivian Nutton.

The theme of this paper is, in part, very familiar. It concerns the transformation of medicine in the Renaissance under the influence of the medical humanists, those scholars who, basing themselves on classical predecessors – principally Dioscorides and Galen – claimed to have brought medicine out of medieval darkness into the bright light of a new age. We are well acquainted with their words and their slogans, their denunciations of scribal perversity and Arabic confusion, their condemnations of therapies misjudged and misapplied, and their exaltations of truth recovered again after centuries of neglect. Their rhetoric is powerful, and almost convincing – at least to the extent that historians of medicine and science have followed their lead in neglecting almost everything between the Black Death and 1490, the year when the humanist demand for a break with the Middle ages was first announced in print. Historians then move quickly on to 1525, the *annus mirabilis* that saw the first edition of the works of Galen in Greek and of the Hippocratic Corpus in Latin translation; and above all, to 1543, the year of Vesalius' great treatise *De humani corporis fabrica*. In three short skips, medicine passes from medieval to modern, from the authority of the book to the authority of observation, from a backward-looking search for ancient and classical precedent to a forward-looking expectation of the triumph of the new science. A new botany, a new anatomy, and a new chemistry, if not a whole new scientific revolution, are created.

It would be going too far to reject this schema all together, or to deny the importance of the three dates, 1490, 1525, and 1543, but historians have rarely bothered to set them in their context, whether social or intellectual. In particular, there has been a tendency to assume that with the discoveries of Vesalius and Fracastoro,[1] to say nothing of Paracelsus, medical humanism had fallen from favour by 1550, having fulfilled . . . its historically necessary role as a preparatory handmaid for higher and more important things. In other words, the writings of the medical humanists, having acted as a sort of alarm clock, can be safely disregarded; their work is over, their travails done. But to consider the literary productions of at least half a century merely as propaedeutic to something in the future is ungracious, some might claim unjust, and this paper sets out to examine what some have thought of as the rise and fall of medical humanism by looking at one centre, Ferrara, and at three successive professors of medicine, Nicolò Leoniceno, Giovanni Manardi, and Antonio Musa Brasavola, whose university teaching spans nigh on a century, from 1464 until Brasavola's death in 1555. . . .

Of the three men the best-known today is Nicolò Leoniceno, the Nestor of medical humanities – I use the phrase advisedly, for he lived from 1428 to 1524, active until the end, and – an example to all – at the age of 94 even securing a grant of 400 lire a year from the university authorities to assist him in completing his translations of Galen. A year later, aged 95 and struck down by a cold that left him hardly able to speak, he was still able to correct his doctor's misinterpretations of a Hippocratic Aphorism and to cure himself by a determined adherence to his favourite diet, good red meat, thick soup, and lots of strong, sweet wine. Leoniceno was, as Joseph Scaliger[2] put it in 1578, the first to link philosophy and medicine with humane letters, and the first to show how men who practised medicine without 'bonae literae' (by which, of

---

[1] Girolamo Fracastoro (c. 1478–1553) was a humanist physician based in Verona in Italy. In 1546, he published an original treatise on the cause of syphilis, which he had earlier described in a poem, in which he claimed that the disease was contracted by seeds or spores that could infect at a distance.

[2] Joseph Scaliger (1540–1609) was one of the most important humanist scholars and writers of the late sixteenth century.

course, Scaliger meant Greek) were like lawyers in an alien court, lost before they even began. It was Leoniceno's trumpet blast in 1490 *On the errors of Pliny and other doctors in medicine* that provoked a Europe-wide controversy which, as every Renaissance scholar knows, dethroned Avicenna as prince of physicians and replaced him and Pliny with Dioscorides, Galen, and Hippocrates. Leoniceno, the friend of Politian and Erasmus, of Linacre and Calcagnini, the collaborator with Aldus and Musurus in the Aldine edition of Aristotle and in their pro-jected edition of Galen,[3] the most important translator of ancient Greek medical texts into Renaissance Latin, not surprisingly finds a place in all discussions of Renaissance humanism. . . .

Given Leoniceno's reputation, it might seem almost impertinent to remark that this fame has been bought at a price. Scholars have become so familiar with Leoniceno that they are in danger of misunderstanding his role and his achievements precisely because of that familiarity. To take only some of the most obvious misunderstandings, the first sixty years of his life are generally passed over in silence – perhaps with good reason, for the only recorded incidents of a trip to England around 1460 are an unhappy visit to Oxford and a brawl in a Dutch bar on the way home. He may then . . . have returned to Padua to lecture on philosophy, and it was as a teacher of metaphysics that he began his teaching career at Ferrara in 1464. But despite his long association with that university, what he taught and when are not entirely clear. The university rolls record payments to him for lecturing on practical medicine from 1464 to 1473, and in 1474 he was paid for teaching moral philosophy. The next year he is down as teaching medical theory, and he appears to have taught this from then on. . . . But curiously, after 1475, although his name regularly appears as one of the *promotori*[4] for medical degrees, almost into his nineties, and although he was in receipt of a salary as a lecturer at the time of his death, we know almost as much about his teaching outside Ferrara as in it.[5] . . .

Our general ignorance of his actual university teaching is partly because what survives of his writings abandons the traditional type of

[3] Nutton refers here to some of the leading lights of Renaissance humanist scholarship. Desiderius Erasmus (d. 1536) was perhaps the most famous intellectual and classical scholar of his day. Linked to him were the classical linguists and humanist scholars, Angelo Poliziano (Politian) (1454–94), the Englishman, Thomas Linacre (c. 1460–1524), and Celio Calcagnini (1479–1541). Aldus Manutius (Manuzio) was the founder, at Venice, of the most important scholarly press in early sixteenth-century Europe. He, along with collaborators like the Greek specialist, Marcus Musurus (c. 1470–1517), was responsible for printing the complete works of classical scholars like Aristotle, Plato and Galen in the refined Greek and Latin of the day.

[4] One who screened and supported candidates for the degree of M.D.

[5] He taught twice at Bologna – in 1483 and 1508–9.

production by a university professor. There are no surviving lectures by him on Galen, Hippocrates, or Avicenna, no medical commentary on a familiar text, no collections of practical advice, no medical *consilia*. Instead his writings often take the form of short essays on topics of wider interest, and are directed as much to a non-medical as to a medical audience.[6] . . . Even when Leoniceno deals with a topic familiar throughout the European medical schools, his method and manner of approach differ greatly from those to be expected of a medical professor. A distinguished series of modern scholars has pointed out the significance for the development of scientific and philosophical method of medieval and Renaissance discussions of the sentence that opens the Galenic *Ars medica*. They have rightly emphasized that it was Leoniceno in 1508 who was the first to explain in print that Galen was not, in this sentence, talking about scientific procedures for investigating particular questions, but merely about how one might organize a subject for teaching purposes, a *didascalia* or *doctrina* in the narrow sense of the word. What they have failed to note is that Leoniceno was almost the only man in the world in a position to make that observation in 1508: the medieval Latin translations were wrong, the new humanist Latin version, just published in 1506, was ambiguous at best, and Galen's original Greek was not available in print. Leoniceno knew Greek extremely well, and he happened to have a Greek manuscript, indeed several Greek manuscripts, of the *Ars medica* in his own possession. More interestingly, the format of Leoniceno's discussion differs greatly from that of his predecessors. . . . In the abundance of its classical documentation it has more to do with the investigations of philologists than with any lecture to a group of medical students.

But Leoniceno's philological interests can be seen earlier, in the part of his life rarely noticed by historians of medicine. Although he had been a court doctor since the 1460s, evidence for his actual treatments is hard to find. Instead, he seems to have been employed by the duke of Ferrara as a translator from Greek into Latin and Italian, first of the Greek historians. . . . In the 1480s his focus as a translator shifts to medicine and science, to the *Harmonics* of Ptolemy, to Euclid,[7] and, above all, to Galen. It is these Galenic translations, eleven in all, that gave him a European reputation to go with that he already enjoyed in Italy, and which embodied, in practical form, the programme that he constantly preached in his other writings. The science that was practised by his

---

[6] For example, his short treatises on syphilis and poisonous snakes.

[7] The work of the second-century AD astronomer, Ptolemy, laid the foundation for the belief that the earth lay at the centre of the universe. The Greek mathematician, Euclid (fl. c. 300 BC), was the pioneer of geometry.

contemporaries, so he proclaimed, was fundamentally flawed, because it relied on a basis of error and mistranslation. Only by a return *ad fontes*,[8] to the original Greek, could one understand properly the meaning (and, all too often, the misunderstandings) of the authorities on whom all relied, and only by accurate translation into Latin could the results of this enquiry be properly communicated to a wider audience. This was a bold claim, and one fully in tune with the humanist circles in which Leoniceno moved.

Its fulfilment demanded three essentials: accessibility of material, energy, and linguistic ability. Energy and linguistic ability Leoniceno had aplenty; before he was eighteen he had by heart Aristophanes, Demosthenes, Euripides, and some Sophocles.[9] But however good his Greek, he could not have done what he did without access to Greek texts; and these, as the catalogue of his library demonstrates, he had in abundance. At his death in 1524 he possessed the largest single collection of Greek scientific, philosophical, and medical writings in western Europe, if not the world. . . . From Padua, from Venice, from Florence, and from further afield, from the private libraries of scholars and those of princes, he begged, borrowed, and bought manuscripts for his own use. . . .

His were manuscripts for use as well as ostenstation. He cites in his writings rare Greek texts, like that of Aetius[10] that have still to appear fully in Greek in print today. His library was an arsenal, and an impregnable fortress; only a handful of contemporaries had even heard of some of the authors he quoted, let alone read them. His claims, usually justified, that previous interpreters, medieval, Arabic, and Roman, had misunderstood the underlying Greek could scarcely be challenged, let alone refuted, at least on the grounds on which he made them. Those who read today the printed volumes of Galen [and others] . . . need to be reminded constantly just how unfamiliar these treatises were in the 1520s, let alone in the 1490s, and just how few manuscripts of Greek medicine, science, and philosophy there were in Italy in the 1480s and 1490s. Leoniceno's demands for a revision of medicine and science rested on what he had in his own library, and, often, on what he alone possessed. Both in his insistence on the supremacy of Greek and, more

---

[8] Literally, 'to the sources or springs'.

[9] Aristophanes (d. 388 BC), Euripides (c. 485–406) and Sophocles (c. 496–406) were celebrated Greek playwrights. Demosthenes (d. 322 BC) was the famous orator of Athens.

[10] Aetius was a sixth-century physician whose main work, *Tetrabiblos*, consisted of sixteen books on a variety of medical topics. His writings were highly esteemed in the Renaissance.

importantly, in having at his disposal the means to fulfil his aspiration for reform, Leoniceno stands by himself. . . .

Primarily, he saw himself as an educator . . . and it was as a teacher reaching out to Italy and Europe through his versions and published *opuscula*[11] rather than as a typical professor that he gained his fame. His style, his aims, and his methods were different from those of almost any other medical teacher of the day. Where he could be criticized, and his opponents wasted no time in so doing, was in his preference for the authority of the Greeks over the needs of medical practice. Alone in his study with his library, Leoniceno might well neglect the information that medical experience alone could bring – and his library is not over-stocked with modern writings on practical therapies.

3.2

Bloodletting in Renaissance medicine

Nancy G. Siraisi, *Medieval and Early Renaissance Medicine: An Introduction to Knowledge and Practice* (Chicago and London, University of Chicago Press, 1990), pp. 136–41.

Of the various therapeutic interventions adopted by medieval and early Renaissance physicians, one of the most common was phle-botomy, or bloodletting. In this short extract, Nancy Siraisi describes the principles behind the procedure and traces its evolution from Galenic humoural theory to the early Renaissance. She also stresses the fact that there was not unanimity among the learned medical pro-fession with regard to the fine details as to how and when it should be implemented which culminated, in the Renaissance, in a heated con-troversy that involved, among others, such famous figures as the anatomist, Andreas Vesalius (for whom, see below extracts 3.3 and 3.4).

The ultimate goal of the treatment of disease was, of course, cure. But cure was not necessarily conceived of as a rapid, immediately recog-nizable return to total health. A more vague and diffuse concept of recovery was the concomitant of the complexional interpretation of health and disease and the similarity between the medical regimen for

---

[11] Small, learned treatises.

sickness and the dietary regimen for health, as well as of actual health conditions that must have involved much chronic illness, weakness, malnutrition, and lasting aftereffects of injuries. The Galenic idea of a neutral state between health and sickness surely accorded with the experience of medical practitioners.[12]

Learned practitioners knew and discussed the fact that the relation between medical theory and medical practice was uneasy and ambiguous, although very few showed any signs of readiness to modify theory in the light of experience. And ... medical practitioners of all kinds had no monopoly on the administration of medical treatment. With or without medical guidance, patients practiced self-help in the form of self-medication, visits to medicinal baths, pilgrimages, or prayer; and religious shrines offering alternative forms of healing were omnipresent. In many instances, any of these endeavors was as likely to be successful – or unsuccessful – as the most skilled medical attention.

Operating within these constraints, practitioners treated mental and physical illness with three main types of therapy, traditionally classified as the three 'instruments of medicine': diet, medication, and surgery. Diet was an important component in the treatment of illness as well as in the maintenance of health; but because dietary principles were essentially the same in sickness and in health, no further discussion seems called for. Surgery, in the sense of treatment by incision, cautery, or physical manipulation, was from the thirteenth century normally relegated to surgeons, barber-surgeons, and barbers, although the division of labor was far from complete. Two minor surgical procedures, cautery and phlebotomy, were, however, frequently prescribed by physicians as part of the treatment for complexional illness. . . .

The use of cautery for complexional disorders (that is, internal complaints such as headache), as distinct from its surgical use for wounds, was predicated on the notion that actual cautery with a heated metal instrument or 'potential' cautery by the application of heated cups or caustic substances to the skin could be used to direct good or bad humors to different parts of the body. Cautery was an ancient technique that probably became more widespread in the medieval West after the influential surgical manual of Albucasis,[13] which devoted much attention to the subject, became available in Latin during the course of the twelfth century.

---

[12] For Galen on health, see extract 1.1 above.

[13] Zahrawi or Albucasis (fl. c. 940) was the little-known Spanish author of a medical compendium that included a detailed section on surgery and surgical techniques, including 200 illustrations of surgical instruments.

Knowledge of phlebotomy was part of medical skill, not only because some medical practitioners performed bloodletting themselves but also because an important part of any physician's task was to judge when and how phlebotomy should be performed. Phlebotomy was unquestionably one of the most frequently used forms of general therapy; presumably its less painful character made it more tolerable to patients than cautery. The principle behind this ancient and long-lived therapeutic procedure was that bloodletting drew off corrupt matter from the body. Each of the four humors, all of which were contained in blood, was capable of being transformed by disordered complexion into a harmful secondary humor that had to be removed if the patient was to recover (or maintain) health. Galen was influential in systematizing and elaborating these concepts as well as so many others.

Simple phlebotomy tracts circulated in western Europe during the early Middle Ages; but when the works of Haly Abbas, Avicenna,[14] and Albucasis and some of Galen's own writings on the subject became available in Latin, they provided much fuller accounts of Galenic theories about phlebotomy and considerably more detailed practical instructions. The Arabo-Latin encyclopaedic accounts formed the basis of subsequent Latin and vernacular treatises on phlebotomy. At least in the opinion of Pietro d'Abano,[15] who reviewed the technical literature on phlebotomy available in Latin about 1300, the Arabic medical writers who transmitted Greek phlebotomy doctrine were somewhat more conservative in their recommendation of venesection than their Greek sources had been. Pietro thought that the difference in emphasis might have been because the Arabs wrote in a hot climate, where the local diseases would be of a kind for which phlebotomy would not be useful. By contrast, the Greeks, although they wrote 'for the whole world and not just for Italy,' provided directions suitable for the robust constitutions found in temperate climates such as that of Italy.

Practitioners could inform themselves from the technical literature as to conditions for which bleeding was appropriate, together with the correct vein to incise for each. Most commonly, blood was drawn from one of three major veins of the arm (named the cephalic, median, and basilic); but other veins were opened for particular conditions – for example, melancholy might call for bleeding from a vein in the forehead. Bloodletting was normally performed by surgical venesection, although leeches were also used on occasion. Textbooks and manuals also gave fairly detailed directions for ligating the arm, making an inci-

[14] For Haly Abbas and Avicenna, see notes 18 and 15 in Part one respectively.
[15] For Pietro d'Abano, see note 28 in Part one.

sion, recognizing and avoiding nearby nerves and arteries, and stemming bleeding. Also provided were rules and recommendations regarding the patient's diet before and after the procedure and appropriate seasons of the year, phases of the moon, and times of day for performing the operation in different types of patients and cases.

Phlebotomy called for the practitioner to exercise both theoretical and practical judgment. Fundamental theoretical issues were whether it was preferable to draw a large quantity of blood at once (removing much noxious humor, but possibly causing the patient to faint) or a series of small amounts and whether it was preferable to bleed on the side of the body nearest or side of the body furthest away from the part afflicted – that is, whether the bad humors should be drawn off directly from the site of the disease or encouraged first to migrate away from that site. The second of these issues, important in the ancient literature and well known in the Middle Ages, took a fresh lease of life in the early sixteenth century under the stimulus of a fuller knowledge of both Greek medical texts and human anatomy and inspired a controversy in which Vesalius was an active participant.

At a more immediately practical level, practitioners had to consider the possible hazards of phlebotomy, hazards of which they were well aware. Routine advice was that small children, pregnant women, the old, and very weak patients should not be phlebotomized. The author of one phlebotomy manual, who wrote probably at Montpellier at some time between 1150 and 1225, firmly repudiated the notion that it was ever desirable to remove such a large quantity of blood that the patient fainted; he frankly gave as his reason fear of the opinion of ordinary people outside medicine. The translator of a Middle English version of the same text made about 1400 added a series of dire warnings about the damage unskilled phlebotomy could do, especially by inadvertently cutting an artery or by causing the arm to become so swollen that death ensued (presumably as a result of the introduction of infection by the knife or lancet).

3.3
Attending a public dissection by Vesalius, Bologna, 1540

Andreas Vesalius' *First Public Anatomy at Bologna 1540,*
an Eyewitness Report by Baldasar Heseler Medicinae Scolaris,
ed. and trans. Ruben Eriksson (Uppsala and Stockholm, Almquist
& Wiksells Boktryckeri Ab, 1959), p. 237.

In this brief extract, we possess a rare first-hand account from a
German student, Baldasar Heseler, describing the radical manner in
which the iconoclastic young anatomist, Andreas Vesalius (1514–64),
performed anatomies for medical students at the University of
Bologna. Eschewing the traditional formula for such performances in
which the professor first lectured from notes or a book while a demonstrator, or *ostentator*, performed the actual dissection of the body,
Vesalius adopted a hands-on approach, combining the two functions,
and using it as an opportunity to show, by close observation of the
body, how his own theory of the body's construction differed from that
of the ancients.

First of all, he [Vesalius] said, I shall show you today how true my
theory about the venesection in pain in the side is, about which there is
today among us great controversy, and I shall demonstrate to you that
the picture which I have published is true and corresponds to this body.
You will see how from the vena cava one branch issues running to all
the ribs and nourishing the whole thorax. He showed us the pictures
which he had published in his little book [*Letter* of 1539] and in his
Tables and he compared them with the present subject, and to be sure,
they corresponded completely. For I saw this with my own eyes, as I
stood quite near. And read this little book, how in pain in the side the
vein is to be cut according to his opinion, contrary to the opinion of the
modern surgeons and also to that of D[ominus] Curtius[16] himself.

---

[16] Matthaeus Curtius or Matteo Corte (c. 1475–c. 1542) was Professor of Medicine at
Bologna and a profound admirer of Galen.

3.4
Vesalius and the anatomical renaissance

Andrew Cunningham, *The Anatomical Renaissance:*
The Resurrection of the Anatomical Projects of the Ancients
(Aldershot, Scolar Press, 1997), pp. 102–16.

In the following extract, Andrew Cunningham seeks to cast a very different light on the origins and significance of the work of the celebrated anatomist, Andreas Vesalius (1514–64). Drawing on the same source cited in the previous extract, he stresses the originality of Vesalius in utilising visual aids in his teaching, and his willingness to criticise the authority of Galen. At the same time, however, he argues that Vesalius' purpose was not to overthrow Galen, but rather to complete his anatomical work or project, which he believed was unfinished at the time of Galen's death. As such, Vesalius is described as a 'second Galen', critical of specific aspects of his master's legacy, but nonetheless indebted to the general principles that lay behind the work of his celebrated forbear.

It is at a series of demonstrations he gave in Bologna in January 1540 that we can best see Vesalius in action before he had his 'blinding flash', as it were. He was invited to Bologna by the students, who still retained the right of organizing the dissection. His reputation had preceded him, but it was because of his reputation as an exceptionally skilled dissector (with an unusual claim about bleeding in pleurisy), not because he was some kind of reformer of anatomy that he was invited. We are most fortunate that a student (a German) took down virtually verbatim notes of this event, including comments on the reaction of the audience. This allows us to see with extraordinary clarity the way in which a public anatomy was conducted in 1540, and precisely what role the dissector was expected to fill. Thus we can see that the event as a whole consisted of:

1. A series of *lectures*, based on the *Anatomia* of Mundinus,[17] given on this occasion by the Professor of Theoretical Medicine, and

---

[17] The *Anatomia* of Mondino dei Liuzzi, a compilation of the surviving works of Galen concerned with the structure of the human body, was written in 1316. It was widely used in medical teaching in the universities of late medieval and early Renaissance Europe, and was frequently printed.

2. In a separate place, and at a separate time, an interlocked series of *demonstrations* of the parts dealt with in the immediately previous lecture, conducted on a series of human and animal bodies.

The lectures were given by Professor Matthaeus Curtius (Matteo Corte, *c.* 1475–*c.* 1542), a grand old man of academic medicine. Curtius had received his own education when the scholastic approach was still the norm. However, when obliged by custom and statute to lecture on the text of Mundinus, Curtius showed himself in anatomy to be just about as up to date in his attitudes as could have been wished. In lecture after lecture he announces his position: that wherever Mundinus had deviated from the strict doctrines of Galen, Mundinus was in error. That is to say, for Curtius the standard of truth was the doctrine in the pristine text of Galen. In this he was as modern as Sylvius or Guenther.[18] However, today Curtius might look to us like an anatomical reactionary and ignoramus, for it was his unlucky fate to have had Vesalius as his demonstrator on this occasion. It was unlucky in two ways. First, Curtius was a participant (as a Modern) in the debate on where to bleed in pleurisy, and had published on it in 1532. Thus he and Vesalius were at daggers drawn on a highly controversial issue. Second, Vesalius was busy transgressing all the boundaries of what a demonstrator should do. He was thus challenging Curtius on an issue of etiquette, respect and authority. And in so doing the 25-year-old Vesalius was to subject the 65-year-old Curtius to the most outrageous public humiliation. The students, of course, loved every minute of it.

Curtius had already given five lectures (covering Mundinus's text up to the peritoneum, the membrane enclosing the organs of the lower venter) before the first of the demonstrations. Meanwhile (though it is not recorded in this student's notes) Vesalius was lecturing on Galen's book *On the bones*. It was only during the course of the third lecture that the first criminal who was to be dissected was executed.

Picture the scene. We are in the middle of the fifth lecture in the church of San Salvatore. The beadle arrives with a message from the students in charge of the demonstration: the body was now prepared for the anatomy.

> And they asked us through the beadle, that after the lecture we should go to the anatomy in good order and without disturbance: for we should all well be able to see wonders which we had not seen hitherto. Dominus Cur-

---

[18] Jacobus Sylvius or Jacques Dubois (1478–1555) was Professor of Medicine at the University of Paris, which he helped to make into a stronghold of Galenism. Likewise, Johann Guinther von Andernach (1487–1574) was a devoted follower of Galen, whose works he helped to translate. He had also taught Vesalius briefly at Paris.

tius likewise asked us to do so. And yet after the lecture we proceeded to the demonstration in great disorder, as the mad Italians do.

The place they rush to, where the body is laid out, is another church, San Francesco. Vesalius has had four banks of temporary staging erected in a circle to create within the church a theatre to accommodate about 150–200 people. . . . The students running the demonstration go in first; then those who had paid 20 sol; then the doctors and the students. At last Vesalius arrives.

> Then Dominus Vesalius began: Domini, he said, you know how the Physicians, both ancient and modern, usually divided the human body: the Egyptians and the Arabs begin from the trunk and the extremities; but Galen, whom Mundinus has followed too, divides it according to the three venters.

Vesalius is obviously beginning to give a lecture of his own. Immediately Curtius interrupts, and requests Vesalius to proceed with demonstrating what he, Curtius, has been lecturing on. Vesalius recovers his ground: 'But, omitting these issues, we shall proceed to our anatomy.' And he does so. In the lower venter he demonstrates the skin, blistering off the outer layer to reveal the inner; then the fat under the skin; then the muscles of the belly, which he has dissected out in readiness. But he cannot resist talking and giving his opinion:

> He showed us two long muscles along the length of the belly, joined together at the lower part by white membranes, but they were more separated at the top end. And he showed us how they ended at the sternum (*os pectinis*), but had their origin from the collar-bone (which could not yet be seen) and not from the shield of the mouth of the stomach as Mundinus says.

Curtius interrupts again: But this is not the opinion of Galen! Vesalius answers:

> No, Dominus, he said, and even if Galen says that, yet we shall demonstrate here that in fact it is so. But, he said, we do not now want to fight with many words.
>
> Then the [student] Rector said, rather uncouthly: Dominus Doctor Andreas, do not be afraid of telling your opinion on these matters, do not fear such fathers [as Galen] (*patres istos*).
>
> Vesalius answered: Later in the anatomy of the middle venter I shall demonstrate that these long muscles begin from os iuguli and not from the mouth of the stomach.

As we can see from the first moments of the demonstration, one thing Vesalius was not afraid of giving was his own opinion – whether it was at variance with that of the Professor, or with that of Galen. But Vesalius,

as the demonstrator, was not supposed to be giving any opinions at all;
it was the job of the lecturer to lecture, not that of the demonstrator.
But there was no stopping Vesalius. Vesalius was beginning to reveal
himself as possessed of a talent, an ego, and a lack of false modesty
comparable only to the great Galen himself.

Right from this first demonstration we can see how Vesalius conceived his task as demonstrator, what he thought ought to be demonstrated and in what order. He had near-ideal conditions here in Bologna,
with three human bodies and several dogs and other animals available
to him over the course of this series, lasting two weeks. He had already
demonstrated the *skeleton*. Now, in and from this first demonstration on
the body what Vesalius is obsessed by is the *muscles*.

> Observe, he said, that all muscles take their rise from bones, beginning
> from sinows (*a nervis*) where their head is, and then ending in tendons or
> cords they are again fastened to bones, in order to effectuate their natural
> voluntary movement in the body . . .
>
> They had killed a dog upon which he showed that the muscles in dogs
> as also in other animals were fastened in quite another way [than in man],
> so that they should be able to run faster. He promised to show us after
> dinner the anatomy of the muscles of one forearm; in the meantime we
> ought to read about them in Galen, *De usu partium* I and II, and *De
> anatomicis administrationibus* I. He had erected his anatomy of the
> bones [i.e. a skeleton] on the table, by means of which he always the better
> demonstrated to us the site of the parts of the body.

Vesalius has brought an articulated skeleton with him, and it is present
at all the demonstrations. He seems to have travelled nowhere without
at least one skeleton for demonstration purposes (he had actually
brought a spare one, plus the skeleton of a monkey, with him to
Bologna, both of which he gave to a friend). Every time he discusses a
muscle or group of muscles, he shows where and how it is connected to
the bones. He has taught the *bones* from the skeleton. And he dedicates
the first corpse to a full demonstration of the *muscles*.

Thus what happens for the first ten days is that Curtius goes on correcting Mundinus morning and evening in his lectures, as he works
through the account of the three venters. When the students come to
the demonstration Vesalius gives a short treatment, but not precisely of
the parts that Curtius has dealt with. Where possible Vesalius does his
demonstration on the human corpse, but where the pertinent parts had
already rotted (such as the intestines), he uses a dog or some other
animal. But the bulk of each demonstration is taken up by the dissection of the *muscles* – that is, things which Curtius had not been dealing
with. First the muscles of the inner forearm:

71

He showed by dissection how these muscles arise from the head of the bones of the forearm with a thin sinew (*nervo*), and how after a long course they end in the hand and the joints of the fingers, how the muscles are situated one over the other in a double arrangement, always four over four, and how the lower ones extend to the first joints, while the upper ones extend to the second and third joints, always passing through the first muscles. This was indeed most beautiful to see.

This, as we shall see, was a very significant place to start. The dissection of these muscles Vesalius was to take as his trademark. Then (demonstration 3) he dissected the muscles of the outer forearm; of the palm of the hand (4); of the face, forehead, jaw, eyes, nose, lips (5); of the shoulders, shoulder-blades, neck and upper arm (6); of the rest of the arm (7); of the thorax (8); of the hip and upper leg (9); of the thigh (10); of the back of the lower leg (11); of the foot (12). He used a dog to demonstrate the muscles that move the neck and head (13) because these had been damaged when the human subject was hanged. The only muscles that Vesalius had not dealt with yet were those associated with the penis, which were too desiccated in the available subject. While waiting for a fresh human body Vesalius devoted the next demonstration to the dissection of a pregnant bitch to show the uterus, and of her unborn pups. With a fresh human body, Vesalius devoted the 15th demonstration to the brain and its parts, including the *rete mirabile* from the brain of a sheep, and the seven pairs of cranial nerves. This demonstration led to the students behaving in a very disturbed manner.

At this point, Vesalius announced that he wanted to proceed to anatomizing the *arteries*, the *veins* and the *nerves*. Unfortunately the Professor of Practical Medicine had sneaked off with the best of the two bodies to initiate a rival dissection. So as this body was 'worthless' . . . Vesalius took it and started on the anatomy of the *three venters* instead. Meanwhile Curtius, steadily following and correcting Mundinus in his lectures, was still at the beginning of the middle venter and had almost reached the lung. Vesalius devoted demonstrations 16 and 17 to the organs of the lower venter and the organs of generation (the subject was male); 18, 19 and 20 to the organs of the middle venter.

Curtius and Vesalius were now, for the first time, in step in what they were treating. And they had now reached the point where conflict was inevitable in what they were teaching. For here they had reached the question of where to let blood in pleurisy. Vesalius gave a demonstration (number 20) to familiarize the students with his point of view; Curtius in response devoted two lectures to a refutation of it, in full scholastic style. But then:

When the lecture of Curtius was finished, Vesalius, who had been present and heard the refutation of his own arguments, asked Curtius to accompany him to the anatomy [the 22nd of the series]. For he wanted to show him that his own opinion was most true. Therefore he brought Curtius to our two subjects for dissection.

Now, he said, excellentissime Domine, here we have our subjects: we shall see whether I have erred. These we now want to examine; and we want to put Galen aside for a while, for I acknowledge that I have said – if it is permissible to say so – that here Galen has erred because he did not know the site of this 'vein without pair' in the human body, something we have today the same as he did.

Curtius answered by smiling, for Vesalius, as he was choleric, was very excited: No Domine, he said, Galen should not be put aside by us, since he always well understood everything, and consequently we also follow him. Do you know how to interpret Hippocrates better than Galen knew?

Vesalius answered: I am not saying that, but I am showing you here in these two subjects the 'vein without pair', how it nourishes all the lower ribs, except the two upper ones in which pleurisy does not occur. For always here – here he knocked with his hands against the middle of the chest – occurs inflammation and pleurisy, not in the two upper ribs. Consequently, as this vein is also distant from the heart, as you see, by three fingers' breadth, it will in pleurisy and all pain in the side always be better to bleed from this vein only; or it ought to make no difference from which part [of the body] blood is let, because the ribs are nourished exclusively by this vein.

Curtius replied: I am no *anatomista*, but there can well be still other veins nourishing the ribs and the muscles besides these.

Where, I ask? Vesalius said, Show them to me.

Curtius said: Do you want to deny the ducts of Nature (*meatus naturae*)?

Oh! Vesalius said, you want to talk about the invisible and the occult – but I am talking about the visible (*de manifestis*).

Curtius answered: Indeed I always deal with the most evident (*de apertissimis*). Domine, you do not understand Hippocrates and Galen well on these matters.

Vesalius replied: It is quite true, because I am not such an old man as you are, etc.

Thus with much quarrel and scoffing they attacked each other, and in the meantime they accomplished nothing.

Vesalius said: Domine Doctor, I beg Your Excellency not to think me so unskilled that I do not know and understand these matters.

Smiling, Curtius said: Domine I did not say so, for I have always said that you are excellent, but I have rejected your false exposition of Hippocrates implying that Galen should have erred in these matters.

Vesalius replied: I acknowledge that I have said that Galen has erred in these matters, and this is evident here in these subjects, as also many more mistakes of his.

Aliud est monstrare, aliud vero est inferre, it is one thing to show, but it is quite another to draw conclusions. This is what they are arguing about, the difference between 'what is visible' (*manifestus*) to the eyes and 'what is most evident' (*apertissimus*) to reason as taught by authority.

Throughout these demonstrations one can see a number of distinctive features of Vesalius's approach. Firstly, as with his first known lecture at Padua, he thinks visually all the time. He is forever picking up a piece of charcoal and drawing on the dissection table; our student reporter remarks on Vesalius doing so on several occasions, copying down the spontaneous sketches into his own notebook. Vesalius also brings pictures into the dissecting theatre: his own Tables, his little book on bloodletting . . . and a book recently published in Marburg by Dryander,[19] with illustrations of the dissection of the brain. So whether or not Vesalius was the artist for his own woodcuts, we can see that he instinctively thought in terms of pictures, diagrams and sketches. He had a pronounced visual sense, words alone were not sufficient for him.

Secondly, in these demonstrations we can see Vesalius having, or progressively acquiring, the courage (or impertinence) to criticize Galen relatively freely. As we saw when he was arguing with Curtius, Vesalius could now claim that comparison with the body revealed '*many more mistakes*' on Galen's part (*plures sui errores*). Yet Vesalius's criticisms are in fact very limited and specific. What he criticizes are *particular* doctrines, claims, statements by Galen (or in the texts ascribed to Galen).

What we have to recognize here is that Vesalius's experience of comparing Galen's texts with the body – the human body – that those texts were about, was second to none. Of the texts, Vesalius is now able to compare to the body, some of them, which had been almost completely unknown to the generation of his teachers, he had got to know from editing them for the press. For the great *Complete Works* of Galen put out by the printer Guinta in Venice in 1541, Vesalius had edited (sometime over the period 1539–40) *On the dissection of the nerves* and *On the dissection of the veins and arteries*. He had also revised Guenther's translation of Galen's *Anatomical procedures* for the same edition. But this work, in Vesalius's case, was not something which could be done simply in a study or a library. Vesalius could not keep away from the practice of dissection; everything he read about in Galen's anatomical

---

[19] Johannes Dryander (1500–60) was Professor of Medicine at Marburg in Germany. He carried out some of the first public dissections in Germany, publishing the result of his researches in his *Anatomia capitis humani* (*The anatomy of the human head*), which first appeared in 1536.

works he wanted to dissect out and see for himself in the body. Thus when Galen writes, as he does at the beginning of *Anatomical procedures*, that one should study human bones at every opportunity and preferably the articulated skeleton, this is precisely what Vesalius does. When Galen writes, in the same place, that one should study every muscle with relation to its origin and insertion (that is, how it is connected to the bones), this is what Vesalius does.

[. . .]

The Vesalius we have discovered so far is a northern youth, a resourceful Fleming, one who had become celebrated as a dissector in Italy, indeed at the most famous school of medicine in the world. He is someone who, by personality, is obviously prepared to criticize his elders (such as Curtius) in public, and his greater elder too (Galen). He stresses to his students the need for *personal engagement* in anatomy, and says that such personal experience is essential for anyone who claims to be a practitioner of medicine, and he puts the evidence of sight and touch above that of logic, custom and authority. All of this suggests that he is precocious, aggressive and intelligent. Yet all the striking and seemingly innovative things we have so far seen in Vesalius's approach to anatomy can . . . be laid directly at the door of Galen himself. For with all his innovations Vesalius was most certainly criticizing neither Galen the anatomist nor the project that Galen had been engaged in: Vesalius was not saying (for instance) that we need to find out about anatomy in some way, or in some terms *other* than those Galen used. Far from it. For the anatomical project of Galen is precisely what Vesalius was following. What he was criticizing was not Galen, nor Galen's project, but the points at which Galen himself had not fulfilled it properly. No one since Galen himself had followed the *practice* of Galen in anatomy as precisely as Vesalius was now doing. And in his grace, skill and expertise in dissecting, in his familiarity with it, in his making the senses the arbiter of truth, in his demanding to see *in the body* the pathways that other people invoked in their explanations, Vesalius was also another Galen. In his confidence in his own skills, his assertiveness, his willingness to criticize other people, Vesalius was another Galen too. From this we can see that Vesalius wanted to be, and felt himself to be, a second Galen.

3.5

Vesalius, *On the Fabric of the Human Body* (1543)

Andreas Vesalius, *On the Fabric of the Human Body*, trans.
W. F. Richardson with J. B. Carman (2 vols, San Francisco,
Norman Publishing, 1999), vol. 1, pp. 87, 378, 382–3; vol. 2,
pp. 147, 150.

The following extracts are taken from an English translation of Vesalius' most famous achievement, *De humani corporis fabrica libri septem* (*On the structure of the human body in seven books*), first published at Basel by the celebrated printer, Joannes Oporinus, in 1543. This work represented a major turning point in medicine. Not only did it systematically critique the received tenets of Galen on human anatomy, but it also did so by recourse to graphic illustrations that owed much to recent developments in Renaissance art. The various extracts included here show another side of Vesalius's work, illustrating as they do the various ways in which he sought to legitimate his radical new approach to anatomy. Thus, he refers to those who have actively encouraged him in his work, his willingness to learn from ordinary artisans and his own dextrous skills in the art of surgery and the use of specialised instruments. They also suggest the highly unorthodox routes that Vesalius was frequently driven to in order to acquire this knowledge.

(i)

The organ of hearing will be more fully discussed later on; this enumeration of the ossicles is enough for now. . . . It is for this reason in particular that *Marcantonio Genua*,[20] most accomplished of musicians and finest ornament among the philosophers of our time, takes the greatest pleasure in the contemplation of the harmony of the organ of hearing; he is a leading professor of philosophy in Padua, fully versed in the erudition of various disciplines, and it is to him that students of the world of nature owe whatever of value they will gain from this undertaking of mine, for it was he who particularly encouraged me to begin it and was throughout an exacting critic. So too was *Wolfgang Herwart*,

---

[20] Little else is known of either of Vesalius' two patrons mentioned here.

an Augustan patrician and rare model of virtue, who deserves to be remembered for his incredible love of literature and of those who study literature, and whose friendship I shall cultivate so long as I shall live because he left nothing undone to the limit of his strength in assisting me toward the completion of my work.

(ii)

[At the cemetery of the Innocents in Paris] we found a rich supply of bones, which we examined indefatigably over a long period until we were able to make a bet with our fellow-students that, blind-folded, we could identify by touch alone any bone which they pulled from the piles over a half-hour period and handed to us. We were forced to these lengths because, though eager to learn, we had no teachers to assist us in this aspect of medicine.

(iii)

I went for a walk with *Gemma Phrysius*,[21] a man with few peers as mathematician and physician, in the hope of seeing some bones. We went to the place where, to the great advantage of students, all who have suffered the death penalty are displayed by the public highway for the benefit of the rustics; and there I came upon a skeleton like that of the brigand which Galen records having seen. The birds had stripped the flesh from Galen's one, and I think they had picked this one clean as well, for a year ago his body had been merely charred and as it were toasted over a straw fire, and, tied to his stake, he had provided the birds with such a tasty meal that the bones were completely bare and bound together solely by the ligaments, with only the origins and insertions of the muscles preserved. This does not normally happen in the case of people who have been hanged; despite a popular impression to the contrary, the birds normally peck away nothing but the eyes, because the skin is so thick, and as the skin remains intact the bones decay inside and are quite useless for teaching purposes. This skeleton was completely dry and completely clean, and I examined it carefully, determined not to lose such an unexpected and long-sought opportunity. With Gemma's help I climbed the stake and pulled away a femur

---

[21] Gemma Frisius (1508–55) was a mathematician and scholar of international renown.

from the hip bone; and, when I pulled at the upper limbs, the arms and hands came away bringing with them the scapulae. The fingers of one hand were missing, together with both patellae and one foot. I took the legs and arms home in several secret journeys, leaving the trunk and head. The thorax was tied with a chain high up, and in order to secure it I allowed myself to be shut outside the city at nightfall; so keen and eager was I to obtain these bones that I did not flinch from going at midnight amongst all those corpses and pulling down what I wanted. I had to climb the stake without any assistance, and it took a great deal of effort and hard work. Having pulled down the bones I took them away a certain distance and hid them in a secret place, and brought them home bit by bit the next day through another of the city gates.

(iv)

First of all one must procure a supply of the cutting instruments which barbers use in shaving hairs, and which are commonly known as razors. Some of these should be sharp, some not so sharp (though you will find that you invariably have more of the latter than you need). The smaller and lighter type should be chosen, though there is no harm in having a few large ones; but you should purchase (or ask the barbers for) a large number, both because in dividing membranes, or tendons and ligaments, they become blunt at the slightest provocation and because, since they are made of very fragile iron, they rapidly become thin, especially if the ones you apply to your task are new and not worn away by sharpening. From some of these, particularly the smaller ones, one may usefully remove the iron knob that prevents the blade from extending beyond the line of the handle, and this should be done as a matter of prime importance when you cannot find any razors constructed with a curved handle, like the ones used by Gallic barbers and those of our own country. The Italians used crude knives with large upstanding hilts or handles, and these hilts tend to be a nuisance in making curved incisions, and they also get in your way and prevent you from bending your hand as you might wish.

To the razors should be added some small knives for cutting pens, some sharp and some not so sharp. Some of these should have a rounded tip and some a long pointed one. The best are those that are made wholly of iron; in the others when we try to cut through transverse ligaments the hilt is easily broken, and the iron blade is rather insecurely fixed in the hilt by resin softened in hot water. Curved knives shaped like sickles should be rejected, as it is usually only the tip that is used in dissection, and as this is bent inward in these curved knives it is hard to insert under the transverse ligaments.

(v)

But the skin can be separated from the fat or the membrane only by means of a large number of incisions with very sharp razors. The butchers can instruct us about this: when they undertake to remove the skin in the armpits they leave the fleshy membrane attached to the animal's body so as not to remove too much flesh. Nor is this the only thing the butchers can teach us; they can also instruct us about the nature of the cuticle when they scorch pigs before shaving them, or rather immerse them in hot water before scraping off the bristles along with the cuticle.

3.6
Fabricius and the 'Aristotle Project'

Andrew Cunningham, 'Fabricius and the "Aristotle Project" at Padua' in A. Wear, R. K. French and I. M. Lonie (eds), *The Medical Renaissance of the Sixteenth Century* (Cambridge, Cambridge University Press, 1985), pp. 206–9.

Hieronymous Fabricius of Aquapendente (1533–1619) was lecturer in surgery and professor of anatomy in Padua for nearly fifty years, from 1565 to 1613. At this time, Padua was the most important centre in Europe for the study of anatomy, its new, permanent anatomical theatre (still in existence) the brainchild of Fabricius. In this article, Cunningham argues that Fabricius spent his whole career engaged on anatomical research in what he terms the 'Aristotle Project'. This he defines as an open-ended research programme designed to discover the true knowledge of causation in the various parts, organs and processes of the animal body. In adopting this approach, Cunningham rejects the traditional view of historians that Aristotle and his Renaissance followers were engaged in an attempt to provide a comprehensive taxonomy and comparative anatomy of the animal kingdom – something distinctively 'backward-looking' when compared to the work of Vesalius and the 'progressive' empiricism of the seventeenth century. Instead, he argues that there were many avenues of anatomical research in this period, not all of them identical to that undertaken by Vesalius in his attempt to become a second Galen (see extract 3.4 above).

In this extract, Cunningham cites extensively from Fabricius' *On the little doors in the veins* (1603), which, he argues, formed part of a much larger work that he elsewhere referred to as his *Theatrum totius animalis fabricae* (*Theatre of the whole animal fabric*). Incomplete at the time of his death, he nonetheless bequeathed to his students, who included William Harvey, a distinctive approach to the work of anatomy in this period which, Cunningham argues, was never solely concerned with the body of man.

In [1603] . . . Fabricius also put into print an account of a discovery he had made as long ago as 1574: *On the little Doors in the Veins*. It is clear that he had discovered these first in the veins of a human corpse he was dissecting: the demonstration of the veins in the human subject was, after all, one of his teaching duties. The illustrations that he provided for this work are confined exclusively to the body of man. Does this work therefore represent a departure from Fabricius' enquiry into the *animal* fabric? Is it an instance of a piece of purely man-centred anatomical investigation? I think not, even though this is how we customarily read it. (Our customary readings are of little use here, however, for we customarily read *ostiolum* as 'valve', which makes nonsense of Fabricius' exposition.) For if we read it in the light of Fabricius' publishing programme . . . we can see that this treatise is indeed of a piece with the other works. Fabricius himself says that it is part of his larger work on the fabric of the whole animal: it is indeed (he says) an example of the format in which he wants the other parts of the *Theatre* to be printed. As it has long been a central text for historians of physiology, *On the little Doors* deserves a more extended discussion here, in the course of which it should be possible to demonstrate how Fabricius treats his discovery as an integral part of his enquiry into the *animal* fabric.

No-one could claim that this short treatise is written in a way which is as systematic as the other treatises we have been discussing (unless it is perhaps constructed on some formal pattern unknown to me). Moreover its topic is somewhat different, for the *ostiola* are not single discrete bounded organs (like the eye, larynx and ear), since they are distributed throughout the body. Nevertheless an analysis of the presentation that Fabricius adopts shows that he does deal with these *ostiola* in a way directly comparable to that in which he had treated the discrete organs in the earlier treatises. What then is he doing? Fabricius refers to his discovery as *res nova inventa*, a 'new-discovered thing', and a 'thing' (*res*) for him is a phenomenon or object with a real material existence. He takes it for granted that it is the role of the natural philosopher to give an account of why such 'things themselves' (*res ipsae*) in the real world are the way they are, and fill the role they do: in other words, to investigate their causes. So this is what he does. It is not enough for him merely to report on the existence of these little structures: as an anatomist it is his role to *explain* them, for nothing less is a proper anatomical account in his eyes. The account he gives of them is as rigorous as anything else in his writings. But (naturally enough) the causes which Fabricius ascribes to the *ostiola* are generated from his underlying understanding of physiology.

So Fabricius quite naturally starts from the understanding that the veins are a system for distributing nutriment to the whole body, nutritive blood continually moving out unidirectionally in the veins to the parts, from the vena cava. The arteries by contrast contain blood with a vivifying role, and are based on the heart, and in them 'a flux and reflux of the blood constantly takes place'. Nevertheless, though the two systems have distinct functions, they both contain blood, and both exist to distribute essentials to the parts: they are both 'canals' of the blood. It is entirely appropriate therefore that they have similar (but not identical) structures. What Fabricius had discovered, in these *ostiola*, are membranes which occur only in the veins, and only in some of them at that. His causal explanation therefore has to be able to account for why there are no *ostiola* in the arteries (why they are not needed), even though the function and structure of the arteries is comparable to that of the veins; and also to account for why the *ostiola* exist in some veins but not others: what role do they fulfil where they are present, and what are the conditions which make them unnecessary where they are absent? His account of the *purpose* of the *ostiola* must be one which answers all these questions in the same terms. And while Fabricius does indeed discuss the occurrence of these *ostiola* in the body of man – where he had in fact first discovered them – his account nevertheless is still of the membranes as they occur in *animals*, with man as a special (or typical) case. Let me offer a simple tabulation of some of Fabricius' prose to bring out some of these points.

Definition: What I am referring to by this name ('little doors'): delicate membranes in the cavity of veins, occurring singly or in pairs, mostly in the limb veins; opening upwards, and having a form like a node in a twig.

Overall purpose: To *delay* the blood, in the interest of the proper distribution and assimilation of nourishment throughout the body.

The *ostiola* are necessary in order
    (a) to ensure that the 'upper' limbs receive adequate nourishment;
    (b) to prevent permanent swelling in the extreme ends of limbs.
No anatomist has discovered them hitherto. Why not? Maybe because
    (a) since the veins are intended for the free flow of blood, anatomists would not expect to find *ostiola* in them;
    (b) they do not occur in arteries;
    (c) they do not occur in all veins (for example the vena cava, the jugulars, the 'outer' veins).
Why arteries do not require them:
        [Arteries have a different role: (a) although they contain blood, the arteries are not concerned with nutrition;]
        [Arteries have a different structure:] (b) their thick walls are unlikely to suffer distension;
        [Arterial blood has a different movement:] (c) in arteries there is constant flux and reflux, rather than predominantly one-way flow.
It was necessary to retard the flow of blood to ensure appropriate delay for aliment to be assimilated. This is shown (observationally) by the *construction* of the *ostiola*.
Why small veins do not need them:
    (a) they contain only a small amount of blood 'and all that suffices for them' for purposes of local nutrition;
    (b) their needs are met by the action of the *ostiola* in the larger veins.
Another need for the *ostiola* in the limbs (where they mostly occur):
        The frequent local motion which is characteristic of the limbs creates local heat; this would naturally draw more blood to the limbs, hence creating
        (a) undernourishment of the principal parts;
        (b) rupture of the limb veins;
... either of which was going to be very pernicious to the whole animal (*toti animali*), given it was essential that the principal parts such as the liver, heart, lungs and brain should always abound most copiously with blood. It was for this reason, I believe, that the vena cava (where it passes through the trunk of the body) and similarly the jugulars, should have been quite destitute of *ostiola*. For it was requisite that the brain, heart, lungs, liver and kidneys – which procure

the conservation of the whole animal (*totius animalis*) – should abound with nourishment, and it was essential that it should not be detained in them even for a moment, both in the interests of replacing lost substance, and of producing the vital and animal spirits whereby life is conserved for animals (*animalibus*).

But if you observe *ostiola* at the beginning of the jugular veins in man, you may say that they have been placed there to detain the blood, so that in the declined position of the head it should not flood into the brain like a river and be accumulated there more than is appropriate.

Enough material has now been presented from this little work for us to see the nature of Fabricius' account. He deals with the *ostiola* as phenomena of the whole animal (*totius animalis*), giving a *historia* of them (number, form, site, distance, and so on), an account of their action, and of their use. And his account is at all points a *general* one. The last passage quoted is of particular interest, for here Fabricius gives the general case of the incidence of the *ostiola* in the jugulars, based on observation: that the jugulars are devoid of *ostiola*; and he gives the general reason for it: that here the blood must suffer no delay since the brain, as one of the principal organs, needs an unchecked supply of fresh nourishment. He then deals with an apparent exception, the case of man, where *ostiola* may be seen in the jugulars. This exception is resolved by relating it to the particular characteristics of the life of this animal. The *general* reason for the presence of the *ostiola* (even here) still holds good: *ad sanguinem detinendum.*[22] But man usually carries his head upright, and the supply of nourishment to his brain is suitably catered for in that position. So, when man bends his head, a rush of blood would occur to the brain: hence the (exceptional) presence of *ostiola* in the jugulars of man, fulfilling a function necessary for the life of this particular animal.

Thus, even in a treatise clearly first inspired by his having discovered the *ostiola* in a human subject, and a treatise illustrated exclusively by pictures of the *ostiola* in man, it can be seen that Fabricius is still dealing with the incidence of the *ostiola* in *all animals*, of which man is but one instance. For him to treat matters in this way was virtually second nature to him, since the investigation of the whole animal fabric was the subject-matter, goal and point of all his research.

---

[22] For holding back the blood.

Part four

Medicine and religion in sixteenth-century Europe

4.1
Luther and medicine

Martin Luther, *Table Talk*, ed. and trans. Theodore G. Tappert in *Luther's Works* (55 vols, Philadelphia, Fortress Press, 1957–72), vol. 54 (1967), pp. 53–4, 102–3, 237.

Martin Luther (1483–1546) was an Augustinian monk and university teacher when he started what became the Protestant Reformation by nailing the 95 theses to the door of the university church in Wittenberg in October 1517. Between 1518 and 1520 his disagreement with the Catholic Church and the pope widened. Luther's hugely influential tracts of the 1520s, such as the *Address to the Christian nobility* and *On the Babylonian captivity of the church*, eventually resulted in his excommunication in January 1521. This signalled the split in Western Christianity, subsequently known as the Reformation. The three extracts below are taken from Luther's *Table talk*. They were not written by Luther himself, but compiled by some of his friends and colleagues from their conversations with the reformer.

(i)

Medicine may be used to cure disease (autumn, 1532)

I believe that in all grave illnesses the devil is present as the author and cause. First, he is the author of death. Second, Peter says in Acts that those who were oppressed by the devil were healed by Christ.[1] Moreover, Christ cured not only the oppressed but also the paralytics, the

[1] Acts 10:38.

blind, etc. Generally speaking, therefore, I think that all dangerous diseases are blows of the devil. For this, however, he employs the instruments of nature. So a thief dies by the sword, Satan corrupts the qualities and humors of the body, etc. God also employs means for the preservation of health, such as sleep, food, and drink, for he does nothing except through instruments. So the devil also injures through appropriate means. When a fence leans over a little, he knocks it all the way down to the ground.

Accordingly a physician is our Lord God's mender of the body, as we theologians are his healers of the spirit; we are to restore what the devil has damaged. So a physician administers theriaca[2] when Satan gives poison. Healing comes from the application of nature to the creature, for medicine is divinely revealed and not derived from books, even as knowledge of law is not from books but is drawn from nature. . . . It's our Lord God who created all things, and they are good. Wherefore it's permissible to use medicine, for it is a creature of God.

(ii)

In his practice the physician needs forgiveness
(summer or autumn, 1533)

I[3] argued in this fashion against medicine. Major premise: He who practices an uncertain art is imprudent. Minor premise: All medicine is uncertain.[4] Conclusion: All physicians are imprudent. I prove the minor premise (that all medicine is uncertain) by saying: First, our bodies are subject to the devil; he can alter and weaken them by his breath. Second, created things are also subject to Satan, and they can infect [our bodies] as if they were poison. Afterward the physician comes, gives the sick man something, and so the patient dies. This is imprudence and impiety.

[Martin Luther] replied, 'It's the devil who kills, not the physician, although it is the physician who administers the medicine. Food can spoil on the table, but it isn't the cook who therefore kills the man who eats.

But what is to be said in answer to all this? Like the study of law, medicine is lacking in general rules and is on this account uncertain. When a physician visits a sick person, doesn't diagnose the illness well, prescribes a drug, and this kills the patient, the physician is certainly the

---

[2] An antidote for poison.

[3] 'I' here refers to Veit Dietrich, the recorder of this conversation with Luther.

[4] That is, imprecise or fallible.

author of his death and is guilty of manslaughter. Nor is it an excuse that, insofar as it was possible, he did with all diligence whatever he was able to do. I reply: It isn't possible for the physician to be excused except through the forgiveness of sins. He must go to this for help. Otherwise, if he acts by his own righteousness, he is of the devil.'

(iii)

Luther's illness and comment on medicine (March–May 1537)

Dr Martin [Luther] left the church when he felt faint during communion, and on his way, he said, 'Yesterday I felt fine, but today my condition is completely changed. It is due to change in the weather. Men are the best and most natural mathematicians,[5] for they quickly feel in their limbs any opposition or conjunction [of stars] and any change of weather.

The devil's also a fellow who can cause sickness. As Peter said in the book of Acts, the sick are oppressed by the devil.[6] Disease doesn't spring only from men's constitutions, and we observe that various medicines have been found to treat one sickness. Although these medicines have helped once or twice, soon they are ineffective. So powerful is the devil that he can alter all medicines and drugs and change what is in the boxes. Accordingly let us pray to the true physician, Christ. When the hour comes, as it must, in which we breathe our last breath, God grant that we may have a cheerful end. Amen.'

4.2

The church, the devil and living saints: the example of Maria Manca

David Gentilcore, *Healers and Healing in Early Modern Italy* (Manchester, Manchester University Press, 1998), pp. 159–60.

The story recounted here is taken from Mauro Pattichio, *Brieve ristretto della vita di Maria Mancha della Terra di Squinzano* (*A short summary of the life of Maria Manca from the territory of*

---

[5] Luther here uses the term interchangeably with astrologers, who used a variety of mathematical skills in charting the conjunction of the planets, etc.

[6] Acts 10:38.

Squinzano), published at Naples in 1769. It was therefore written a century after the death of the subject of the book, Maria Manca (1571–1668). Pattichio was a local man, educated by the Dominicans in the nearby town of Lecce. It is probably fair to assume that this work formed part of an attempt to have Maria canonised (made a saint), and that it was supported and promoted by the local Dominicans.

To explore how the devil was believed to operate in early modern Catholic society, let us turn to [the case of] Maria Manca.

Manca was born in 1571 in the town of Squinzano, near Lecce. Married at the age of nineteen to a local patrician, she was widowed four years later, and made a vow to God to remain chaste and never remarry. However, a local tradesman – a repairer of windmills – fell blindly in love with her. When Maria told him of her vow to God, the tradesman, Lupo Crisostomo, realised he would have to employ other means to win her love. He thus turned to a local cunning man for a love philtre, which consisted of some powder sprinkled on a mushroom, Maria's favourite food. Brought to her that evening for supper, she ate the mushrooms and soon felt the burning passions of love. Her hagiographer[7] refers to its 'burning in her guts'. She immediately went out to find Crisostomo, arriving at his house late that night. When he answered the door she told him that her mill needed repairing, to which he replied that it was her brain that needed repairing. The whole town was soon gossiping about the affair and Maria's relatives decided that she would have to marry him in order to save her honour. The love philtre allows the hagiographer to account for Maria's breaking of her vow and subsequent remarriage, unusual events in a candidate for canonisation. But more importantly, it explains the terrible torments that were soon to afflict Maria, after the death of her first child. Demons had been introduced into her body through Crisostomo's spell and started to cause havoc. They began by beating her and causing her terrible visions at night, including a 'black Ethiopian' and 'most shameless embraces and a hundred and a thousand dirty and foul acts.' Visions like these were regarded as real manifestations of the demonic presence.

The physical manifestations began after the death of her second child, immediately after birth. Comparing her to Job, Maria's hagiographer describes her torments:

> By reason of the fever having left almost by accident her most worn-out body, which resembled a corpse, having almost nothing more to consume,

---

[7] One who writes biographies or lives of saints; in this case Mauro Pattichio.

she soon saw herself covered with wounds, abscesses, gangrene and with the most dreadful pains, which tormented her with all their power all the time, without ever letting up. She offered her most gentle limbs to the knife, flame and every other similar and most painful remedy with a most exemplary and incomparable constancy, but the surgeon worked in vain, because he was incapable of finding a remedy and cure for the grievous diseases of Hell. The wounds grew more cruel in such a way that her most delicate flesh rotted, so as to generate nauseous worms, and these ulcers emanated such a pestiferous stench that whoever came to visit her, fled at once from her presence and held her in abomination, like a plague victim.

Seeing her suffering, Crisostomo asked forgiveness and took her to the Greek Rite church in Lecce, whose priests were believed to be expert exorcists. They concluded that she was possessed but could not liberate her of the demons. The same negative result was obtained by Catholic priests who performed exorcisms repeatedly over the next nine months. Crisostomo even went back to the cunning man who had cast the original spell, but he said he was unable to undo it. From this point on, Crisostomo was miserable and melancholic, developed pleurisy and died.

After the medical practitioners and exorcists, Maria offered her ailments up to God, allowing the hagiographer to exercise his descriptive skills once again:

> Her disease having become harsher and she herself having become a dungheap of putrefaction, a centre of filth and a sink of rot, overwhelmed by unbearable pains, eaten alive by worms, held in abomination, abandoned and shunned by everyone, in imitation of Agatha,[8] she held up her wounds to the Celestial Doctor and, scorning human industry, placed all her hope in him.

Meanwhile, her habit of going to a tumbledown chapel outside the town and praying to an image of the Virgin and child there eventually paid off. One day a young woman appeared to her and gave her a carnation, telling her to take it to a certain church in the nearby town of Galatone. The rumour of her divine favour spread and the clergy arrived at once to perform an exorcism, taking advantage of what seemed to be a propitious moment. A demon announced he would depart her body the following day on the way to Galatone. Maria was thus finally liberated, vomiting the charm: 'a round bone the size of one of the larger *tari*

---

[8] St Agatha, a Sicilian saint, was reputedly tortured for her Christian faith. Among other things she is supposed to have had her breasts cut off, but was then miraculously healed after witnessing a vision of St Peter.

coins, perforated in the middle with a piece of string and a few hairs at the tip'.

4.3

Paracelsus on the medical benefits of travel

Paracelsus, 'Seven Defensiones, the Reply to Certain Calumniations of His Enemies. The Fourth Defence: Concerning My Journeyings' in his *Four Treatises*, ed. H. E. Sigerist (Baltimore and London, Johns Hopkins University Press, 1996), pp. 24–9.

Paracelsus (1493–1541) wrote his *Seven defensiones* in 1538, after he had settled in the Austrian province of Carinthia, having spent the previous decade travelling. The *Seven defensiones* forms the first part of what subsquently became known as the Carinthian trilogy, the second part being *On the errors and labyrinth of the physicians*, and the third entitled *On the origin and cause of sand and stone*. The work itself was a response to Paracelsus's many detractors and enemies, particularly those in the medical faculties of the universities of Basel, Leipzig and Vienna, with whom he had repeatedly clashed. It was not published, however, until more than twenty years after the author's death.

It is necessary that I answer for my journeyings and for the fact that I am resident nowhere. . . . I have to exonerate myself in some measure to you, since I am so much harangued to, to vex me and ridicule me too, because I am a wayfarer and as though I were therefore the less worthy. No one should take it amiss, if I should complain about this. The journeys which I have thus far made have profited me much, for the reason that no man's master is in his home and none has his teacher in the chimney-corner. Thus the arts are not all confined within one's fatherland, but they are distributed over the whole world. Not that they are in one man alone, or in one place: on the contrary, they must be gathered together, sought out and captured, where they are. . . . Is it not true, art pursues no man, but must be pursued? Therefore do I have authority and reason to seek her, and not she me. Take an example: If we would go to God, we must go to Him, for He says: Come to me. Now since this is so, we must go after what we want. Thus it follows: if a man desire to see a person, to see a country, to see a city, to know these same places and customs, the nature of heaven and the elements, he must go after them. For, for them to go after him, is not possible. Thus the way for anyone who would see and experience something is that he go after the same and competently enquire; and when things go best, move on to further experiences.

[. . .]

[W]hat can be testified without sight? Did not God allow Himself to be seen with the eyes, and does He not call us to witness that our eyes have seen Him? How then should an art or anything else renounce the testimony of the eyes? I have sometime heard of those experienced in laws, how they wrote in their laws that a physician should be a wayfarer: this pleases me greatly. The reason is that diseases wander hither and thither throughout the breadth of the world, and stay not in one place. If a man wish to recognise many diseases, let him travel: if he travel far, his experience will be great and he will learn to recognise many things. . . .

[. . .]

. . . It shows great perception in man that man is reasonable enough to seek the gifts of God where they lie, and understands that we are obliged to go after them. If then there is an obligation here, how can one despise or spit upon a man who carries it out? It is true, those who do not thus, have more than those who do: those who sit in the chimney-corner eat partridges and those who pursue the arts eat a milk-soup. The corner-trumpeters wear chains and silk: the wanderers can scarcely pay for ticking.[9] . . . I think it praiseworthy and no shame to have thus far journeyed cheaply. For this I would prove through nature: He who would explore her, must tread her books with his feet. Scripture is explored through its letters; but nature from land to land. Every land is a leaf. Such is the *Codex Naturae*;[10] thus must her leaves be turned.

[9] A bed for the night.
[10] The book of nature.

4.4

The religion of Paracelsus

Charles Webster, 'Paracelsus: Medicine as Popular Protest' in
Ole Peter Grell and Andrew Cunningham (eds), *Medicine
and the Reformation* (London and New York, Routledge, 1993),
pp. 64–74.

In this article, Charles Webster argues that Paracelsus' writings, be
they medical or non-medical, should be seen as closely integrated, and
furthermore as part of the pamphlet literature of the age, which frequently espoused a radical social and religious agenda. Webster also
argues that we cannot understand the medical ideas of Paracelsus
unless we consider them in the context of the popular, protest literature of the Reformation.

Paracelsus painted a portrait of a Church almost totally overtaken by
idolatry and seemingly vanquished by Satan. Yet even in the prevalent
darkness the word of God carried forward the Christian message, and
revelation was available to all those amenable to the inspiration of the
Holy Spirit. Through this medium Christ himself was an active, living
force, rather than merely a past historical example.

The purity of Christ's message, Paracelsus believed, had been undermined by the academic theologians over the centuries. This old learning, embedded in the Old Testament and classical learning, he
associated with flattery ... and corruption. Christ, he argued, had
replaced the Old Testament by the New Testament. The new should
therefore sweep away the old. Christ was therefore associated by
Paracelsus with spirit, youth, vitality and power. The old religion was
dead and earthbound. Paracelsus boldly announced that the tenure of
the corrupt priesthood was over and he conducted a fierce diatribe
against virtually every aspect of current Church practice, including
most of the popular targets, such as indulgences, pilgrimages, religious
orders, and taxes. The whole system was condemned because instead
of faith springing from the heart it substituted trivial tokens of religious
observance, which were exploited by the privileged classes to the
detriment of the poor.

[. . .]

Paracelsus [stressed] the fundamental beneficence of the deity. Notwithstanding our fall from grace in the Garden of Eden, God had endowed the earth with ample resources to satisfy all human needs. These gifts were freely available to those pursuing their vocation in the spirit of genuine liberality.

High among God's blessings were the riches of medicine. . . . Christ undertook to feed the thousands, heal the sick and the insane, restore the sight of the blind, and indeed to raise the dead. These signs and wonders, frequently reiterated in the gospels, were guarantees of the powers allotted to the righteous.

Scientific knowledge was of course universally available, but Paracelsus argued that true insight into nature was restricted to those Christians genuinely subscribing to the apostolic faith. It was not suggested that spiritual enlightenment provided some direct revelation of the truths of natural philosophy. Post-lapsarian men and women were destined to live by hard work. Achievement of higher moral standing constituted a necessary precondition for determining that their labour would be rewarded by genuine knowledge, power over nature, and useful arts. Paracelsus repeatedly contrasted the dead knowledge contained in scholastic sources, signifying no more than the print from which it was composed, with the vital and productive knowledge stemming from the light of nature.

Every person was granted complete freedom, either to make responsible use of God's gifts or to abuse their privileges, by falling victim to such vices as intolerance, false pride or avarice. . . .

Fundamental to the expression of liberality was disinterested pursuit of the interests of the least privileged members of the community, the 'poor neighbours' as they were designated. In the eyes of God all were equal, bound together in universal brotherhood. In this context Paracelsus made repeated reference to the injunction of the Psalms: 'blessed is he that considereth the poor'.[11] Also the gospel laid down a firm obligation of Christian duty to feed the hungry, give drink to the thirsty, clothe the naked, or take care of the prisoner, the sick and the stranger.

Paracelsus wrote particularly harshly against those who squandered their liberality on drinking and gaming in low company. He wrote at length on the improper and improvident use of God's bounty. . . . The Lord was ever vigilant to detect hypocritical avoidance of Christian responsibility to the poor. Communities guilty of this vice would be

[11] Psalms 41:1.

deprived of the access to useful medicine, and indeed fresh plagues would be visited on them.

Any doctor taking up a court position or assuming civic office was judged guilty of betraying his obligation to use his knowledge for the common good. Fine dress and social status were regarded as pretentious surrogates for effective practice. The doctor was invited to learn from the sweaty worker or sooty miner, rather than the religious and secular orders, with all their distinctions of dress and obsession with hierarchy. Since academic education, status and wealth led to intellectual sterility and moral corruption, Paracelsus was forced to the conclusion that the greater merit resided in the lower orders, especially the skilled artisans. . . . The apostles were recruited from among the common people. Paracelsus believed that Christ's judgement on this matter could be taken as a sign of the intrinsically superior capacity of the common people to attain apostolic purity.

Hypocrisy served the purposes of the Devil. Neglect of the solemn obligation to serve the poor paved the way for regression into vice and ostentatious living, the ultimate expression of this tendency being relapse into idolatry. This marked the final accomplishment of the cunning wiles of the Devil.

. . . The worship of idols was associated with the corruption of values and the persecution of the saints.[12] Corruption was detected by Paracelsus at all levels in the Church. Even the seemingly innocuous hermits wandering about in the forest, or the monks behind the thick walls of their monasteries were chastised for engaging in useless or impoverished works of mercy. Their faith and works were useless because they sprang from authority rather than the heart. Such errors were magnified with ascent in the hierarchy of the Church.

The papacy was attacked for embodying the institution of corruption. Lavish ceremonial feasts, elaborate dress, ornament, jewellery, silver, statues and paintings were castigated as manifestations of pagan idolatry. . . . The vices of self-indulgence were intruded into the centre of religious life. Secular elites and church hierarchy had thus become united in a common way of profligate life. Religious and secular organizations were bound by rules and orders which stemmed from humans rather than from God.

In order to sustain their affluent existence the idolaters, like ants, were covetous and avaricious. Thereby they exploited rather than assisted their poor neighbours. Even their acts of charity were without

---

[12] By saints, Paracelsus refers here to all those who were redeemed in the eyes of God and not just the select few, ordained and canonised by the papacy.

real content. Even when cried up with trumpets and bells, their liberality was inspired by the Devil, as for instance the unction administered by priests, or the salves of the doctor, all of which were worthless to the poor. False prophets, false apostles and false doctors were no better than the Pharisees or Anti-Christs, all of whom would be subject to the eternal damnation at the Day of Judgement. . . .

. . . The revival of medicine was presented as a major feature of the process of renewal which would take place during the final age when the Church was reformed. In the new age of the spirit[13] a general amelioration of life would take place. This would allow fulfilment of God's declared intention that the human race should overcome its sins and enjoy a long life. God had endowed nature with marvellous powers, but this knowledge had become neglected and lost. By following Christ's example it was now within the capacity of doctors to recover these skills and apply them for the benefit of those with the greatest need. By this means the art of medicine would reproduce the miraculous cures recorded in the New Testament.

Paracelsus aimed to replace the prevalent 'theory' of medicine derived from the ancients with a new theory, which he also called the 'religion' of medicine. Galenic medicine is dismissed as a redundant scholastic exercise. The construction of abstract systems and discussion of recondite issues of causation was attacked by Paracelsus as a refuge from the more important priorities of medicine.

The 'highest religion' of medicine required the intensive investigation of stones, roots, plants and seeds, in order to reveal their powers. Paracelsus appealed for diseases to be treated as species with distinguishing characteristics, just as other natural species. Species of disease were to be identified and given an appropriate name. Each disease was then capable of being combated by a specific cure or arcanum.

[. . .]

The writings of Paracelsus conventionally classified as scientific and medical are strikingly different from their counterparts produced by the medical establishment. Paracelsus avoided the commentaries, compendia, consilia, pandectae or systematic expositions beloved by his medical humanist contemporaries. His writings contain few traces of the stylistic conventions cultivated in learned circles. The individual works of Paracelsus are generally short, simple in structure, impressionistic in

---

[13] This is a reference to a popular sixteenth-century apocalyptic expectation whereby the Day of Judgement would be preceded by a golden age (the age of the spirit) lasting for a thousand years.

style and wide-ranging in their coverage. Their titles pronounce bold and radical objectives. Often the title-pages include a Latin short-title, sometimes making the connection with some medical classic which Paracelsus aimed to supersede, but the text is entirely in the vernacular, following the vigorous, polemical and sometimes coarse style of the pamphlet literature. Paracelsus made few concessions to humanistic refinement. . . .

Although virtually none of the scientific and medical writings of Paracelsus were published during his lifetime, the works prepared for publication bear many of the hallmarks of the protest literature. . . . The connection with the protest literature is particularly indicated by the intrusion of religious and social comment into the scientific works. Indeed the entire edifice of his scientific and medical writing is built on an explicit theological infrastructure, and this is emphasized by the frequency with which scientific tenets are linked to biblical quotation. Indeed the Bible is virtually the only literary source acknowledged by Paracelsus. This overt biblicism is a further feature of the protest tracts.

[. . .]

The *Defensiones septem*[14] contains a particularly passionate defence of the direct and combative style of his writings. Paracelsus boasts that his manner is rooted in the habits and customs of the simple country people among whom he has lived and journeyed. . . . He aligned himself with the itinerant journeyman,[15] dressed in coarse homespun cloth, fed not on figs, mead or wheaten bread, but on cheese, milk and oatcakes. Journeys among the fir-cones in the relentless search for knowledge was the only sound way to experience. The only way to understand nature was to tread its books with one's feet. This unpretentious and humble path to learning was repeatedly contrasted with the bankruptcy of the learned doctors whose culture was inimical to sound learning and effective medical practice. Academic physicians were caricatured on account of their fine dress, fondness for jewellery, and effete habits. . . . Instead of following the example of Christ and the apostles and practising out of love for their poor neighbour, the learned practitioners practised for selfish gain. . . . Their practice could not be fruitful unless they gave away their wealth and abandoned practising for profit. . . . Although Paracelsus made few overt comparisons, both from style and content of the critique of the medical profession, the reader would

[14] See the previous extract.

[15] Following a period as an apprentice, every artisan continued to practise their trade as a journeyman, travelling from place to place in search of short-term employment prior to setting up as a master in their own right.

readily have made the connection with the anticlericalism of the protest tracts.

Readers would also have recognized the strong apocalyptic over-tones of the *Defensiones septem*. Paracelsus opened his first defence by stating the conflict between the new and old theories of medicine. The old theory was discredited, not only because it was corrupted by gen-erations of scholastics, but also because it was in principle irrelevant to different geographical circumstances and the special characteristics of the new age or latest monarchy, which was characterized by unprece-dented social and economic change, greater population pressure and new diseases, all of which called for a new form of knowledge and much greater level of inventiveness than had previously existed.

God provided for the cure of diseases and other human needs in each preceding monarchy, but corrupt manners prevented exploitation of the abundance of nature. The example of Christ, which had itself hith-erto been disregarded, provided renewed guarantee of reaping the full benefits of the light of nature. ... Only the regenerate would be endowed with the full gifts of knowledge, which were implicit in the system of Paracelsus, and which constituted 'a new medicine appropri-ate to the present Monarchy'. For those guided by the precepts of humil-ity and love for their neighbour, God would provide a cure for every disease, even diseases which the learned physicians claimed were incurable.

[. . .]

The epistemology outlined by Paracelsus was modelled on the empiri-cal procedures of craftsmen. This form of knowledge was called *Expe-rience, Experiment* or *Erfahrenheit*. The *Labyrinthus*[16] outlined the way in which empirical methods could be pursued on an organized basis, to embrace all aspects of nature. The total system was called Magic, the descendant of the knowledge possessed by the wise men who travelled from the East to pay homage to the infant Christ. By con-trast with the fictitious entities and dead knowledge of the academics, letters, words, sentences, etc. of empirical data could be constituted into living books, giving an insight into the real elements and species of nature. This system would reveal the whole course of disease and enable cures to be matched with diseases. In searching for appropriate analogies, Paracelsus concluded that the seeds of plants, their growth

[16] The *Labyrinthus medicorum*, or *Maze of the physicians*, was a small work written by Paracelsus consisting of eleven short chapters, which provides a detailed exposition of his ideas on the origins and nature of medical wisdom.

and development, provided a model for the understanding of disease, which should replace humoral theory. Therefore the medical practitioner should follow the wisdom of the farmer and abandon the fictions of the Galenists. The system of magic would reveal signatures which would appropriately link cures and diseases. This form of magic was possessed by the peasant rather than the physician.

The above body of knowledge based on sound precepts of theology was called the 'theology' or 'religion' of nature. While the knowledge through the light of nature was ascertained empirically, Paracelsus emphasized that acknowledgement of faith through the light of the Holy Ghost was a necessary precondition for the proper realization of the light of nature. The Doctors who lacked faith in God, the Trinity, and who failed to imitate the example of Mary and the saints, were destined to fall into vice and neglect their duty to the poor. Only those who loved God and followed the path of righteousness would be granted their share of the benefits of nature. If this duty was neglected no benefits would be forthcoming. At the Day of Judgement those who had failed to abide by the injunction of Christ to help the needy and who had cherished their treasure on earth would face their punishment. Paracelsus appealed to the academic physicians to abandon their vices and turn to the light of nature. Otherwise there would be no escape from the labyrinth in which they were entrapped.

... It is impossible to avoid the conclusion that the religious framework and social criticism [of Paracelsus' writings] were essential and integral. Paracelsus linked his critique of the medical establishment with the anticlericalism of his time, and he self-consciously presented his own alternative system as a natural extension of the form of scriptural piety which commanded wide assent in reforming circles. By drawing on the modes of expression developed in the vernacular tracts, Paracelsus evolved a formula capable of appealing to a wide audience. The mood of social protest and apocalyptic tone cultivated by Paracelsus induced a sense of the heightened urgency of his message. His tracts therefore directed a potent blend of religious and technical argument against the medical establishment. His success as a propagandist is confirmed by the intense efforts made by the medical elite to suppress his work. Consequently, a variety of adverse circumstances prevented the immediate publication of the majority of his writings. Nevertheless his editors discovered a remarkable level of continuing demand for these works. Thereby Paracelsus succeeded posthumously in his mission to draw medicine into the centre of the Reformation stage. The relevance of the Reformation as a religious and social context to the genesis and reception of the ideas of Paracelsus must be taken into account in the evaluation of his location in the history of medicine. . . . Any realistic assessment of Paracelsus must recognize the unity of his vocation as apostle, prophet and healer.

4.5

The Christian physician in time of plague: Johan Ewich

Johan Ewich, *Of the Duetie of a Faithfull and Wise Magistrate, in Preserving and Delivering of the Common Wealth from Infection, in the Time of the Plague or Pestilence . . . newlie turned into English by Iohn Stockwood Schoolemaister of Tunbridge* (London, Thomas Dawson, 1583), fols 13v–15r.

Johan Ewich was appointed town physician in Bremen in 1562. His work on the plague drew on his personal experiences of a serious outbreak of the disease in Bremen in the mid-1560s. It was first published in Latin at Neustadt in 1582. In the same year, he also published a devotional tract on plague in German, *Die pestilenz, ob sie eine anfaellige Seuche sei, und inwiefern ein Christenmensch ihr weichen moege* (*The plague, whether it is an infectious disease, and whether a Christian is allowed to flee it*) (Basel, 1582). John Stockwood, the Heidelberg-educated, puritan master of Tonbridge School in Kent, was the author of numerous tracts. His translation of Ewich's work appeared just one year after the publication of the original at Neustadt.

These therefore appoynted Preservers (as I tearmed them) by the common consent of the Senate or bench, and by ye assent of the Citizens (if neede be) the firste thing of all, that they shal think they ought to see unto, shalbe, that they provide the common wealth of Phisitions, Chirurgians, and suche as they commonlye call Apothecaries, such as for yeares, fame, experience, honestie of manners, virtue, and the feare of God, they shall iudge to bee best lyked and fitte. . . . And these being hyred for a convenient stipend, & bounde by o[a]th unto the common wealth, that they take no occasion to start away, for feare of the sicknesse greatly increasing (such is man his weakenesse) they must severally everye one of them bee put in minde of their office: namelye, that manfullye shakinge off the feare of death, they lustilye imploye them selves to approve their faithfulnesse and service both unto God and man: considering that God is the beholder and iudge of the things which they doe, howsoever they may be hid from the com[m]on people unskilfull in the arte. If they doe anye thing through errour or deceite, that it shal[l] not be unpunished: but if they shal[l] behave them selves in their office diligently and faythfully, that then they shall receyve a farre greater rewarde after this lyfe, then can of men in this world be payd unto them. *Well shall it go* (saith the Psalmist) *with that man, which faithfully dealeth with the sicke: for at what time hee him selfe shall suffer any trouble, the Lorde in like manner will helpe him.*[17]

The Phisition privatelye must bee put in mind by the preservers, that he often consider, how great an hope of al[l] men he taketh upon him, whereby all the Citizens will have him in admiration, and reverence him as it were some God, sent downe from heaven. Also how great good wil[l] he shal[l] winne among the men of all degrees, who with good successe shall use his helpe, and be healed: and how notable a name he shall get amongst others which shall not be forgotten, no not after death. For albeit the unthankfulnesse of some be verye great, especiallye towardes Phisitions: yet many will bee so bounteous, that with their lyberalitie, they will bounteously recompence, that which others of covetousnes foreslow to doe. That it is the part of honest men to have more regarde of their duetie then of gaine, and rather to seeke and have an eie unto the health of the Citizens, (wher[e]unto a Christian phisition ought to referre and apply all his labours) then either unto promotion or riches. And therefore that he shew him selfe gentle and curteous unto al[l] persons, that he afoord the poore not onely his service, but also his monnye according to his abilitie: and that of the rich he receive the rewarde, whiche they give him with such modestie and chearfulnesse, that he may seeme to love the gifte for the mens sake, and not the men for the gift sake: that ambition and the wicked desire of having, beecommeth bragginge and vaineglorious Thessalians[18] and Paracelsians, not suche as are desirous of their owne health, or the health of their Citizens: But rather let them studie night and day, that whatsoever is profitable, whereby with his arte, he may from so daungerous an enemie preserve and cure those that are committed to his truste and charge, let him use the same betimes, and wisely in the feare of God, that hee may so neere as may be, come unto that point, speedily, safely, pleasantly (wherein doth consist the whole office of a wise & godly Phisition).

[17] Ewich probably refers here to Psalm 41.
[18] The people of ancient Thessaly were renowned for their magical cures.

4.6

Protestantism, poor relief and health care in sixteenth-century Europe

Ole Peter Grell, 'The Protestant Imperative of Christian Care and Neighbourly Love' in Ole Peter Grell and Andrew Cunningham (eds), *Health Care and Poor Relief in Protestant Europe 1500–1700* (London and New York, Routledge, 1997), pp. 50–60.

Until recently most historians have argued that the changes to poor relief which were introduced from the beginning of the sixteenth century, such as lay control and administration, the creation of a common chest, etc., were brought about by the rapidly changing socio-economic conditions of the sixteenth century. This article, however, argues that the role of the Reformation and Protestantism was seminal in providing a rationale for the changes which took place and the speed with which they were introduced. It also points to the particular significance of health care in the new Protestant church orders of the towns and cities of northern Europe.

For Protestants charity became a Christian obligation within the civic, Christian Commonwealth. 'You shall love your neighbour as yourself' became the Protestant rationale for charity, as a consequence of and proof of faith and grace. Thus the role of the voluntary poor such as the mendicant orders was obsolete if not downright negative. Solely by removing them and the confraternities Protestantism cannot but have improved the chances of the impoverished sections of the laity.

A number of historians have correctly emphasised that the reward motive in connection with good works continued to play a part in Protestant charity, but it did so with a significant difference. Where Catholic charity was performed with the certainty of reward in the afterlife – being claims already underwritten by the church – Protestant donors had no such guarantees, and their hope of reward could never be more than a pious hope, which found continuous expression in a religious context where clerical middlemen no longer existed to ease the Christian individual's troubled journey towards salvation.

Because Protestant charity became solely a civil obligation towards the Christian Commonwealth, it focused on the living, and on the present as opposed to the hereafter. It treated the poor as subjects, as unfortunate Christian brethren and sisters who had justifiable expectations

100

of assistance from their Christian community, which in turn had the right to make its own demands on its poor. This . . . differed starkly from the rationale of Catholic charity which continued to be preoccupied with the salvation of the donor's soul in particular, and to treat the poor as objects, even after the post-Tridentine reforms.[19]

Without the Reformation the centralisation and increased accountability of poor relief which took place in the sixteenth and seventeenth centuries would have been unimaginable. . . .

The optimism which characterised the early reformers during the first years of the Reformation quickly evaporated. It proved much harder to convert the majority of the people than they had expected, even where the Reformation was strongly backed by government. Similarly, the reformers' high hopes for the reforms of charity and poor relief met with some early disappointments, as can be seen from Luther's letter to Spalatin[20] where he pointed out that the reforms in Leisnig (1523) had not been as successful as he had hoped. But these examples do not necessarily mean that the Reformation and the reforms of poor relief failed, only that the reformers' expectations were too great. . . .

[. . .]

The single most influential Protestant reformer of poor relief and health care provision in Northern Europe was undoubtedly Luther's friend and collaborator, Johannes Bugenhagen. Bugenhagen, born into a burgher family in the small town of Wollin in Pomerania in 1485, came to dominate the reforms from 1520 onwards. Where Luther started, Bugenhagen followed. His influence in the region we are concerned with is demonstrated not only by the six church orders he helped draw up, starting with Braunschweig in 1528, Hamburg in 1529, Lübeck in 1531, Pomerania 1535, Denmark in 1537–39, and Schleswig-Holstein in 1542; but also by his public letters to the people of England and Livonia in which he defended Lutheranism.

Bugenhagen's contributions to the social reforms are generally considered to have been insubstantial and mainly pertaining to the administration of poor relief, with one exception: the division of the common chest into two chests, one exclusively for the poor, the other for salaries of ministers and teachers and expenses for the upkeep of churches. This was done in order to make it easier for the Protestant preachers to

---

[19] That is, the reforms initiated as a result of the Council of Trent (1545–63).

[20] Georg Spalatin (or Burckhardt) (1484–1545) was a German humanist and private secretary to Elector Frederick the Wise of Saxony and a former student of Luther's.

exhort their congregations to give liberally to the poor without being accused of acting out of self-interest, secretly trying to increase their salaries. . . .

With regard to the reform of poor relief, its detailed administration, the definition of the deserving and undeserving poor, and antagonism towards begging, Bugenhagen added little to what Luther and others had already advocated. Instead, his contribution was in the area which we label health care provision. . . .

For Bugenhagen health care provision became as essential a part of a proper Protestant church order as the reform of poor relief had originally been for Luther. The attention these issues received in Bugenhagen's church orders centred around four main points: baptism, midwifery, nursing and hospitals. Even if there may have been a considerable local input in these orders, Bugenhagen's awareness of and emphasis on these matters appears to have increased over time. . . .

Baptism

The Protestant reformers in their ambition to demolish the sacramental power held by the medieval Catholic Church, decided to retain only two of the sacraments, the eucharist and baptism, and then only in a strongly modified form. Apart from the changed importance attached to baptism, it was no longer considered absolutely necessary for salvation, and unbaptised children were no longer consigned to limbo. The reformers also cleansed the ceremony of what they considered unnecessary and superstitious practices. . . . What remained was the cleansing and salvation of the soul through the 'living water', as mentioned in the Bible.[21] . . . This stress on the spiritual cleansing of the baptised child shifted the focus away from the sacrament (as absolutely necessary for salvation) and its significance for the hereafter, towards the living child. . . .

In some parts of Northern Europe, most likely as a consequence of the cold climate but probably also encouraged by the evangelical movement, it had become common practice to have children baptised swaddled as opposed to naked, with water poured only over their heads. As far as I can see, this practice was first recorded in the new Protestant Church Order for the territory of Hadeln near Bremen which was issued in 1526. It stated that children should be baptised by having water scooped over their head three times and added: 'In winter the sexton shall heat the water in a dish and put that in the font. Because baptism

---

[21] John 4:10–11; 7:38.

is for healing not harming'. Bugenhagen evidently accepted this practice. . . .

[. . .]

A slightly different description can be found in the Danish Church Order of 1539. Here it is stated that children should be uncovered, but only that water should be scooped or poured over them three times, without specifying whether or not it should be applied to the head solely. However, it states that the guiding principle was to be the health of the children. If at risk from bad weather or disease the children should remain swaddled, because 'it was children's welfare not their harm which was sought through baptism'.

[. . .]

Thus for Protestants the significance attached to baptism lessened. No longer was it considered absolutely necessary for salvation and the afterlife. Instead, the emphasis shifted away from the dead rite towards the living receiver, as prominently demonstrated in the growing concern for the health of the child.

Midwifery

As was the case with the reforms of poor relief, the first attempts to regulate midwifery had already started in some German cities towards the end of the fifteenth century. For doctrinal reasons alone it became important for Protestants to supervise midwives, not least because of their central role in emergency baptisms. Bugenhagen accordingly included separate sections about midwives in his church orders. In the Braunschweig Church Order Bugenhagen emphasised that the midwives were to be educated and visited by the local minister or superintendent in order to make sure that they were of sound doctrine, while a group of 'honourable and wise women' appointed by the magistracy should make sure that only upright and honest women were licensed as midwives. Apart from these doctrinal and moral concerns, however, the Braunschweig Order is primarily concerned with providing a reasonable and reliable service for the Christian community in Braunschweig. It wanted to remedy the shortage of qualified midwives which affected poorer families in particular. It stated that it was a Christian obligation for the community to provide enough qualified midwives, supported by the common chest, covering all sectors of the town. Poor women should enjoy their services free of charge while women who were not destitute should continue to pay. . . . In his *Visitation-Book*, Bishop

Peder Palladius[22] encouraged women to pay good midwives generously, and town councils to exempt them from all taxes. Furthermore, Palladius advocated the practice already known from Germany whereby 'honourable women' exercised control over the appointment of midwives. This system has been interpreted as a municipal way of controlling a 'profession' which was predominantly recruited from the lower classes. This may have been the intention in some German towns, but for [Palladius] the motivation would appear to have been the ambition to secure the best possible care for pregnant women:

> And the eldest and most excellent Danish women in the parishes or in the town should inquire whether or not she (the midwife) is good at her office, before she is allowed to attend any Danish women, otherwise everything is lost. . . .

> Who wants to have his child killed, who wants his wife ruined, how many are those who have been destroyed by evil and ungodly midwives? Accordingly, it is of the utmost importance, for men as well as women, that the midwife is a good, learned and pious woman, because no-one wants to see any of his nearest ruined.

This increased concern with the physical care of mother and child was not unique to Palladius and Denmark, but was a characteristic element of Protestant care. . . .

Nursing

A further example of Bugenhagen's deep concern with the obligation of the properly reformed Christian Commonwealth to provide care in the community can be found in his attempts to establish some form of nursing service. In the Church Orders for Braunschweig and Hamburg a paragraph was inserted which specified that the ministers should keep a register of the names of all the women who were maintained in the hospital and of all those who received regular support from the common chest. These women were obliged to nurse the sick, except when they had small children of their own or sick members of their immediate family. It was underlined that these women were to be remunerated either from the common chest, if the patients were poor, or by the patients personally.

---

[22] Peder or Peter Palladius (1503–60) was the first Lutheran bishop of Zealand in Denmark. He matriculated at the University of Wittenberg in 1531. A pupil and friend of the leading Reformer, Philip Melanchthon, he received his doctorate in theology from the University of Wittenberg in 1537. Palladius then returned to Denmark where he collaborated with Bugenhagen on drawing up the first Danish Protestant Church Order of 1537–39.

However, should any of these women refuse to undertake such duties they were to be excluded from the hospital and from regular pay-outs from the common chest. In this Protestant version of the Christian Commonwealth the poor not only had a rightful claim on assistance from the local community, but also an obligation to contribute to society.

Similarly, in his advice for the administration of the common chest in the Church Order for Pomerania (1535), Bugenhagen emphasized that the deacons should never spend all the money in the chest, but hold something in reserve for the poor who fell sick suddenly or who were about to give birth. . . .

Hospitals

Initially Bugenhagen's church orders appear to have concentrated exclusively on the need to establish plague hospitals. This is hardly surprising since Johannes Bugenhagen had recent and personal experience of a serious epidemic in which, among others, his sister had died. Together with Luther, Bugenhagen had remained in Wittenberg during 1527 when plague raged in the city for six months in order to minister to his congregation and to lecture to his students.

In Braunschweig the plague hospital was to be placed outside the city, while in Hamburg it was to constitute a separate part of a new, large hospital, but in all cases it was to have a number of separate chambers for the plague-stricken to make sure they did not infect each other. These hospitals were to be supplied with a salaried nursing staff in times of plague. The common chest was also to pay for food, beds, medicine and other necessities for the patients. The Braunschweig Order indicated that when the patients' families or masters did not meet the expenses incurred, the costs should be borne by the common chest. It emphasised that only heathens would incarcerate plague victims without providing for their physical needs, underlining that their isolation also served to protect the healthy. However, in the Hamburg Order, issued the following year, it had become a 'Christian obligation' for the victims' masters and families to pay the costs in order not to put unnecessary strain on the public purse.

Considering that syphilis or pox, which first appeared in Europe in 1495, seems to have spread with particular speed in the decade leading up to 1520, it is understandable that it should receive special attention in some of Bugenhagen's church orders. The need for a separate pox hospital is first mentioned in the Church Order for Lübeck issued in 1531. Pox also featured eight years later in the Danish Church Order.

Concerning hospitals, the Danish Order specified that the sick should be isolated in separate rooms in the hospital, according to their type of disease, in order to prevent diseases from spreading, especially in cases which were feared to be of an epidemic nature. Pox, which was here considered a curable disease, was given a special mention. The Order emphasised that the town physicians should do their utmost to cure syphilitics and other sick, against payment, 'in order that the poor are not only kept alive, but are helped to improve their health as much as possible'.

Syphilis was evidently of great concern in Northern Europe in the 1520s and 1530s. . . . [W]hen Peder Palladius identified the deserving poor for his readers, he wrote:

> But if you want to see who receive your charity, then, when you are in Copenhagen on some other business, go to the hospital of the Holy Spirit, which is in the centre, where you will find the door open and walk along one side of the hospital and then the other and you will see how many poor alms-receivers lie in these beds from all over Zealand, whose noses, eyes and mouths have been eaten away by the pox, and whose arms and legs have rotted away through cancer and pain and still rot by worms and maggots, none of whom will ever be cured.

The horror of such a visit was intended to remind the visitor of his own good and, importantly, undeserved fortune, thus encouraging him to show greater charity towards his less fortunate neighbours.

Undoubtedly, there were several aspects of these hospital reforms which had already been introduced elsewhere well before the Reformation, both in Italy and southern Germany. Thus Bugenhagen would have found plenty of support from Christian humanists . . . for his ambition to forbid wealthy pensioners buying themselves old-age care in the hospitals. Similarly little or nothing would have separated the Protestant reformers from Christian humanists concerning the administration of hospitals. Where funds proved insufficient, despite attempts to retain donations previously given to the Catholic Church, for the new, Protestant establishments, reformers as well as humanists agreed that lay government had an obligation to step in.

Let me conclude by emphasising that by seeking to re-insert the Reformation into the story about early modern innovations in poor relief and health care provision, I am not arguing that Protestantism alone brought about these changes, or that social and economic factors were of little or no consequence, but only that the Reformation was responsible for the speed and to some extent for the nature of these changes. . . .

In other words what concerns me here is not the early Reformation *per se* in a chronological sense, but early rather in a generational sense.

Thus it is of little consequence whether the Reformation was Lutheran or Reformed in character, or if it took place in the early sixteenth or a century later, but whether the reforms were driven by a strong sense of religious urgency and a commitment towards establishing a new Christian Commonwealth. This often had a strong millenarian tinge which might occasionally serve to revive a Protestant urge for reform which was seldom sustainable for more than a generation.

Thus it was Protestant reformers such as Johannes Bugenhagen who gave much needed urgency and theological justification to these reforms. Built into their reformation of church and state was the ambition to create a Christian Commonwealth which possessed the proper institutions for providing for the sick and the poor. For them, this consisted of a reciprocal arrangement whereby the Christian community had an obligation to look after its destitute members with the aim of helping them once more to become valuable members of society, while the poor, on the other hand, were obliged to undertake some form of service to the community, if need be, and, if they were not already fully committed looking after their own, destitute families. By nature, such arrangements imposed a degree of social control on the poorer members of society. Perhaps historians of the post-Foucault era have made too much of the control side of these reforms and forgotten the care aspect, which, after all, was the motivation which caused so many of the Protestant reformers to emphasise the importance of reforms to poor relief and health care provision in their church orders.

4.7

Rules for ministering to the sick in the Maggiore Hospital, Milan (1616)

P. Mario Vanti, *S. Giacomo Degl'Incurabili di Roma nel Cinquecento. Dalle Compagnie del Divino Amore a S. Camillo de Lellis* (Rome, Tipolitografia Rotarori, 1991), pp. 139–41. Translated by Silvia de Renzi.

This is an extract from the comprehensive rules for the Order of the Ministers of the Sick at Milan's Maggiore Hospital, dating from 1616, and entitled *Rules observed by our brethren in the Maggiore Hospital in Milan, to serve the poor infirm with every perfection.*

The ministers of the sick, also known as the Camillans, were an order founded by Camillo de Lellis (1550–1614) in the mid-1580s. They began their service in Milan in 1594.

Rules for the corporal nurse brother

1. First of all he should carefully provide the poor with food, and restore them according to what the doctor orders in the morning, and at the established times.
2. As soon as the sick arrive in his ward, he should put them to bed without any delay, using clean sheets; and he should take those with scabies in the same wheelbarrow. Then he should add the names of the sick to the list of confession.
3. He should distribute the plums, oranges and broth at the time indicated by the doctors.
4. He should mark out those with the flux (*flussanti*), dropsy, and those vomiting or in pain (*pontura*).
5. In the evenings, before the poor eat dinner, he should make his rounds, seeing who suffer from severe fever last; then he should put their names down in the list for the nurse on duty, also noting what they should receive. If somebody is seriously ill and they have not received the Holy Oil, he should add their names to the list.
6. In the mornings, when the doctor comes, he should inform him in detail about everything, including what happened during the previous day.
7. When he has put the sick to bed, he should ask them about their illness at that time, and if they have been given a purge, at what time their fevers occur, so that he can give them the food earlier, and inform the doctor.
8. On Sundays he should receive four towels and four aprons from the caretaker (*consegniero*), and he should return them when they are dirty. And he should do the same on Thursdays.
9. When he needs distilled confections or anything else from the apothecary, he should ask the barber in his ward for them.
10. When lunch time or dinner time is approaching, he should warn the brothers in order that they might lay the tables.
11. On Wednesdays and Saturdays, room mates should take turns and sweep their rooms.

[. . .]

Rules for the assistant corporal nurse brother

1. His main concern should be to make sure that, in the absence of the corporal nurse brother, what he has ordered should be performed.
2. When the nurse brother is in, he should not put any of the poor to bed, neither should he distribute anything to the sick without permission of the above mentioned nurse brother.
3. Before the poor eat their lunch and dinner, he should give them what is necessary to wash their hands, warming up the water in wintertime, and he should cover everyone's small table with a cloth (*mantini*).

[. . .]

Rules for the spiritual nurse brother

1. His main task will be to prepare the poor and make them ready to receive the holy sacraments, that is Penance, Communion, the Holy Oil. Therefore, as soon as the sick are in bed, he should prepare them.
2. When he sees that a sick person is worsening in the ward, he should urge them to confess (*facci le proteste*), and should inform the Father priest about the Holy Oil, remembering to make sure the sick can gain the Plenary Indulgence through the Medals;[23] and if somebody is dying, he should give them the Cross, the book to commend their souls to God, the vessel with the Holy Water and lit candle, and he should be the first to assist them for an hour.
3. He should teach the Lord's Prayer, the Hail Mary, the Credo and the Ten Commandments to those in his ward who do not know them.
4. When it is necessary, he should prepare the table for the Holy Communion and the Holy Oil for his ward.
5. When the assistant corporal nurse brother gives the poor what is necessary to wash their hands, he should bring the towels and give spoons to everybody, counting them when the meals are over.
6. In the morning when he is on ward duty, he should freshen up the mouths of the poor, cleaning their tongues, and distribute the chamber pots for urine.
7. When Holy Communion is to be given in the ward, the night before he should warn the poor who are to take communion that they should not drink after midnight, and he should check that they have

---

[23] Devotional objects.

thoroughly confessed, so that in the morning they can reconcile themselves well.

8. On the days when nobody in his ward is taking Holy Communion, he should make the beds of the poor with the assistant corporal nurse brother.

9. On all the holy days of obligation, he should warn the poor by waking up those who are asleep, so that they can prepare for Mass.

Rules for the assistant spiritual nurse brother

1. He should make sure that the lamps in his ward are lit, and keep them clean. In wintertime he should also put the tallow candles in the middle of the ward. He should also remove the chamber pots of the poor and, when they are washed, return them to the storeroom.

2. He should ring the bell for the examination of conscience in the evening following the day he was on duty, and keep it going for a quarter of an hour; he should then put the clock and the bell back in the window for those who are on duty the same night.

Part five

Chemical medicine and the challenge to Galenism: the legacy of Paracelsus

---

5.1
Paracelsianism in England: Richard Bostocke (1585)

R[ichard] B[ostocke], *The Difference betwene the Auncient Phisicke . . . and the Latter Phisicke* (London, Robert Walley, 1585), sigs A5v–A7r, H6v–H7v.

Richard Bostocke (d. 1606) was a lawyer and member of Parliament during the reign of Elizabeth I. He was a student at St John's College, Cambridge, and was admitted to the Middle Temple in 1551. In the work from which the following extract is taken, Bostocke was one of the first Englishmen to publicly espouse the advantages of Paracelsianism over the traditional therapeutic methods of the followers of Galen.

And (O most mercifull God) because the heathnish Phisicke of *Galen*, doth depende uppon that heathnish Philosophie of *Aristotle*, (for where the Philosopher endeth, there beginneth the Phisition) therfore is that Phisicke as false and iniurious to thine honor and glory, as is the Philosophie. For, that heathnish Phisicke (O God) doth not acknowledge the creation of man, whereby it doth not rightly knowe why he is *Microcosmus*, or little worlde: which is the cause why they neither knowe his diseases rightly, neither provide medicine for him aptly, nor prepare it fitly, neither minister it accordingly. This heathnish Philosophie and Phisicke, doth attribute thy workes (O God) to heate, colde, and such causes, which it calleth falsely naturall . . . and whereby in seeking for like cure in such defects, their Phisicke must needes erre, in not seeking helpe at thy handes, nor praying to thee, nor give thankes to thee: No more doth that heathnish Philosophie and Phisicke acknowledge, that all seedes did receive by thy divine worde the power of multiplying, of transplantation, the essence and properties: of which, all Philosophie, Phisicke, and Alchimie doth consist: Therefore they must needes erre, both in the cause & effects of thinges in the great worlde and in the little world.

[. . .]

And because they understand not, that deseases doe proceede of the mechanicall spirites and tinctures of impure seedes ioyned to the pure by thy curse, O iust God, therefore they seeke not their medicines in the pure seedes. And because (O mercifull God) the heathnish Phisicke and the heathnish Philosophie doth not acknowledge, that it is thy power and vertue that bringeth forth all thinges that growe, and that thy working power doth preserve and maintaine all thinges: and that it is thy curing vertue that helpeth and cureth all deseases, greefes and infirmities, by such meanes as it pleaseth thee, or without: therefore they cleave fast to their false imagined naturall causes and meanes of helpe, forgetting thee: whereby many of them become Atheists. And because the heathnish Phisick of *Galen*, doth not knowe how thou (O God) hast ordeyned all thinges in unitie peace and concorde, therefore it seeketh the cure in dualitie and contraritie. To bee short, because (O most merciful God) the heathnish Phisick doth not knowe that the purest, best, and medicinable parte of each thing is in his Center, therfore it neither doth seeke, neither have his favorers learned, nor doe knowe, how to finde that pure parte, nor to separate the pure from the impure. . . .

[. . .]

[Paracelsus] was not the author and inventour of this arte as the followers of the Ethnickes phisicke doe imagine . . . no more than *Wicklife, Luther, Oecolampadius, Swinglius, Calvin,*[1] &c. were the Author and inventors of the Gospell and religion in Christes Church, when they restored it to his puritie, according to Gods word, and disclosed, opened and expelled the Clowdes of the Romish religion, which long time had shadowed and darkened the trueth of the worde of God. And

---

[1] John Wycliff (d. 1384) was an English cleric, theologian and founder of the Lollards, a heretical group whose theology was similar to that later adopted by the Protestant reformers of the sixteenth century. Joannes Oecolampadius (1482–1531), Ulrich Zwingli (1484–1531) and John Calvin (1509–64) were the leaders of the Protestant reform movement in Basel, Zurich and Geneva respectively.

no more then *Nicholaus Copernicus*,[2] which lived at the time of this *Paracelsus*, and restored to us the place of the starres according to the trueth, as experience & true observation doth teach is to be called the author and inventor of the motions of the starres. . . . Neyther was any Countrey or people at any tyme tyed and fast bound to one kinde of Salve, Oyntment or Medicin, but it was lawfull and needefull for men to search and find out, and to adde better to that was in use, and to altar the same, though it were unlike and contrarie to that was before used. So that latter ages have alwayes added somewhat to the former and newe diseases require newe Medicins. And so much the rather, for that by the Ethnickes phisicke, old and common diseases have not their certeine remedies, as the Goute, the Leprosie, the Dropsie, the falling sicknesse, nay now and then the Quarteyne and blacke Jaundies. . . . Therefore true searche and true proofe by him [i.e. Paracelsus] made and revived, and true principles by him restored, are and ought most ioyfully of others to be embraced & folowed.

5.2

Sanitising Paracelsus: the Paracelsian revival in Europe, 1560–1640

Hugh Trevor-Roper, 'The Court Physician and Paracelsianism' in Vivian Nutton (ed.), *Medicine at the Courts of Europe, 1500–1837* (London and New York, Routledge, 1990), pp. 79–84, 87.

In this important article, Trevor-Roper discusses the various ways in which the radical and iconoclastic image of Paracelsus and his teachings was shed in the years after his death, thus allowing for the rapid spread of his medical teachings throughout northern Europe. Among other important factors, he stresses the close relationship between Paracelsianism and Protestantism, but above all points to the crucial role played by the princes of northern Europe – especially in Germany

---

[2] The Polish cleric, mathematician and astronomer, Nicholas Copernicus (1473–1543), was the author of *De revolutionibus orbium coelestium* (*On the revolution of the heavenly bodies*) in which he proposed that the earth and the other planets circulated the sun. It was published in 1543, the same year in which Vesalius' ground-breaking *De humani corporis fabrica* first appeared.

– in providing a protective environment for the medical followers of Paracelsus to pursue their research and publish Paracelsus' works.

Paracelsianism is one of the great intellectual phenomena of the sixteenth century. In retrospect, we see it as a medical phenomenon, but in its origin it was much more than this. Though its permanent result was medical – the insertion of chemistry into medicine – it began as a total movement, a philosophy, a new *Weltanschauung*, with revolutionary implications. Seen in his context, in the intellectual history of his time, Paracelsus was a kindred spirit, and a rival, to his contemporary, Martin Luther. Both were products of the spiritual crisis of Germany in the sixteenth century, and they shared many German, and many personal, characteristics. Like Luther, Paracelsus was a violent, intemperate man, of strong language and rough manners, and he addressed himself primarily to the German world: he wrote in German for Germans. His medical teaching was the application, within his own special field, of a general philosophy, indeed cosmology, which far transcended that field; and this philosophy, he claimed, as Luther claimed for his, was true Christianity, restored to its original purity, free at last from the corrupt incrustations of the Middle Ages. In Luther's eyes, that corruption came from the paganism of the Roman church; in those of Paracelsus, it came from the paganism of Aristotle and his medical disciple Galen.

Philosophically, and in its political implications, Paracelsianism was far more radical than Lutheranism – at least than Lutheranism after the German Peasants' Revolt of 1525. It had a revolutionary messianic content which it never entirely lost. . . .

This revolutionary content of Paracelsianism must not be forgotten even if we are concerned only with its medical application; for it affected the reception of its medical teaching. It alarmed the established classes, just as the initial revolutionary content of Lutheranism had done when it became apparent in the Peasants' Revolt. So long as Paracelsian medical ideas were inseparable from their revolutionary premisses, they were bound to be suspect to conservative rulers. On the other hand, if they could be separated from those premisses, and judged, and vindicated, purely empirically, the grounds for suspicion were taken away. The external history of Paracelsian medicine – the history of its dissemination – is thus, to a large extent, the history of its disengagement from Paracelsian cosmology: a disengagement which (combined, of course, with its proven effectiveness in some cases) rendered it acceptable among the conservative classes. That separation was never absolute: there were always occasions when Paracelsianism returned, as it were, to its revolutionary roots. But this was not the Paracelsianism patronised by princes – except in those cases (for there were some) when princes themselves became revolutionary.

The effective dissemination of Paracelsian ideas and practices began in the generation after the death of their author in 1541. Paracelsus himself seems to have shown remarkably little interest in the publication of his works. A wild, disorderly charismatic genius, perpetually on the move, he scattered his ideas and his manuscripts without apparent concern for their preservation. However, his disciples treasured these documents as declarations of saving religious truths, or at least as manuals of profitable medical practice. They published the truths, or some of them, and they applied the practice. However, since both the truths and the practice were heretical, they inevitably ran into opposition: the religious truths were suppressed by the religious establishment, the medical ideas and practice were opposed by the medical establishment. For Paracelsianism, as a medical system, was a doctrine for the depressed classes of the medical world, for the apothecaries and surgeons. It was an affront to the traditional establishment, the Galenist physicians organized in colleges and faculties. Thus, from the start, patronage was necessary to overcome this opposition.

Where could such patronage be found? It could come from variable sources. There was the private patronage of rich individuals. There was the patronage of city corporations: many German cities appointed a Paracelsian physician as their *Stadtphysicus*.[3] Other such physicians were maintained, just as heretical chaplains could be, in private households of the nobility. Still others maintained themselves by general practice – but precariously, at a low social level, always at the mercy of the established medical corporations which had the right to expel unqualified practitioners from the cities of their jurisdiction. And then there were the armies of warring Europe. Paracelsus himself had been an army doctor, and so were many of his followers. The battlefield was perhaps the greatest laboratory for the new experimental science of Paracelsian surgery, as were the city slums for the Paracelsian apothecaries, the physicians of the poor.

Thus, in the generation after Paracelsus, in spite of official disapproval, his ideas circulated. They circulated mainly in the German world, to which they were addressed; and because they were apparently disorderly and certainly revolutionary, they were taken up, vulgarized, and distorted by a host of so-called 'spagyrists' – empirics, not to say quacks, who gave them a bad name. However, even in those

---

[3] Town physician.

years, thanks to certain enthusiastic disciples, they made their way in lay society, and here and there they even won the attention, and favour, of that most valuable of all protectors (as Luther knew), a prince.

For obviously, for any heresy, the ultimate protection, at that time, was princely power. A Renaissance prince could defy the entrenched authority of a medical faculty or corporation. He could give protection against the law. He could pay for the publication of books and guarantee them against censorship. He could provide resources – a laboratory, a professorial chair in his private university, a team of researchers, international contacts. And he could also provide power, wealth, and fame: to be in charge of the health of a prince, to have protected him against assassination by poison . . . to be also . . . his alchemist, capable – at least potentially – of creating wealth by chemical transmutation, was a responsibility which, of itself, brought in rewards. . . .

The part played by the princes in the fortune of Paracelsianism began, naturally enough, in Germany. Paracelsus himself was far too independent a character to acknowledge any patron. . . . However, in the years after his death, his disciples found princely patrons, and soon the fashion spread from court to court. Royalty has often shown a preference for unconventional doctors; the princes of the Renaissance were themselves, in many respects, radicals: intellectual heretics, innovators not traditionalists in practice; and anyway, Paracelsianism itself, thanks to its commentators, was coming to meet them. In the generation after the death of the Founder, we find it quietly disowning his revolutionary ideas and exchanging his disordered peasant clothes for a more courtly dress.

One of the first, perhaps the first, prince to take up Paracelsianism was the great humanist and patron of printing and the arts, Ottheinrich, Duke of Neuburg, afterwards Elector Palatine and head of the senior branch of the house of Wittelsbach. His court physician was Adam von Bodenstein, who had been converted to Paracelsianism by his own experience and became the first great propagandist of Paracelsus, publishing over forty of his works. Ottheinrich also had chemical interests. He employed a chemist, Hans Kilian, who made a large collection of Paracelsian manuscripts. These were stored in the Elector's castle of Neuburg on the Danube, and remained there after 1545, when the Elector was driven out of his little Danubian principality and forced to take refuge in the Palatinate, at Weinheim on the Rhine.

The Elector was driven out because he had become a Protestant. From the beginning, the heresy of Paracelsianism was closely linked to the other new heresy of Protestantism. It was, or became, a heresy within that heresy. The connection was not exclusive, however. Sometimes family tradition was stronger than doctrinaire consistency. The junior branch of the Wittelsbach family, the ducal house of Bavaria, would also become patrons of Paracelsianism. Indeed, at the end of the century, it was a younger son of that family, Ernst von Wittelsbach, Elector of Cologne, a vigorous politician of the Counter-Reformation,[4] who would finance the first publication of the complete works of Paracelsus. That was a remarkably bold step in 1590–1605, when the Catholic Chuch was condemning all forms of Platonism, hermeticism, and so on. However, the Elector of Cologne was a powerful prince and could afford to be eccentric. The editor of this great edition was the Elector's court physician, Johann Huser, a Paracelsian from Breslau; and he based it on the 141 volumes of manuscripts which Ottheinrich had collected and which had remained at Neuburg. He was just in time, for within a few years the growing opposition of the Roman Church would reach its climax and the works of Paracelsus would be put on the Roman Index. Later, when the Wittelsbach Palatinate had fallen into pious Roman Catholic hands, Ottheinrich's great collection would be solemnly burnt.

Ottheinrich also employed, as librarian and physician, a German doctor from Danzig, Alexander von Suchten. It was while at his court that Suchten too became a Paracelsian – indeed, the most distinguished of the early Paracelsians. Afterwards (in 1554) Suchten was employed as *Archiater*, i.e. chief physician, by Sigismund Augustus, King of Poland; but his religious views got him into trouble in Poland – he had already been condemned in Rome and deprived of his canonry of Frauenberg – and he returned to Germany and published his offending Paracelsian works at Basel. . . .

The year 1570, when Suchten published his first volume, may be taken as the year when Paracelsianism became respectable. It was then that Paracelsian books began to come out in a steady stream, presented not in barbarous German but in civilized Latin, addressed to, and sponsored by, learned men. In 1571, the venerable Winther von Andernach, the teacher of Vesalius, having been converted by one of Paracelsus' disciples at Strasbourg, published his *De Medicina Veteri et Nova* [*Of the ancient and new physick*], in which he announced his respect for 'the new medicine'. Even more important, in the same year a Danish physician, Peder Sorensen, *alias* Severinus . . . published at Basel his

---

[4] The movement within the Catholic Church aimed at winning back Protestants after the breach initiated by Luther in the early sixteenth century. Among the various measures adopted by the papacy in the Counter-Reformation struggle against Protestantism were the creation of new, militant orders such as the Jesuits, or Society of Jesus, and the creation of the Papal Index, which censored publications that were thought to undermine the true faith.

Idea Medicinae Philosophicae [*The concept of a philosophical medicine*]. This was an academic presentation and vindication of Paracelsianism. Severinus had studied Paracelsianism in Germany. Now he went back to his native Denmark and was appointed court physician to the King of Denmark – a position he was to hold for thirty years. There he became an important person in an important court of the northern Renaissance.

[. . .]

Paracelsianism was a complex system of thought, unsystematically expressed, imperfectly published, and often misunderstood. It was open to different interpretations according to time, circumstance, and inclination, and by 1570 these differences were becoming apparent. In particular, it was becoming clear that if it was to capture the royal court, it must shed, or at least suspend, its revolutionary content – or rather, escape from its revolutionary context: its religious and ideological messianism, its insistence that the Prophet Elijah was to return – *Elias Artista*, Elijah as alchemist – to create a new 'chemical' transformation of the world. We may observe that, in the whole of the sixteenth century, it was only the medical and never the specifically religious works of Paracelsus that were published: these circulated in manuscripts, but, until the nineteenth century, they remained the private possession of obscure German sects, and it is only since the end of that century that they have been published. Of course Paracelsus' religious views emerged incidentally in his medical works; but there they could be taken or left at choice. Meanwhile, his medical ideas became detached from his total philosophy and could be absorbed piecemeal into more orthodox medicine.

5.3

Challenging the medical status quo: the fate of Paracelsianism in France

Allen G. Debus, *The French Paracelsians: The Chemical Challenge to Medical and Scientific Tradition in Early Modern France* (Cambridge, Cambridge University Press, 1991), pp. 48–51, 53–5, 56–9, 65, 84–5, 88–91, 93, 94–5, 100–1.

In this extract, Allen Debus, whose pioneering work on the reception of Paracelsianism in Europe has led to a major reassessment of its place in early modern medicine, explores the fate of Paracelsus' legacy in France. Here, the conflict over the recognition of the worth of chemical medicine was long and bitter. Debus demonstrates that acceptance of the new medicine was not solely down to medical or scientific debate. At the heart of the conflict between French Galenists and Paracelsians were issues relating to the organisation and status of the medical profession in the capital, Paris, as well as competing religious and political affiliations.

In 1593 Henry of Navarre ended a long period of civil war by taking Paris, a military and political event that had unexpected medical and chemical results. The French physicians who were interested in the work of Paracelsus and the application of chemistry to medicine were almost all Huguenots. These protestants, many of whom had been in exile for more than twenty years since the St Bartholomew's Day massacre[5] felt that they could to return to France now, even to Paris itself. If they were aware of the hostility of the Parisian Medical Faculty to chemistry and the Paracelsians (and they surely must have been), they must also have known that the new king, Henry IV, favoured the new medicine. Even the ill-fated Roch le Baillif had been appointed *médecin ordinaire* to Henry III, and chemical physicians were being welcomed to the service of the rulers of the principalities of Europe at a time when they remained anathema to many of the medical schools on the Continent.

In 1594 Jean Ribit, sieur de la Rivière (ca. 1571–1605), a Huguenot, was appointed first physician to the king. Critical of the many unlearned Paracelsists he had met on his travels throughout Europe, Ribit de la

---

[5] The St Bartholomew's Day massacre of French Protestants took place on 24 August 1572.

Rivière nevertheless had a genuine interest in the new chemically prepared drugs, which seemed to offer much for the future of medicine. Ribit's appointment was symptomatic of change in the new reign, so it is not surprising to find him appointing chemists as royal physicians. The two most prominent were Joseph Duchesne and Theodore Turquet de Mayerne (1573–1655). . . . Mayerne . . . was of Huguenot stock; his parents had fled to Geneva after the St Bartholomew's Day massacre, and it was there that he was born. He attended Heidelberg and then Montpellier, which was becoming a center for Paracelsian and chemical medicine. There he took his medical degree in 1597 before moving to Paris where Ribit de la Rivière obtained a post for him as *médecin ordinaire* to the king, as he had earlier done for Duchesne. Mayerne proceeded to organize a series of lectures on chemical medicine for surgeons and apothecaries (1599) and quickly became widely known as one of the foremost proponents of the new medicine.

It should be noted that the chemical physicians associated with the court were developing into a formidable medical group. . . . Before the reign of Henry IV there were on average some fifteen to twenty-five physicians for the king and another five to ten for the members of the royal family. With the accession of Henry of Navarre the post of *médecin ordinaire* was established to assist the *premier médecin*. These two physicians then arranged for the appointment of eight regular physicians, who served by quarter [i.e. for 3 months], plus fifteen consulting physicians for the king alone. This total of twenty-five for the king and ten or more for the royal family is comparable to the number of physicians in the Parisian Medical Faculty. If one takes into account the fact that the *premier médecins* of Henry IV and Louis XIII were interested in chemical medicine and sought to expand their own medical establishment, we can see the basis for a serious clash, relating to both authority and method.

The controversy was exacerbated by the changing tone of the chemists. . . . [M]ost of the chemical works published in France prior to 1600 dealt primarily with the internal use of chemical preparations, and the anger of the Galenists was directed primarily at the compounds of metals and minerals.

Significantly, it was Joseph Duchesne who added a new dimension to the debate. . . . [I]n 1603 he published a new work, this time on theoretical medicine [which contained] a strong plea for the superiority of chemical medicine. It appeared at a time when both chemistry and the medical establishment surrounding the king seemed to threaten the Parisian Medical Faculty. . . . Although there had been almost continuous debate between the Parisian Medical Faculty and the chemists for forty years, Duchesne's work of 1603 sparked a new debate that was to continue into the third quarter of the seventeenth century and was to have an undercurrent of medical politics in addition to the question of theoretical orthodoxy.

The opinions of Duchesne that were so offensive to the members of the Parisian Medical Faculty were primarily expressed in the *Liber de priscorum philosophorum verae medicinae materia* of 1603 and the *Ad Veritatem Hermeticae medicinae ex Hippocratis veterumque decretis* of the following year. Here was to be found a defense of chemistry, the new remedies, and a chemical interpretation of nature and medicine. As in his earliest works, Duchesne did not reject the ancients, only their modern disciples. . . .

[. . .]

Duchesne called the Galenists of his day dogmatists and contrasted them with the spagyrists. The dogmatists, he said, turn to Galen 'and as if by a royal edict where the sentence is firm and without doubt, pronounce that contraries cure'. But the spagyric chemists place their faith in reason and experience rather than books. They seek the internal essence of bodies. . . .

Although Duchesne was no more a blind follower of Paracelsus in 1603 than he had been a quarter century earlier, it is clear that he approved of many concepts that were generally accepted by the Paracelsians. Like them he based his cosmology on the Creation story in Genesis in which God played the part of a divine alchemist:

> We holde by *Moses* doctrine that GOD in the beginning made of nothing a *Chaos*, or Deepe, or Waters, if wee please so to call it. From the which Chaos, Deepe, or waters, animated with the Spirits of God, God as the great workemaister and Creator, separated first of all *Light* from *Darknesse*, and this *Aetheriall Heaven*, which wee beholde, as a fifth Essence, or most pure Spirite, or most simple spirituall body. Then hee divided Waters, from Waters; that is to say, the more subtill, Aiery, and Mercuriall liquor, from the more Thicke, Clammy, and Oyely, or Sulphurous liquor. After that, he extracted and brought forth the *Sulphur*, that is to say, the more grosse Waters, from the drye parte, which out of the separation standeth like salte, and as yet standeth by it selfe apart. . . .This was the worke of God, that hee might separate the Pure from the Impure: that is to say that he might reduce the more pure and Ethereal Mercury, the more pure and inextinguible Sulphur, the more pure, and more fixed salte, into shyning and inextinguible Starres and Lights, into a Cristalline and Dyamantine substance, or most simple Bodie, which is called *Heaven*, the highest, and fourth formall Element.

Salt, sulfur, and mercury were for Duchesne the active elements. . . .
'There are three principall things mixed in every Naturall bodie: to wit,
'*Salte, Sulphur*, and *Mercurie*. These are the beginnings of all Naturall
things'. As in alchemical tradition, these three principles were not our
modern laboratory reagents but were sophic substances 'which never-
thelesse hath some conscience and agreement with com[m]on Salt, Sulphur, and Mercurie'.

Constantly seeking triads, Duchesne compared the *tria prima* with
body, soul, and spirit 'for the body is attributed to salt: the spirit to Mercurie: and the soule to sulphur: everyone to their apt and convenient
attribute.' These principles also had more recognizable attributes. Mercury 'is a sharpe liquor, passable, and penetrable, and a most pure &
Aetheriall substantiall body'; sulfur 'is that moyst, sweet, oyly, clammy,
original'; salt 'is that dry body, saltish, meerly earththy, representing the
nature of *Salt*'.

[. . .]

Duchesne's medicine was dominated by his acceptance of the macro-
cosm-microcosm analogy and the search for chemical analogies. The
distillations and condensations that he recognized in the atmosphere as
the causes of rain were the same as those that caused catarrh in man.
By analogy he reasoned that in the microcosm the true source of wind,
sleet, and snow is the condensation of mercurial vapors, which in man
cause ringing in the ears, paralepsy, apoplexy, and similar illnesses. In
short what we learn of one world must be acceptable to the other.

Duchesne insisted that all those who accepted the Galenic dictum
that contraries cure would 'never easily finde out a remedie for sicknesse,' and that, indeed that was not the true meaning of Hippocrates'
words. Rather, like cures like and the best medicines are those prepared by chemical means. The preparation of medicines was the main
use of chemistry, not the transmutation of base metals to gold. . . .

Duchesne insisted that he was not a Paracelsian. For him, chemical
medicine was the true medicine of Galen and Hippocrates. He affirmed
that the principal object of his *De priscorum philosophorum* concerned the Galenic *materia medica*, and he sought primarily to embellish Galenic remedies with some chemical ornaments 'plus beau, plus
riche & plus utile'. He wrote that Paracelsus should not be given full
credit for this chemical philosophy because he was only one of many
who had taught it over the centuries, going back to the greatest antiq-
uity. At the same time Duchesne was convinced that there were new
diseases in the seventeenth century that had been unknown by the
ancients, and new remedies were required for them. Because these new

diseases were often localized, it was imperative that all true physicians be well traveled. In no other way could they learn of these current medical problems.

If Duchesne did not consider himself a Paracelsian, others did, and the reaction of the Parisian Medical Faculty to his works was swift. The elder Jean Riolan (1539–1606), censor of the faculty, produced in 1603 an *Apologia pro Hippocratis et Galeni Medicina* [*An apology for Hippocratic and Galenic medicine*]. . . .

[. . .]

Duchesne was defended in print by his protégé and friend, Theodore Turquet de Mayerne . . . in which he insisted that the use of chemically prepared remedies should not be considered an attack on the ancients. However, Mayerne had been spreading his views on chemistry in a series of lectures to young surgeons and apothecaries, and his defense of Duchesne was considered highly offensive by the members of the faculty. . . . In a decree against Mayerne, the Parisian Medical Faculty declared that he was:

> unworthy of practising medicine because of his rashness, his impudence, and his ignorance of the true principles of medicine. [The Medical Faculty] urges all physicians who practise medicine wherever they may be to distance themselves from Turquet and to reject similar opinions. . . .

Those who did not adhere to this decree would be deprived of their university degrees and the privileges of the academy and would be expelled from the Order of the Doctors Regent. . . .

Turquet left for England in 1606 and was incorporated M.D. at Oxford. He was to become physician to both King James and Queen Henrietta Maria as well as president of the Royal College of Physicians. There he became interested in the long-delayed pharmacopoeia of the college. He pressed for its publication (1618) and was largely responsible for the inclusion of chemical preparations in the volume.

[. . .]

A persistent problem for the medical faculty was Petrus Palmarius (Pierre Paulmier) (1568–1610), a Parisian physician and a member of the faculty who wrote in support of the faculty while advocating the use of chemical medicines. As early as 1591 he had been censured for proposing to give a course on spagyric chemistry to apothecaries, and in August 1603 an *arrêt*[6] was issued against him. Six years later he pub-

---

[6] Writ of arrest.

lished his *Lapis philosophicus Dogmaticorum* [*The philosopher's stone of the Dogmatists*], in which he wrote of the superiority of the ancient medical authors and their modern supporters and at the same time defended the use of chemically prepared drugs, insisting even that antimony could be used internally for very difficult cases. Predictably Paulmier was condemned by the faculty. He was banned from the faculty and ordered not to be reinstated for at least two years, and then only after asking pardon for his offenses.

[. . .]

Although the Paracelsian chemical philosophy was well known to present a chemical interpretation of the universe that was opposed to Galenic medicine and to Aristotelian philosophy, the debate in France until about 1625 centered on medical and pharmaceutical problems, particularly the medicines derived by chemical means from metals and minerals. The broader cosmological problems became a matter of greater concern in ensuing years.

[. . .]

In the fourth decade of the [seventeenth] century a new champion of chemicals arose in the person of Théophraste Renaudot (1584–1653). A protestant, he had taken his degree at Montpellier where he had matriculated in 1605. It would have been impossible for him to have attended Paris, where proof of one's Roman Catholicism was required. Unlike many others, after receiving the licentiate, which permitted him to practice, he had gone on to take the doctorate (12 July 1606). After a period of travel he returned to his home, Loudun, where he married and set up his practice.

At Loudun Renaudot became aware of the problems of the poor, and at this time (1611) he met Armand-Jean du Plessis de Richelieu, later to be named cardinal. The following year (1612) Richelieu called a meeting in Paris to discuss the problems of the poor. Renaudot was invited and while there he was given the title of royal physician in reward for offering his ideas on poor relief to the Crown. In 1618 he was given the additional title of *commissaire des pauvres du royaume* [commissioner for the kingdom's poor]. These were honors that did not require his attendance at court, and Renaudot remained for most of the year at Loudun. Nevertheless, it seemed wise to convert to Catholicism, which he did sometime before 1626, when he finally moved to Paris. As a royal physician he was able to set up practice even though the Parisian Medical Faculty tried to enforce its right to limit physicians in Paris to its own graduates. He became an active supporter of Richelieu, who saw to it that Renaudot's titles were reconfirmed. . . .

In Paris, Renaudot was in a position to establish his Bureau d'Adresse (1630 or perhaps a year or two earlier), which he hoped would go far to solve the problems of the poor. In part this was a clearing house for the unemployed, who could register and hope to find a suitable employer. . . . In addition to this practical function, the Bureau d'Adresse provided medical assistance. Free medical consultations were being provided to the poor as early as 1632. At first this service was confined to medical consultations on Tuesday afternoons, when the physicians would examine patients, prescribe treatment, and refer them to a physician who would treat them gratuitously. In addition Renaudot inaugurated a system of low-interest loans to aid the poor; a printing shop that published the *Gazette* (1631), one of the first French newspapers; and a long-running series of conferences which are of interest in reference to the development of European scientific academies.

[. . .]

There is little doubt that Théophraste Renaudot had already become an important figure in the realm. He had been trained first as a physician and thought of himself as such. His degree was from Montpellier, and many of his assistants at the Bureau had similar academic ties. They all had an interest in chemistry and often prescribed antimony to their patients. Because of these factors, Renaudot and his medical activities were viewed with alarm by the members of the Parisian Medical Faculty.

The medical community at Paris – other than the court physicians – was for the most part quite . . . conservative. . . . Lectures at the medical school were based on Hippocrates, Galen, and the 'other princes of medicine'. The medical faculty itself extended far beyond the two professors (until 1634) of medicine to include all the medical doctors in the city; and . . . these were usually limited to graduates of Paris. In this way the members of the professional medical community were also members of the educational community.

The Parisian Medical Faculty claimed that only their graduates could practice throughout France; the practice of those who had been trained elsewhere was, or should be, limited only to the towns in which they were trained. With the exception of the royal physicians, the medical faculty strove to keep the medical community free from 'foreign' influence, which meant that even graduates of Montpellier were forbidden to practice in Paris. . . . Montpellier was suspect not only for its long interest in chemical medicine but also because it accepted protestant students. The Parisian Medical Faculty also attempted to maintain its authority over the surgeons and apothecaries of Paris, who understandably resented the interference.

It was during the 1630s that Renaudot was giving free medical advice at the Bureau d'Adresse from ten to twelve o'clock every weekday morning. His medical staff was composed of physicians from non-Parisian schools, many of whom were protestants and advocates of chemical medicine. It seemed to the members of the Parisian Medical Faculty that their power was being directly challenged.

A series of swift-moving events brought the matter to a head. For fifteen years the faculty had been at work on a pharmacopeoia, the *Codex pharmaceutique*. One of the approved purgatives contained antimony, *vin émétique*. This had been accepted by a committee headed by Hardouin St. Jacques, dean of the Parisian Medical Faculty. The question of whether this approval had been given properly was to plague the members of the faculty for decades and was a source of embarrassment to those members who opposed chemical remedies, especially antimony.

At this time the two sons of Renaudot, Isaac and Eusèbe, were medical students in Paris. Seeking to injure the father through his children, the faculty forced them to sign a disavowal of their father's activities in order to pass the first grade (1638). This hardly affected Théophraste who had furnaces built at the bureau (September 1640), so that chemicals could be prepared there, and soon after obtained permission to build new facilities for the Bureau d'Adresse. Renaudot was at the height of his power. He employed foreign-trained (non-Parisian) physicians whom he could license to practice throughout France through his power as *commissaire général des pauvres*; he attracted students of the Parisian medical school to his weekly conferences, students who would learn there of chemical medicines; he had obtained the right to set up his chemical laboratories; and he had a program of free medical consultations, which could serve as a teaching clinic. Furthermore, he had widespread support among the apothecaries and surgeons, whom he treated as equals.

To extend the program of medical advice Renaudot prepared *La présence des absens*, a medical form that described symptoms and could be completed by anyone and sent to the bureau. The bureau staff would then diagnose the patient in absentia and make recommendations for treatment by mail. This made the bureau truly a medical center for the entire country, and of course, it was considered to be one more affront to the Parisian Medical Faculty. . . .

[. . .]

Three weeks after Renaudot had obtained permission to build furnaces at the bureau, he was officially informed by the medical faculty of the injunction against foreign physicians in Paris. On 3 November 1640 Guillaume du Val became the new dean . . . and one of his first acts was to set up a commission to investigate the activities of empirics in Paris, especially Renaudot. For the next three years Renaudot and his adversaries waged a pamphlet war [much of which] concerned the history of the two chief medical schools, Paris and Montpellier, and the validity of their rights and privileges. Also of concern to both parties was the history of the use of chemical medicines both before and after the decree of 1566 against antimony. The Parisian Medical Faculty insisted on its right to grant permission to practice in Paris, and they remained firm in their opposition to chemical remedies, especially all forms of antimony. . . .

[. . .]

Early in 1643 a new dean of the medical school, Michel de la Vigne, sought and obtained the support of the University of Paris in their process against . . . Renaudot. At this point Louis XIII died (May 14), and the medical faculty called for injunctions against all of Renaudot's activities. The court was now controlled by Anne of Austria, who was opposed to Richelieu [who himself had died in the previous December] and all his supporters. In August the suit against Renaudot was transferred from the Conseil du Roi to the prévôt of Paris. With this transfer Renaudot had essentially lost his case.

In a final effort Renaudot appealed to the queen . . . but on December 9 he and his associates were ordered to cease their activities.

A public session of parlement was held on 1 March 1644. Five lawyers represented Renaudot, his sons, the University of Montpellier, the Medical Faculty of Paris, and the University of Paris. Chenvot, representing the faculty, attacked chemical medicine as no better than traditional medicine and as a system that ran the risk of killing some patients. He attacked Renaudot personally, noting that he had graduated too young by Parisian standards. Furthermore, he had created disorder in the medical profession. He was a protestant from Loudun, a town noted for devils. His given name was Théophraste, recalling . . . Theophrastus Paracelsus, the originator of the chemical heresy in medicine. Beyond that, Renaudot was ugly and had a misshapen nose – unfortunate in a profession in which handsome practitioners were expected to inspire their patients. The legality of all his titles and offices were also questioned.

Renaudot's lawyer argued that scientific ideas were not proper for a legal case. More to the point was the argument that all of Renaudot's privileges had been accorded through the Conseil du Roi and that is where the case should have been settled. But Renaudot no longer had significant support at court. Anne of Austria was hostile to him, and Richelieu's successor, Mazarin, was indifferent.

An *arrêt* of parlement demanded that Renaudot return his letters patent for the establishment of the Bureau d'Adresse. ... He was allowed to keep his title as *maître et intendant général des Bureau d'Adresse de France*, but the title alone was meaningless. He was forbidden to practice medicine in Paris, but he was allowed to continue his publishing activities: The *Gazette* had been useful to the crown and it could remain so. On the other hand, the value of the public medical consultations he had established were recognized by an *arrêt* ordering the medical faculty to establish charitable consultations for the poor.

[. . .]

Although the Parisian Medical Faculty was triumphant at the humiliation of Renaudot in 1644, the victory did not last long. The old defenders of Galen led by Jean Riolan the younger and Gui Patin were aging, and the younger members were inclined to accept antimony and other chemical remedies. The cure of Louis XIV in 1658 with *vin émétique* signaled the end of the conflict, and antimony quickly became a fashionable cure among the wealthy. When antimony was proposed as an approved medicine in 1666, only ten percent of the assembled Parisian Medical Faculty opposed the motion.

5.4

Helmontianism and medical reform in Cromwellian England: Noah Biggs (1651)

Noah Biggs, *Mataeotechnia Medicinae Praxews. The Vanity of the Craft of Physick* (London, Giles Calvert, 1651), pp. 77–8, 136, 161–2, 193–4, 198, 200–1, 213–14, 216–17, 219, 221.

Of Noah Biggs, the author, nothing is known. The work excerpted here, however, is an important one since it represents the first full-length treatise in English in favour of the new medical theories of the Flemish iatrochemist, John Baptista van Helmont (1579–1644). Indeed, much of the work contains direct translations from the Latin edition of van Helmont's collected works, published posthumously in 1648. The bulk of Biggs' treatise is given over to a comprehensive assault on the theoretical and therapeutic rationale of Galenism. At the same time, Biggs, in true Helmontian fashion, rejects the philosophical principles upon which Paracelsianism was based, as well as its belief in cure by similars. Helmontianism proved highly popular in England in the 1650s, and there is much evidence in the language of the extract demonstrating a close link between the religious and political outlook of the new Cromwellian regime and the medical reformism of Biggs.

... But it may be made appear unto ample satisfaction by the consent of experience, *that laxatives do not take away the noxious humours, or any disease lodg'd in them*. Then, that there are no *such things* in *Nature*; nor was ever this *meridian of humours* ever touch'd or come nigh to, by those, who, *Drake-like*, have compass'd the whole *Globe* and round of *Nature* ... but hangs onely (like castles in the aire) in the *Eutopia* of *vulgar* Physitians brains, or in the narrow creek of their *base-born* books, and no where else: neither do any diseases *respond* or goe a *pilgrimage* to lodge in the *New-found-Land* of *Americall* or *Prestor-John* humours.[7] Then also, that whatsoever the *Catharticks* profligate, banish, and cast out from the *Independency* of our vitall *Oeconomy*, is not one of the three humours which they say offends, is become malignant, and endeavours to settle a commission of array[8] [. . .] but is onely the honest *round-head*, a true and peaceable Common-Wealth's-man, the *bloud* who is chosen and ordain'd to be one of the *Keepers* of the *liberties*, *life* and *health* of our bodies, now slain by the *laxative* medicine, and sacrific'd as a *Holocaust* on the *Altar* of its virulency and *poison*.

[. . .]

We now willingly come ... to arraigne and examine the naturalities of the other universal main pillars of curing, namely *phlebotomy*, *fontanells* or *issues*, and *Dyet*, as three other props of healing, which being shaken, the whole edifice falls downe of its own accord as rubbish, and being taken away, Physitians do desert their patients, having no remedies but such as *purging* and *bloud-letting*.

[7] Prestor John was a mythical European king who was thought in the Middle Ages to rule in parts of the Orient or Africa.

[8] At the beginning of the first English civil war (1642–46), the royalists sought to raise troops in the counties by issuing commissions of array.

[. . .]

[Of blood-letting] [i]t's true some forreign excrements may perturb the bloud in the veins . . . to wit the surplusage, or mean retinue as well of their own, as another *digestion,* but never the Lord chief Treasurer of life, the *bloud.* Because according to scripture, *it is the seat, the chamber and magazine of life.*[9] If therefore the grand seigniour himself, the life, cannot preserve his own throne and Treasury in the metropolis or Royaltie of the veins, from the invasion or treacherous undermining of that petty Rebell, corruption, from becoming Competitor or Tenant thereto, when then will he keep it? And how can it be ever free from the same? And also if the life cannot save harmles & keep indempnified from the charge of putrefaction, the bloud, *custos vitae,*[10] in which she sits enthron'd, and growes and encreases in glory and vigour, how will then the bones be preserved?

The veins therefore are ordain'd by the high court and Councel of Heaven to be Lord Commissioners deputed to keep the bloud from corruption: because the life is confermented to the bloud of the veins, and therefore both are cast out by the lease of ejectment of bloud-letting; they both together have their current through the sluice of *phlebotomy,* and make their *exit* at one door, the orifice of the vein. Under this question therefore the glory and destination of Nature doth come to ruin: or the whole course of healing hitherto ador'd by Physitians.

[. . .]

. . . For let those eares that have the patience to hear, and the openesse to receive truth, know, That when Physitians see they have afforded no benefit to their patients, by the lavish expences of the laudable juices of the body, and the diminution of natural vigour, when *bloud-letting, purging, cupping, rubbing* . . . and other grievous and ineffective remedies have done no good; they at length remit them to the sober rules of *Diet* . . . and so leave them by the painfull use of *fontanells,* and reiterated moderate *purges,* to spin out the weak thred of their remaining life, *Diaetetice,* by a medicall, that is, a miserable course of diet.

[. . .]

How many *non-Conformists* are there to the *Kitchin Canons,* who do repudiate the rules that is prescribed them, will be no *obsequious* dietetical slaves, will *observe no bounds,* and yet often *recover* and are well?

---

[9] Biblical justification for the view that the 'life' or soul was present in the blood was based on a reading of Genesis 9:3–4.

[10] The guardian of life.

[. . .]

But diet after sicknesse, or under *convalescency*, is also wonderfull troublesome, if not in vain: seeing nature now is willingly very diligent, and greatly busied about other matters. For in severity of truth a *medicall course of diet*, and Kitchin operations, cannot but accuse the defect of a sufficient remedy, and so an implicite confession of a false and treacherous sanation. Let Physitians no more attempt by these fruitlesse meanes, to dreigne the hopes, bodies, veins, strength, and purses of the sick; but let them cure as they ought, and becomes them, worthy their name and profession, and as nature moves and enclines, and if not goe along with, yet to follow her, for the security and assurance of restauration.

It is not to be scrupled that the omnipotent and wise Creator saw and judged all things that he had made to be good. That is, whatsoever he had ordained for food, was good. And whatsoever he had decreed to be poison, was good poison, qualified to its purpose. For else the poor man, might with much right, and justly complain, that God in his distributions and largesses had dealt very unequally and lesse fatherly to him, because he had denyed him the means which should recover his health; for being poor, he was incapable to answer the costly and sweet lipped rules of *diet*.

[. . .]

We are ashamed seriously not for [our] own individual *singularity* and *egoity* so much, as for the sake of our Neighbour and Brother, that Physitians are so carelesse, and seem to study only for lucre or gain; and what it should mean we professe not to know, unlesse it be of divine ordering that the schools shall so long grope in the darke, and stumble, till they are got clear and have quitted themselves like men from the errors of the *Ancients*, and come to sharpen their own Axes and Coulters[11] at the forge of Nature. These things have been sooner, and rather found out by our eyes, then thoughts and meditations: yet at this *bone cape* we would willingly touch and unlade our mind to the notice of the sonnes of wisdome, that the errors and ignorances which have been here discovered by familiar and pregnant demonstrations, have not bin sucked and elaborated . . . out of . . . the poison of somes dotages and uncertain principles . . . as from an inward teaching of the mindes heightning and enlightning by an invisible and yet sensible glorious emanation of *light, truth, God, Intellect* and *Intelligible* objects. For they have not come in at a crevise or hole of the *door*, or opened

---

[11] Iron blades, used in plough shares.

themselves by little and little, and entered *gradually* into our mind, so as that we have conceived, meditated, and found them out one after another. For if in this *Discovery* one thing after another had come to our knowledge, we should have esteemed the whole progresse to be the enfeebled and *wier-drawn inductions* of Reason, and phantasie obtruded in the species of *Intelligibilities*.

Lastly, we have one thing more to propound and examine, which we have thought worthy a general notice, and cannot let pas[s] undiscovered, that is, the two general intentions and indications of healing, promoted and abetted by the *schools* and most *practicioners* in Physick in the whole world, namely, by *contrariety* and *simility*. Some attempt to scale the Fort royal of diseases, and rout them in their strong holds *per contraria*, and so by *Contentions, strifes, jarrings* and *clashings* endeavor a *mutiny*; then comes the *Crisis*, as they call it, in diseases, whereby judgement is given of the *victor*, either the disease or Nature to o'recome. This plausible and stupid Doctrine . . . easily pleases all, who are prone to runne into the way of sloth. . . . All the schools of the Christian world have taught and subscribed to this, *that Contraries have their remedy from Contraries*. By which truly every excesse (marked with the *nomenclation* of a *disease*) should be reduced into perfect *symmetry*. As if a medicine should not worke *Physically*, but *mechanically, mathematically* or *demonstratively* only.

[. . .]

To what hath been said of *Contraries*, that there is no intentions in *Nature* of *contrariety* in those things, in whom there is no pretension of *hatred, variance, victory,* or *superiority*, we add; that *unity* is not contrary to *Duality. Nor upwards to downwards*, nor *high* to *low*, nor *East* to *West* are not contrary. Nor is the *right* ear contrary to the *left*, although opposite. . . . Nor is *Generation contrary* to *corruption*. So likewise neither *great* is contrary to *little*, nor *straight* to *crooked*. When one & the same may be now small now great, straight & crooked. The same is to be said of *sweet* and *bitter; hard* and *soft: heavy* and *light: sharpe* and *blunt* . . . or *white* and black. The like is to be said of *water* and *fire: Heat* and *cold.* . . . So that it appears these things are *limitable, alterable,* & by themselves not regarded, and so not fit for principles; and therefore no *contrariety, hatred, discord, warre,* strife of *victory* or *superiority* in natural things, but that they act without *intention* or *precognition* of an end: and so . . . let it be a certain *Analogy* shining rather in *effects* and *causes*, then in the direction of the creator, or distinction of ends: because that they are deprived of proper sense, election, intention of acting, and precognition of ends: The schools therefore and Physitians are exceedingly out of the way who will admit only those as remedies of *diseases*, which by a hostile contrary property, encounter and warre against them, as if there were a power of *sense* and an arbitrary power of *Election* in them.

Others go more amicably to work, and cure *diseases* by *simility*. *Paracelsus* himselfe hath too effeminately stooped to this opinion, and saies, that all *Sanation* must be shut up and finished by *assimilation*. . . . And although *simility* doth proximely include *familiarity*, and *facility* of *reception* and entertaining the remedy . . . yet the abettors hereof know not that these are not *Agents* sufficiently indowed, nor capable or requisite to *Sanation*. . . .

[. . .]

Others there are again who think to make medicine out of the *Chymists* Ternary of new principles, *Sal, Sulphur* and *Mercury*; and thereby think themselves *Natures* . . . imitators. To this do many of this Age subscribe: but it is to be wished that they did know otherwise, and might come to learn that digestion of Nature never tends to those three principles, and that we never are nourished by them. . . .

Happy sure was he constellated, who knew how to take away diseases both safely and readily on the shoulders of *crude simples*. For it is the primitive method of healing noted in scripture. That the Highest had created medicine out of the Earth.[12] . . . We have alwaies greatly esteemed the destination of God in the vertues and gifts of *simples*: forasmuch as he hath endowed them with excellent qualifications, natural, specifick and gifted to an end, without *contrariety* or *simility*. Yet in this *Panegyrick* of *simples*, we do not vilifie, or detract from the due praises of *Pyrotechny*: but well serves onely for a lecture to those, who admit nothing but those three *principles* . . .

But when a disease hath all ready entered the borders of life, and hath risen to some height . . . and hath almost fatally foiled *Nature*, then there is required higher medicines, of a more noble *Entelechie*[13] then those which *Nature* produceth of her own accord. . . . And to speak freely what cannot be concealed, and will daily break out more and more, all this is to be accomplished by the exact benefit and exquisite operations of *pyrotechny*.

---

[12] Ecclesiasticus 38:1.
[13] Perfection.

5.5

A new threat to medical orthodoxy: the Society of Chemical Physicians (1665)

George Thomson, *Galeno-pale: or, a Chymical Trial of the Galenists* (London, R. Wood, 1665), sigs A2r–A4r; pp. 19–20, 48–9, 55, 103–6.

George Thomson (c. 1619–76) was a Helmontian physician and one of the leading figures in the attempt to overthrow the established authority of the London College of Physicians through the creation of the Society of Chemical Physicians in 1665. Having served the royalist cause in the civil war, he subsquently removed to Leyden, in Holland, where he proceeded M.D. in 1648. Shortly after, he rejected Galenic therapeutics and became an admirer of the Flemish physician, Jan Baptista van Helmont. He remained in London during the plague and gained some fame by anatomising the body of a plague victim and living to tell the tale. In this short extract, he seeks to defend the chemists from the slur of their enemies that they lack learning and the requisite social graces required for a physician.

Epistle dedicatory to Gilbert Sheldon, archbishop of Canterbury

Among the many *Moecena's* of *Hermetick Philosophy*, I conceive none more fitting to protect the *Medicinal Verities* here set down, then your *Grace*; who hath been pleased to express very much kindeness and love for this Noble Art, to the no small encouragement of the Professours thereof. And all things duly pondered, where can *Chymical Physick* better shelter it self against Maligners and Opposers of it, then under the wings of *Divinity*, on which it ought to attend as an Hand-Maid? yea, there should be a Synergie, and conspiration of all Arts and Sciences to advance *Theology*, which makes the better Part of us happy.

[. . .]

Certainly there is no better way to attain this then by *Spagyrick Philosophy*, which separates . . . what is Hurtful and Superfluous in every *Concrete*, from the profitable, pure, and sincere; bringing it to such an Entelechie and Excellency, that it is able to display that radiant Virtue which God hath implanted in it for the good both of Body and Soul. And were this course closely followed, and generally countenanced, those rebellious and enormous Vices of the Minde, too grassant[14] at this day among us, which in great part arise from the Feral, Anomalous, unheard of Prodigious, and untractable Diseases of the Body, might in some measure be reformed; and certainly if there be not some timely prevention ... most of our Posterity is like to be born diseased.

Now at length finding that they have strived in vain against truth, by their obloquies and false suggestions still kicking against a prick; and finding they cannot obscure the bright beames of Pyrotechnical Philosophy, they take now another supplanting course, and of a sudden will all become Chymists; but *Galeno-Chymists*, as monstrous and Anomalous as a Centaure or Syren: and hereby they think to blear the eyes of the world, to make them believe, that their Method sweetens all our sharp Vitriolate Medicines, allayes all our Corrosives, fixes all our Mercurial Preparations; and in short, makes all safe and sound, which otherwise would be destructive in our fingers. Thus they still juggle with, and delude the world, still protracting and spinning out the time, very unwilling to part with ease, gain, and honour, notwithstanding thousands suffer by their indirect practice, e're they will come in quietly, and sincerely submit to the truth, for the good of the Nation. . . .

[. . .]

Did the World rightly understand what destruction of mankinde hath been made by this Sanguinary way of curing Diseases in all Ages, since this prodigal emission of Blood came first in use . . . it would . . . utterly abominate any such Physician, or such a pretended remedy.

How happy may those Nations be reputed in this particular, (witness their Longaevity and Sanity above ours) whom Nature hath so well instructed, as not to part with this precious treasure of Life, unless against their wills through some violent separation of the connexed parts. And certainly were we but governed by Nature, which intends all things for its own preservation, and never erres therein, unless interrupted or put by its scope through some transverse contingent, we would by no means admit of this Bloody course for a Cure; being sufficiently convinced, that this Solar Balsom the pure Blood . . . the subject and material foundation of Life, is never exterminated or cast out of the Body by Nature, unless extimulated[15] through some exasperating and hostile matter that is gotten into it.

---

[14] Prevalent with evil intent.
[15] Provoked; incited.

[. . .]

Away then with this detestable lavish Phlebotomy, that hath destroyed more than Tobacco or the Sword together, may it be banished the Court, City, and Countrey, nor ever be depended upon hereafter in this Island, or any of His Majesties Territories, for the cure of any difficult Disease; but let it be confined and inflicted as a feral Plague upon all those that delight in Blood, and hate our Gracious Sovereign, and all his loyal Subjects.

[. . .]

Never was there a more *just, honest, desireable*, and *useful* Enterprise set upon in this Nation, then an endeavour of some Chymists to purchase an Influence and favourable Countenance from our *Sovereign Lord the King*, that thereby we might be authorized and encouraged to meet together, and consult (without interruption) about some expedite and effectual way, for the regulating and reforming those present enormous Abuses in this excellent *Spagyrick Science*; and for the prevention of the same for the future; and that we might joyn our forces for the meliorating, and advancing of that Art, which in despite of all Adversaries, will in some short time manifest it self to be Queen Regent in Physick. Moreover, seldom hath there been any Design more generally countenanced and animated by the learned Nobility, and ingenious Gentry of *England*, then this.

But such hath been our fate, that some malevolent ill-disposed persons (as well from within as from without) have both maliciously and ignorantly cast such rubs in our way, that we have been disappointed from attaining that end, for which his Gracious Majesty hath professed to have no small kindeness.

That therefore every *Inquisitive* man may in part receive some satisfaction, what hitherto hath obstructed our business, we certifie him, that some of us have been overseen at first in admitting among us certain very illiterate persons, that were . . . mock Chymists, no whit exercised in *Anatomy* and *Botanicks*, inexpert in the History of Diseases, their *Efficient* and *Material* Cause, their *Event*, or any *Cure*, of which they could give any Philosophical reason: These have been among us . . . foul blots and disgraces, presumptious Boasters, heady and high-minded, intruding themselves to our disturbance; whereby our subtil supplanting enemies have taken advantage to defame us, representing us to the world a company of Fanaticks, falsly suggesting that we went about to tread under foot all Learning, and to introduce a meer Empirical way of Practice in Physick, with such blasting language, contrived on purpose to diminish our *Repute* and to disenable us from atchieving that which would prove so useful to the world; that they may the better establish their pretended *Polyarchical Government* in the *Galenical* way.

That these Aspersions therefore may be taken off, and no more reflect upon us to our prejudice, who profess our selves Philosophers by the Fire; we freely declare, that we are *Philomathêis*, hearty lovers and promoters of Learning, and shall never go about to derrogate from *Schools* and *Academies*, but shall vigorously defend them so far as truth will admit; and shall be ready to censure him that pleads for *Amathie*, or illiterature in the Body *Natural*, disposed (if ever opportunity be offered to him) to stand up for *Anarchie* in the Body *Politick*. And we are resolved upon mature thoughts, never to joyn with such, that (disclaiming against *Schollarship*) go about to lay the foundation of such an *Illustrious Art*, upon the sandy foundation of some wilde and extravagant Notions, that they have picked up by chance. . . . For whosoever enters upon *Pyrotechnic*, ought to have beforehand some general knowledge in the Nature of things, and to acquire some infallible *Axioms* and *Theorems* delivered to him, by those that have been most expert; which how any one can attain to, without a competent knowledge in the Scholastick Languages, we are much to seek. And certainly *Helmont* never thought a *rude* and illiterate person destitute of any previous *Theory*, a fit Agent to aspire to the Mysteries of this profound Science.

5.6

Defending the status quo: William Johnson and the London College of Physicians (1665)

William Johnson, Α'γυρτο-Μα'ζιξ. Or, some brief animadversions
upon two late treatises . . . Galeno-pale . . . [and] . . . The poor
mans physitian (London, T. Mabb, 1665), pp. 6–8, 67–9.

William Johnson was appointed chemist, or laboratory assistant, to the College of Physicians in London some time in the late 1640s. Much of his time was spent in defending the College from the accusation that it was a haven of medical conservatism. Among others, he rebutted the claims of Noah Biggs (see previous extract) and Nicholas

Culpeper who characterised the College, and its members, as reactionary and disinterested in expanding medical services to the poor. He also published a plagiarised version of a well-known dictionary of Paracelsian terminology by Martin Ruland. His response to Thomson in 1665 was along much the same lines as his earlier apologias. Using measured language, he nonetheless hinted at the anti-intellectual, anti-social and radical intent of the Helmontians rather than addressing the deep-seated medical concerns raised by the College's opponents (including their departure from the city in droves during the plague).

Thus, the more plausibly to deceive all that are not capable of enquiring into the Mystery of their Trade, but yet may be apt enough to avoid them as Up-starts; they range themselves under the banner of *Vanhelmont*, whose Name having made a considerable noyse in the World, they think sufficient to silence such as should question their Knavery; but their ignorance does not a little appear in the very choice of their Patron, for had I been of their Council, I would have suggested to them a more Ancient and Stouter Champion, whom *Helmont* himself ownes, *Theophrastus Paracelsus*, who was the first, not that dissented from *Galen*, but that made any considerable improvement in Chymistry; for it is not to be questioned, but that He and *Vanhelmont* through their ingenious labour in the fire, made discovery of many Rare and Excellent Medicines; but neither of them buried *Galen* in the ashes, wholly laying aside, as these men would have the World believe, his sober Rules and Prescriptions; and this ingenuity of theirs hath been abundantly requited by that Esteem, which hath been paid them by most learned Physitians since their time, but especially those now of the Colledge, (who for many years last past in all the Universities of *Europe* have carried the vogue).

[. . .]

Let any Judicious man but look back, and compare the practise of our Worthy Physitians for Twenty Years last past, with the preceding times, and he must confess Chymistry, and its Improvement has been their great care, and constant study; that pitch, to which this Noble Art is now advanc't, is ow'd to them, and if it ascend yet higher, the same hands must lend their assistance. . . .

[. . .]

'Tis Evident, and something I have said before to the same purpose, but here I must repeat it, that the beginning and rise of Fame to Paracelsian or Hermetical Physick proceeded from some particular Physitians of the Colledge; whil'st the Quacks and Mountebanks of these times, as they never are wanting in that case, impudently assume to themselves, the repute of those beginnings, and from time to time, have continued the same cheat; So that, whenever any Chymical Medicine by the practise of the Colledge began to get Credit, the Empiricks lying at the catch, have made it their business, either really to steal the Receipt, or, which is all one for their Design, to counterfeit the Medicine; and then in their Bills posted in every Corner of the Streets, they confidently impose upon the World a false Affirmation, which is, that by their great Travels, and long Study they have produced these Excellent Secrets for the benefit of their Country. Thus by such shifts, they have all along crept into the Opinion of the Common People, in whose Inclination ther's never wanting a readiness to joyn with irregularity, rather than to adhere to any thing, that carries the face of Order and Authority.

Notwithstanding these subtil insinuations, they could never have gotten such a Repute in the World, but that they Politickly made an advantage of the Factious Principles then abounding in the Common People of our late Unruly times, when the Common Interest was to be carried on by crying down Humane Learning; then these Illiterate Fellows spit in the face of all the Liberal Arts and Sciences. And, as at that time, in point of Divinity, the Fanaticks of that Faction bawling against Learning, as Idolatrous, and Superstitious, yet to delude the World, and better to carry on their Design, made use of necessitated persons, that were Scholars, and of Jesuites[16] too, who (though for another End and Interest) were ready to be transformed into the shape and habit of Coblers, or any other mean Mechanicks, pretending hereby they Preached by the Spirit. The same Tricks and Devices have been continually used by our Fanaticks in Physick, who as well knew the current of those Times, did run in opposition to all Just Authority: But they will find their case to be different, and the modesty of those Discreet Men rewarded, who chose rather to let such snarling Whifflers go on, as things inconsiderable, then appear contentious with such, who by their own growing Enormities (now Justice is in the hand of the Proper Legislator) will prove their own Destruction.

---

[16] The Jesuits, or Society of Jesus, were widely blamed in Protestant England for every major calamity to befall the country including the Great Fire of 1666.

Part six

Policies of health:
diseases, poverty and hospitals

6.1
Fighting the plague in
seventeenth-century Italy

Carlo M. Cipolla, *Fighting the Plague in Seventeenth-Century Italy* (Madison, Wisconsin and London, University of Wisconsin Press, 1981), pp. 51–64.

Carlo Cipolla was one of the major social and economic historians of early modern Europe. In this short extract, he describes how the magistrates of Pistoia, near Florence, set out to combat the plague in 1630–31 when it struck the region. A distinctive feature of the response of the Italian city-states, from the 14th century, was the use of quarantine and a highly organised administrative system and personnel. However, as the dispatches of the physician placed in charge of the lazarettos suggests, the measures adopted were always likely to prove insufficient in the face of a major outbreak.

Unlike Florence and Leghorn, Pistoia did not have a permanent health board. Thus, about the middle of April 1630, when horrible news kept flowing in about the ravages caused by the plague in northern Italy, the General Council of the city appointed six gentlemen to the position of Health Deputies. Understandably, the first measure taken by the newly appointed Deputies was the creation of a sanitary cordon around the city: guards were stationed at the gates and restrictions were placed on the movements of people and merchandise. Toward the end of April the Health Deputies of Pistoia received an ordinance issued by the Central Health Magistracy in Florence, in which the Florentine authority recommended that, as a preventive measure, all cities of the Grand Duchy keep their streets as clean as possible. That was wise, and the Deputies of Pistoia acted accordingly.

The instructions and advice from the Florentine Magistracy were both numerous and continuous and covered much ground. But the Health Deputies of Pistoia did not want to risk overlooking any measure that could be of some use, and thus on April 30 they consulted with four of the five local physicians. . . . All that the physicians could recommend was a prohibition on silkworms and on the production of raw silk within the city. Silkworms produced foul odors, and since the doctors thought miasmas were the cause of the plague, it is not surprising that they regarded silkworms with suspicion. . . .

In the course of time the Health Deputies took other drastic measures. On July 19, on the advice of the local physicians, they resolved that no sick person would be admitted into the city unless he had previously been seen by one of the local doctors. On July 28, they expelled all foreigners, mountebanks, and Jews from the city, and on September 4 they renewed the ban on 'all those foreigners who are not subjects of the Grand Duke, with the exception of those who have home and family [in Pistoia].' The idea was to relieve the crowded conditions within the city walls. At the end of July the Deputies refused to extend the annual livestock fair which was then taking place in Pistoia, and on August 16 they closed the city 'to all beggars and all poor people afflicted with any kind of disease.'

The Deputies were not lacking in diligence. On August 23 they resolved 'that each one of them would go and visit the houses of Pistoia, especially the houses of the poor; and in the case they uncovered filth or anything whatsoever offensive to cleanliness, they would be empowered to have the filth removed and to instruct the inhabitants to keep their homes as clean as possible. Moreover, if they were to find rotten wine, they could dispose of it.' . . . In the same vein, on September 4, the Deputies decided to discuss with the Bishop the possibility of having the fonts in the churches emptied of holy water for fear that it too could spread the contagion.

[. . . On] September 10, all movements of people and merchandise to and from Florence were absolutely prohibited. However, weighty economic interests stood in the way of the public health requirements. Pistoia and its territory were one of the main suppliers of wine to Florence, and at the time of the grape harvest it was customary to bring the old wine to Florence in order to make room for the new wine in the cellars of Pistoia. The prohibition of September 10 had to be temporarily suspended only a few days after it had been decreed; the gates were temporarily reopened and people of all extraction swarmed back and forth between Pistoia and Florence.

The Health Deputies grew increasingly nervous. They sensed that the circle was closing. On September 12 they wrote to the Grand Duke that 'so far Pistoia and the surrounding countryside have enjoyed perfect health,' but considering the general situation, they felt they had to take 'stronger preventive measures, proportionate to the current perils.' They estimated that public health expenditures would cost the city administration some 1000 scudi a month, and they therefore requested the authorization to borrow 9500 scudi in case of need. . . .

On September 19, the plague was identified in nearby Prato. The circle continued to close, and the Health Deputies of Pistoia prepared for the worst. On the twenty-seventh they set up a pesthouse in a building two miles outside the city gates, on the road to Lucca, and they appointed Dr. Stefano Arrighi, physician, and Master Francesco Magni, surgeon, to serve there. The two men were instructed to set up residence outside the walls of the city. The physician would receive a salary of 10 lire a day – that is, 43 scudi a month – while the surgeon would receive 15 scudi a month – that is, approximately one-third the physician's fee. Additional compensation was granted to both men for the use of a horse.

Then the circle closed. On the eighth of October the plague was reported in one house in Pistoia, and two days later another house was declared infected.

The Health Deputies were not medical men. They were administrators, and the proper and efficient use of the funds available was one of their main concerns. On the same day that the first case of plague was uncovered in Pistoia, they resolved to deposit all their present and future funds with the Rospigliosi Bank of Pistoia, and they agreed that all expenditures by the health board would have to be made not in cash but through the bank on the orders of at least two of the Deputies. Two days later, in order to provide for the urgent expenditures which would not suffer any delay, and at the same time to maintain constant and prompt information on the financial situation, the Deputies appointed a *Provveditore* (general manager) in the person of Nofri Nencini.

[. . .]

[T]he local Deputies were supervised by a General Commissioner, the Marquis Cavalier Luigi Vettori, who had been sent to Pistoia from Florence. Judging by his correspondence, Signor Vettori was an unusually diligent and meticulous man. Toward the end of the epidemic which struck the territory under his jurisdiction, he addressed a statistical report to the Health Magistracy in Florence which is admirable both for the information it contains and for the clear form in which it is presented. The Magistrates in Florence were impressed, and while thanking Signor Vettori for the report, they complimented him by recognizing that 'it was done as it should be – namely, with punctual precision.'

[. . .]

[A] lazaretto had been set up outside Pistoia on September 27. From the records of the health board we learn that a private house was first locked up in Pistoia on October 8, 1630. In all likelihood, the first patients arrived in the lazaretto on that same day. What they found – or better yet, did not find – is reported in a letter which Dr. Arrighi hastened to dispatch in alarm that very same day to the Health Deputies: 'Nothing we need is here; there are no bandages for bloodletting nor cloth for dressing tumors, and there are no attendants'.

That was just the beginning of the ordeals. By October 23, the Deputies were confronted with the fact that 'the number of patients at the lazaretto keeps growing to such an extent that there is no room in it for all of them.' Hard pressed, the Deputies hurriedly resolved to requisition 'all houses situated in the same block as the lazaretto, as well as the houses facing it'; they also resolved to order twelve more beds for the hospital, and to make provisions that patients who recovered be promptly dismissed and sent to a convalescent home in order to make room for new patients in the lazaretto. The resolutions were good, but the epidemic, though not particularly violent, kept running ahead of the Deputies. Whereas during the month of October, 31 patients were admitted to the pesthouse, in November the number rose to 141. On November 25, the Deputies resolved to look for another building to set up a second lazaretto. They were still searching when they received a dramatic message from Dr. Arrighi on December 1:

Here the sick continually increase in number, and medication is lacking. We have sent repeated requests to the *Provveditore* and to the Hospital del Ceppo for cupping glasses, black soap, *conconi*[1] for bloodletting, and other things, but nothing arrives, whence it follows that the disease undergoes little respite.

The general situation is very much affected by this, and the patients cannot be dismissed with the rapidity one would hope for.

Regarding linen and blankets: most of the beds are without sheets and have few blankets.

[1] Large bowls, made of terracotta, used in bloodletting.

143

> Regarding beds: the patients are five to a bed, to the detriment of the con-
> valescent who, because of close contact with contagion, suffer relapses.

The following day, December 2, the Deputies decided to turn to charity
and 'go around in the city and collect blankets, mattresses, linen
clothes, woolens, and other things to be used in the service of patients
and attendants in the pesthouse.' They also resolved that of the belong-
ings seized in the homes of the people who had died of plague, 'those
which were not burned ought to be sent to the pesthouses.' The measure was not an orthodox one, but scarcity left little room for orthodoxy.
While the growing number of patients created one set of problems for
the Deputies, the growing number of deaths created another. On
December 2, in addition to the other resolutions, the Deputies decided
to enlarge the cemetery next to the pesthouse, hire more gravediggers,
and buy more lime. . . . On December 12, Dr. Arrighi sent another dramatic message from the lazaretto:

> Twenty people, both men and women, are at the pesthouse waiting to go
> to the hospital at Capo di Strada [the convalescent home], but there are
> [new, clean] clothes for [only] six men and six women. I beg you to see to
> it that the rest of the clothes arrive so that they may all go to Capo di
> Strada.
>
> The number of patients in the pesthouse is increasing and there is no
> longer any place to put them, as they are lying four or five to a bed.
>
> We need vesicants[2] and oils, and the Hospital del Ceppo says they have no
> more. And we also need straps to tie down patients who go out of their
> minds. . . .

The Deputies were caught between the Devil and the deep blue sea. On
the one hand, with the epidemic rampant, they were worried that not all
infectious cases were being reported or detected or that not all persons
infected with the plague were being hospitalized. On the other hand,
they were alert to the crowded conditions at the lazaretto and were
worried that people suffering from ailments other than the plague
would be admitted to the pesthouse. On November 4, 1630, they notified
doctors, surgeons, and barbers that all medical men had 'to report *in
scriptis* [in writing] to the Chancellor [of the health board] all patients
whom they treat daily and declare the nature of their ailments.' On the
twenty-sixth of the same month, they resolved to hire a doctor and a
surgeon to visit all those in the city afflicted with suspicious ailments.

---

[2] Ointments or plasters used to raise blisters on the skin and thus provide an outlet for noxious humours.

Obviously, the Deputies were most anxious to detect all cases of infection and dispatch the infected and their contacts to the pesthouses. However, on December 6, they decreed that no sick person could be admitted to the pesthouse unless he had been seen by the lazaretto physician, Dr. Arrighi, who had to ascertain that the patient was actually suffering from the plague.

Dr. Stefano Arrighi was a young man of thirty years. He was the youngest among the five physicians living in Pistoia, a bachelor, and in normal times served as the community physician – all, undoubtedly, reasons why he was chosen for the dangerous and unenviable assignment of serving in the pesthouse. Judging from his correspondence, the young doctor was a compassionate and very dedicated man. In June 1631 he was still alive, and he wrote a report to the Health Deputies on the regimen and treatments he used for the patients in the pesthouse:

> These poor wretches come to the pesthouse when the disease is far advanced, whence follows that they are extremely weak in regard to both their vital and animal forces. Consequently, I consider it good to refrain from blood-letting and giving purgative medicine, but recommend rather that immediately and then every other day they be given an ordinary enema.
>
> Let them be fed with meals of good meat and eggs, withholding wine from them and giving them instead distilled spirit mixed with water.
>
> I recommend rubbings and cupping glasses morning and evening, and when spots show on the skin they should be scarified[3] for the first time.
>
> It should also be arranged that fragrant herbs sprinkled with vinegar be kept throughout the hospital. And above all great care should be paid to cleanliness and purity.

[3] Incised.

6.2

Plague and the poor in early modern England

Paul Slack, *The Impact of Plague in Tudor and Stuart England*
(London, Routledge & Kegan Paul, 1985), pp. 295–307.

Paul Slack is the author of numerous works on social welfare and
social policy in England in the two centuries after the Reformation. In
this extract, he discusses the reaction of the masses to the prohibitions which local and central government tried to impose on the
people in time of contagion, and he stresses the minor role played by
medical concerns in the attempt of the authorities to maintain law and
order during time of plague. Plague was first and foremost a social
issue, and measures to bring it, and those who contracted it, under
control formed part of a wider concern of the governing classes in
early modern England with the need to impose greater restrictions on
the freedoms of the poor and diseased.

Opportunities for mutual support and consolation were severely cur-
tailed by the restrictions which local and central governments tried to
impose on popular behaviour and popular assemblies during epidemics. . . .

Not everyone wanted to attend church [at such times] but secular
assemblies were also banned by authority. The feasts of companies
were stopped. So were feasts after mayoral elections, which often
extended beyond the oligarchy and were intended, as it was admitted in
Winchester, 'for the maintaining and preserving of love and unity among
the citizens and rejoicing one with another'. The postponement of the
Lord Mayor's Show and the celebration of James I's coronation in 1603
must have caused resentment in London. Prohibition of popular games
and efforts to close down alehouses, which frequently occurred during
a plague, were still more provocative, removing as they did the com-
monest convivial occasions which might have preserved some sem-
blance of normal social intercourse.

There was strong resistance. In Nottinghamshire men gathered
'unlawfully' to play football in the middle of an epidemic. In Winchester
crowds assembled for 'their habitual bullbaiting and other unlawful
exercises' in 1593. Restrictions on normal meetings in Norwich
inevitably led to 'unlawful assemblies' in the fields close to the town.
There was an obvious incompatibility here between policy and social

146

reality, just as there was when town councils closed down schools but tried at the same time to prevent children playing in the streets. There was also a bland refusal to comprehend popular mentality. Aldermen and councillors could not understand the men in York who met to drink at night 'in these heavisome times of the infection'; they fined them.

The interference of government was most deeply resented when it disturbed the customs surrounding death itself. . . . The enormous number of deaths during an epidemic produced orders which sought to alter established habits. Lack of room in the churchyard led one London vestry to forbid burials in coffins in 1593, although other local authorities insisted on this practice in order to avoid contagion. When graveyards were filled literally to overflowing, and the 'noisome stench' from them seemed an obvious cause of miasma, burials there could be stopped altogether. New burial grounds were hurriedly licensed in London, especially in 1665, sometimes without consecration. In the provinces, churchyards were sometimes guarded from contamination even more jealously: the churchwardens of Chelmsford stationed armed watchmen on the bridge to prevent corpses being brought from the suburb of Moulsham to their normal place of burial by the parish church. From the 1540s plague corpses had been refused entry to churches and carried straight to the grave; and the logical conclusion was reached in 1666, when the government's new plague orders forbade the burial of plague victims in ordinary churchyards altogether. . . .

Above all, the government imposed stringent restrictions on attendance at funerals. The national orders of 1578 prescribed the burial of the dead only at dusk, and suggested that ministers officiating should 'be distant from the danger of infection of the person dead, or of the company that shall bring the corpse to the grave'. By 1665 there were regulations in several towns shortening the knells which summoned people to funeral services, and limiting the number who might be present at funerals and burial dinners to the immediate family and a dozen or even fewer 'next neighbours'. There were similar controls on attendance at weddings, christenings and childbirths, but crowds at funerals were clearly thought to present the greatest public danger. In 1603 the city marshal of London, an official normally charged with the apprehension of vagrants, was told to keep the number of people present at plague burials down to six. He found it an impossible task. 'The meaner sort' continued to accompany the dead, and attacked the officers who tried to stop them. . . .

. . . Funeral ceremonies fulfilled important social functions and indispensable psychological ones. The elaborateness of a knell, the numbers present at a burial, and the lavishness of a funeral dinner, all marked the social status of the deceased and reconciled his friends and relations to his death. Attendance at funerals was also a public demonstration of communal defiance against plague. . . .

. . . In 1630 poor mourners were driven away by force: they returned and ignored the risk of infection. Eleven trumpeteers were thrown into Newgate[4] in 1636 for marching behind a colleague dead of the plague, 'with trumpets sounded and swords drawn'. In 1665 the Privy Council[5] was still doing everything in its power to stop neighbours and friends following coffins to burial, including having prohibitions read in every church. The comments of Pepys[6] and others about the 'madness of people of the town, who . . . come in crowds along with the dead corpses', show that the effort again failed utterly. On this point the new public-health policies had come into conflict with ingrained social habits and deeply respected moral obligations, and they had been defeated.

[. . .]

Popular behaviour could carry several meanings at once. The inmates of pesthouses in Worcester and Aylesbury who ripped up fences and gates and used them as fuel, simply needed something to keep them warm; but the women who burned down the pesthouse in Salisbury in 1627 and in Colchester in 1631 were engaged in a demonstration at once as direct and as complex as that of the rioters who demolished hedges in the sixteenth century and Dissenting meeting-houses in the eighteenth.[7] The Salisbury arsonist had been incarcerated in the pesthouse herself; in part she expressed the feelings of the inmates. She had other supporters too, however. The erection of the house had been opposed by a crowd of local residents, led by their landlord, Alderman Matthew Bee, who feared that infection would spread to them. Motives in the Colchester case were equally mixed. The pesthouse was burned down, before any epidemic had begun, by a woman who lived next-door; she was no doubt afraid of contagion when there were rumours that plague cases were to be sent there. But she had also been told that she would herself be shut up if the pesthouse was used, and she and her relatives

[4] A notorious prison in London.

[5] The permanent executive body of government in early modern England which consisted of the most senior officers of state, and the monarch who appointed them.

[6] The famous diarist Samuel Pepys (1633–1703) who, as a senior official in the Navy office, stayed in London throughout the plague of 1665–66 and observed its progress and decline.

[7] Hedges were attacked by the rural poor who saw the process of enclosure as a threat to their traditional way of life; after 1689, dissent from the Church of England was legally tolerated, but those who built their own chapels and places of worship remained the object of much popular hostility throughout the eighteenth century.

and neighbours protested against the injustice of this. In short, pest-houses were hated as symbols of plague as well as of plague-controls: to attack them was to attack infection and isolation at one and the same time.

This confused but powerful perception of oppression and menace animated the crowds who appeared in the streets of plague-stricken towns. It was not just pesthouses but the whole paraphernalia of public-health regulations which aroused popular antagonism. Every new form of government interference was opposed because it seemed allied to, and as threatening as, the disease itself. Just as Londoners forced their way past an Essex watchman who asked them for certificates of health in 1665, so Dutch sailors rioted in Plymouth and Yarmouth in 1635 when attempts were made to quarantine their ships. In Colchester in the plague of 1626, a crowd gathered in St John's Fields and one man said 'before the next fair there would be another course taken for watchmen'. He might have wished for another course for infection too, but his anger was transferred to a more manageable and better-defined target.

[. . .]

In the absence of help or encouragement from the top, respectable arti-sans and junior officials, those caught in the vital middle ground between magistrates and citizens, took the lead in disturbances. . . . [W]atchmen and constables [often helped] to undermine the regula-tions they were supposed to enforce. . . . The rank and file, however, were often women. A 'troop' of women supported Matthew Bee in Sal-isbury; the arsonists there and in Colchester were widows; and women were conspicuous in the crowds at London funerals. In 1630 the wives of two tailors in St Martin's Lane, Westminster, abused the justices and encouraged others to break out of their houses; two widows supported them. Two women – both of them dressed as men – led an unlawful assembly one night in Exeter in 1625.

Wives and widows were, of course, more deeply involved with the care of the sick and the support of their neighbours than men; and they may therefore have clung more tenaciously to those social habits and ideals which plague regulations threatened. For, as with food riots in which women also took a leading part, one element in plague distur-bances was the defence of traditional social norms and traditional neighbourly obligations, however inarticulately perceived. The five York men who were reported to the town council twice in a fortnight for visiting their sick friends showed their views by their actions. It was left to outside observers to put them into words: the poor thought it a

149

'matter of conscience' and a 'Christian' duty to visit their neighbours when they were infected. . . .

[. . .]

Central and local governors were preoccupied during epidemics with concepts, not of neighbourliness, but of 'order'. The word was constantly reiterated in documents concerning plague, in contexts which show that it carried two meanings: command and direction, on the one hand; tidiness, peace and quiet, on the other. The same word covered both because they were inseparable: one followed from the other. Thus the classic text of authority, the national plague *Orders* of 1578 and after, ended with a resounding condemnation of the fact that the queen's subjects had previously been left in 'very disorder . . . for lack of direction'. The London regulations of 1583 were endorsed: 'Orders to be set down of the Lord Mayor for repressing of disorders.' Thomas Lodge's treatise of 1603[8] expanded on the 'order and policy that ought to be held in a city during the plague time', while a proclamation of the same year asserted that plague had spread throughout the realm 'through lack of order' – in both senses.

[. . .]

[D]isorder and unruliness of all kinds were commonly conceived to be both physical and moral sources of disease. In Cranbrook [in Kent] in 1597 plague could be seen in a house 'out of which much thievery was committed', in the home of 'a pot companion and his wife noted much for incontinency',[9] and in inns and alehouses, 'places then of great misorder: so that God did seem to punish that himself which officers did neglect'. It was carried by 'lewd women' into York and Hitchin, and spread in a 'lawless alehouse' in Hampshire and Somerset. Preachers' association of plague with the 'sin of the suburbs' and of the poor, and their attacks on idle vagrants, drunkards, alehouses, plays and popular games, therefore supported magistrates whose public-health regulations included control of precisely the same people and assemblies. That was one reason why religious interpretations of plague were welcomed even by authorities who were anxious about their fatalistic

---

[8] The popular writer, Thomas Lodge (d. 1625), was the author of *A treatise of the plague* (London, E. White, 1603), a translation of a French work that had originally appeared forty years earlier. A well known figure in literary circles in Shakespeare's London, Lodge turned to the practice of medicine some time around 1596, proceeding M.D. at Avignon in 1600 and incorporated as an Oxford M.D. two years later. He had a highly successful and lucrative practice in London.

[9] Incontinency here refers here to a lack of sexual self-restraint, a common theme of early modern preachers.

implications. The quest for godly discipline could give powerful support to the administrative battle against plague. It is important to recognise also that the relationship worked the other way: the need to control plague could justify a whole programme of social and moral reform. The two imperatives were never separated. Public-health policies were part and parcel of a general drive towards greater social control.

The connection was closest in the minds of Puritan magistrates, for whom even attempts to limit funeral knells and funeral crowds during epidemics had a moral and theological purpose. The 'reformation' which [the Puritan magistrates] Sherfield and Ivie wished to push through in Salisbury after the plague of 1627 was paralleled elsewhere. The mayor of Plymouth wrote to his counterpart in Exeter in the same year, after both cities had been devastated by plague, expressing the hope that they might 'by reformation of ourselves and as far as in us lies of the people in both places, provide that the like or greater judgement may be prevented'. Robert Jenison similarly wanted to make Newcastle and other towns 'Cities of God' in order to avert his 'overflowing scourge of plague'. Less godly magistrates would not have used the same language. Yet they would have agreed with many of the practical implications of reformation. In London, for example, the threat of plague was used to justify the repression of brothels, taverns and poor tenements[10] which 'pestered' the suburbs with 'disorder and uncleanness'. Mayerne's treatise on plague[11] presented to Charles I in 1631 began with the premise that 'order is the life and soul of all things'; and it made it clear that plague was a threat brought by 'unprofitable and wasteful' vagrants, by 'idle and naughty' assemblies and alehouses, in short by the 'unruly, base sort of people'. . . .

These reactions were not confined to magistrates: they were the property of many of the polite and respectable who felt themselves threatened by infection. If the poor did not derive an aggressive consciousness of social divisions from the differential incidence of plague, the rich certainly did. It was from them that outbursts of what might reasonably be described as class prejudice came. Some of the citizens of Oxford complained in 1603 that the increase of plague was due to 'the most lewd and dissolute behaviour of some base and unruly inhabi-

---

[10] The erection of unlicensed buildings or tenements, poorly built and overcrowded, was a constant cause of complaint in early modern London.

[11] Sir Theodore Mayerne (d. 1655) was a Huguenot who became physician to James I (1603–25) in 1611, and subsequently to his son, Charles I (1625–49). The treatise referred to here was in fact a report which Mayerne submitted to Charles' government in 1631. It is particularly interesting since it contains one of the first references to the idea, subsequently proved correct, that the plague was carried by rats.

tants'. Twenty householders in Chester had thought the same thirty years earlier. A tavern and a bowling alley were sources of infection offensive to 'many better minded neighbours' in Westminster; so were 'divers poor nasty people' who should be moved 'out of their hovels to the sheds, there to air their bedding as also themselves'. By 1665 it was axiomatic that the poor should be blamed for a disease which was demonstrably not socially random. If it spread beyond them it was due to the 'carelessness of the common sort of people' and 'the incorrigible licence of multitudes'. . . .

Justices of the peace could not have ignored this combination of empirical observation and social prejudice, even if they had wanted to. Like the aldermen of Norwich in 1603, they had to listen when the 'better sort of people' were 'much grieved and offended that the under sort would not be stayed nor by the magistrates restrained'. Their response was the public-health programme [which] marched forward in step with the poor law. Its recipes – pesthouses and household support – were akin to the workhouses and outdoor relief prescribed for the idle and impotent. The Act of 1604 treated the disorderly sick as vagrants, and one of the first charges on municipal finances during an epidemic was often a whipping-post. . . .

This view of plague as part of the broader problems of poverty and disorder unquestionably strengthened the resolve of governors in the pursuit of novel policies. It helps to explain why they persisted with the isolation of households despite intellectual uncertainties, despite the financial and administrative costs it imposed, and despite the fact that in the end its critics alleged that the policy was ineffective, even perhaps counterproductive. It appealed because it was consistent with other endeavours which brought greater government interference in everyday life and sought control through order and rule. By the beginning of the seventeenth century plague was recognised as one element in that generalised threat which the rough 'poorer sort' presented to the respectable sections of English society; and the measures taken against it were primarily intended to defuse the danger. In a real sense, therefore, the effort to control infection was secondary. In adopting plague orders local magistrates were motivated by a less precisely focused but unshakeable conviction that social problems as a whole demanded firm treatment.

6.3

Medical advice in time of plague:
Stephen Bradwell (1636)

Stephen Bradwell, *Physick for the Sicknesse, Commonly called
the Plague* (London, Benjamin Fisher, 1636), pp. 5–11.

Stephen Bradwell (fl. 1630s) was the son of a London physician by the
same name and the grandson of the celebrated Elizabethan physician,
John Banister. In addition to *Physick for . . . the Plague*, he was the
author of *Helps for Suddain Accidents* (London, 1633), which pio-
neered the idea of the first aid guide. Like his father, he was frequently
in trouble with, and prosecuted by, the College of Physicians in
London and was thus not part of the capital's 'medical establishment'.
Here he discusses 'putrid' or physical plague which he contrasts with
'simple' plague – a disease that emanated directly from God and for
which there was no cure.

This *Putrid Plague*, is . . . *venemous*, which is granted of all both Physitians and Philosophers. Now by *Venom* or *Poyson*, we commonly
understand some thing that has in it some dangerous subtle quality that
is able to corrupt the substance of a living body to the destruction or
hazard of the life thereof. This working is apparent in this *Sicknesse*, by
his secret and insensible insinuation of himself into the *Vitall spirits*, to
which as soone as hee is gotten, he shewes himselfe a mortall enemy,
offering with suddaine violence to extinguish them. His subtle
entrance, his slye crueltie, his swift destroying; the unfaithfulnesse of
his *Crisis*, and the other *Prognostick signes*; and the vehemencie,
grievousnesse and ill behaviour of his *Symptomes*, all being manifest
proofes of his *venemous quality*. For in this Disease the *Seidge*,[12]
Urine, and *sweat*, have an abhominable savour, the breath is vile and
noysome: Ill coloured *Spots, Pustles, Blisters, swellings*, and *ulcers* full
of filthy matter arise in the outward parts of the Body: Such as no super-
fluitie or sharpnesse of Humors, nor any putrifaction of matter (without
a *venemous qualitie* joyned with it) can possibly produce.

But though it may thus by the Learned be acknowledged to be *Venemous*; yet it is by many of the *Ignorant* sort conceited not to be *Infectious*.

---

[12] Obsolete form of siege: excrement.

To satisfie such, I define *Infection* or *Contagion* to be *That which infecteth another with his owne qualitie by touching it, whether the medium of the touch be Corporeall or Spirituall, or an Airie Breath.* Of this there are divers *Diseases* that are *infectious*, though not so deadly as the *Plague*. As for Example, *Itch* and *Scabbinesse*, *Warts*, *Measels*, *small pox*, *the Veneriall Pox*; these by rubbing, and corporeall touches doe *infect*: Also *soare Eyes* doe by their *Spirituous beames infect* other eyes: And the *Pthisick* or putrified Lungs doe by their corrupt breath infect the lungs of others. But the Plague infects by all these wayes, and such sicke bodies infect the outward Aire, and that Aire again infects other Bodies. For there is a *Seminarie Tincture* full of a *venemous quality*, that being very thin and *spirituous* mixeth it selfe with the Aire, and piercing the pores of the *Body*, entreth with the same *Aire*, and mixeth it selfe with the *Humors* and *spirits* of the same Body also.

For proofe of this, we see by daily experience, that Garments, Coffers, nay walls of Chambers will a long time retaine any strong sent,[13] wherwith they have beene fumed. Now the *Sent* is meerly a *Qualitie*, and his *substance* is the *Aire*, which is also the *Vehiculum* wherein it is seated and conveighed. So does the *Pestilent Infection* take hold, though not sensibly (for the strongest Poysons have little taste or smell) yet certainly; as experience testifies: for *Garments*, and *Household-stuffe* have beene infected, and have infected others. As *Fracastorius*[14] tels of a *Furred-Gowne*, that was the death of 25. Men in *Verona*, *Anno* 1511. who one after another wore it, thinking still they had ayred it sufficiently. And if *Alexander Benedictus*[15] may be beleeved, *Feather-beds* will keepe the *Contagion* seaven yeares. Other experiences we have also of *live Poultry*, which being applyed to the *soares*, are taken away dead, having not been wounded, crushed, nor hurt any whit at all. And many that have beene Infected, have plainly perceived where, and of whom they tooke it.

But (say some) then why is not one infected as well as another? I have eaten of the same dish, drunke in the same cup, and lyen in the

---

[13] That is, scent.

[14] Girolamo Fracastoro or Hieronymus Fracastorus (1478–1553) was a Veronese physician and humanist and the author of *De contagione et contagiosis morbis curatione (On contagion and the cure of contagious diseases)* (1546) in which he proposed the novel argument that contagious diseases were transmitted by tiny spores or seeds that became attached to clothing.

[15] Alessandro Benedetti or Alexander Benedictus (1450–1512) was Professor of Practical Medicine and Anatomy at Padua from 1490, where he established an important centre for anatomical study. His complete works were first published at Basel in 1539.

same bed with such sicke ones, and that while their Soares were running: yet never had so much as my finger aking after it.

To this I answer, there may be Two speciall *Causes* for this. The first and Principall *Cause* is the *Protection of the Almighty*, which preserves some as miraculously as his *Iustice* strikes others. . . .

And secondly, every *pestilent Contagion* is not of the same nature, nor hath equall conformity with every *Constitution, Age*, or *manner of Living*: For some *Contagion* is apt to infect onely the *Sanguin complexion*, some the *Cholericke*, some the *Phlegmaticke* onely: Some *Children*, some *Youths*, some those of *Ripe age*, some *Antient people*; some the *Rich*, and other the *poore* onely. . . .

And first those are most apt to be *Infected*, that have *thin Bodyes* and *open pores*; and whose *hearts are* so *hot*, that they need much attraction of Aire to coole them.

Also, they whose *Veynes* and *Vessels*, are full of *grosse humors*, and corrupt juyces (the *venemous matter* being thicke, and therefore unapt to breath through the pores) their *putrefaction* is increased by the inward heat, and so driven to *malignitie*; and thence onward to a *Pestilent qualitie*. Hence those bodies that are moist and full of *Phlegmaticke* humors, whose veines are straight (and therefore apter to intercept then entertaine those well well [sic] concocted juyces that would make the purest Bloud) and the thicknesse of whose skin denies the transpiration of excrements: these are easily poluted and infected.

And such are *Women*, especially *women with childe*; for their bodies are full of excrementitious humors, and much heat withall, which is as oile and flame put together. Also *Virgins* that are ripe for marriage, are apt to receive infection, and being once stricken, seldome or never escape without great meanes. . . .

Also *young Children*, in regard of their soft, tender, and moist bodies; and likewise because they feed on moister meats, and feed with more appetite then judgment.

Likewise, the more *Pure and delicace Complexions*, whose bloud is finer and thinner then others, is so much the more apt to receive mutation: and the *Contagion* insinuates it selfe into all the humors; But first and most easily into *Bloud*; *Choler* next, more slowly into *Phlegme*, and most rarely into *Melancholy*.

[. . .]

On the other side *Gluttons* and *Drunkards* . . . can never be free from crudities and distemper'd bloud; which easily takes infection: As *Hippocrates* testifies, when he sayes: . . . Impure bodyes the more they are nourished the more they are endangered.

155

Poore people (by reason of their great want) living sluttishly, and feeding nastily and unwholsomly, on any food they can with least cost purchase, have corrupted bodyes, and of all others are therefore more subject to this *Sicknesse.*

6.4

Healing the poor: hospitals in Renaissance Florence

Katharine Park, 'Healing the Poor: Hospitals and Medical Assistance in Renaissance Florence' in Jonathan Barry and Colin Jones (eds), *Medicine and Charity Before the Welfare State* (London, Routledge, 1991), pp. 31–9.

In this important study of the hospitals of Renaissance Florence, Katharine Park aims to show that the old image of the medieval hospital as a place of last resort where the poor went to die is outmoded and erroneous. Using a range of archival evidence, she suggests, on the contrary, that the city authorities were increasingly concerned to provide the 'deserving poor', if acutely sick, with high quality medical care. In the process, she also refutes any suggestion that the early modern hospital was becoming an instrument of social control. Patients freely entered the hospitals of Renaissance Florence and more often than not were discharged after a short period in better health than when they entered.

By 1400 there were four [hospitals for the sick poor] in the city: Santa Maria Nuova (founded in 1289); San Paolo (thirteenth century); San Giovanni ... (1377); and San Matteo ... (1389). ... All were relatively large institutions: the last three had places for between fifty and seventy-five patients, while Santa Maria Nuova normally housed between two and three hundred. Unlike the leprosarium, they were not places for isolating or warehousing the sick; all four paid salaries to a professional medical staff that included physicians, surgeons and pharmacists. Santa Maria Nuova, for example, employed two (male) doctors in the fourteenth century, three in the early fifteenth, four in 1450, and ten in 1500. By 1376 it had a fully equipped pharmacy on the premises. The doctors were assisted by a resident staff of laymen (*servi*) or laywomen (*servae*), who had donated their possessions to the hospital, taking a vow of obedience and assuming the hospital's grey habit with its emblem of a red and green crutch. Both men and women acted as nurses in their respective wards, while the women also attended to the monumental task of cooking, cleaning, and laundering for the hospital's hundreds of dependants. In addition, several women – probably drawn from among the *servae* – were described as doctors (*medicae*).

The dramatic rise in the number of doctors employed by Santa Maria Nuova over the fourteenth and fifteenth centuries reflects less an increase in the number of its patients, which seems to have remained generally stable, than an elaboration of the medical services it offered. We can appreciate this change by comparing two documents: the hospital statute from 1374 and the statute sent to Henry VII of England shortly after 1500.[16] Although it referred to medical treatment in the hospital, the former concentrated on religious and moral prescriptions – sacraments, religious offices, duties of the priests, restrictions on male visits to the women's part of the hospital, and so forth. The latter, on the other hand, while still emphasizing these aspects of the hospital, also reveals a fully formed and highly developed system of health care. It describes the hospital as divided into two main wards, for men and women. The male ward alone housed a hundred double beds made up with mattresses, bolsters, pillows, linens and covers, and numbered to identify individual patients. The hospital employed a full-time pharmacist, with four apprentices, as well as a staff of ten doctors. The three most junior lived and worked in the hospital in return for room, board and clinical experience. They were supervised by six senior physicians, described as 'the most illustrious in the entire city', who came every morning to examine the sick, listen to the reports of the nurses, and issue prescriptions for the care of each patient. Special classes of patients – including the mentally ill 'from physical causes', those with head wounds, and those with skin lesions – were isolated from the general wards and from each other. The last two groups were treated by a seventh senior doctor, a surgeon, who came to the hospital for two hours each morning and evening.

As the statute makes clear, the patients in Santa Maria Nuova, except when brought unconscious to the hospital, presented themselves voluntarily for admission and were discharged in the same way. During their stay in hospital they received free medical care in the form of food, drink and medications prepared especially for them and identified by

[16] Henry VII (1485–1509) requested the document because he wished to emulate its precepts in his foundation of the Savoy Hospital in London.

the omnipresent bed number. Furthermore, the hospital not only served the poor, although this was its primary mission, but also received sick pilgrims, as well as patients of higher status who could not be cared for at home, either because they were travelling or because they had chosen to enter the hospital as part of a religious vow. . . .These patients were lodged in eight individual bedrooms with a fireplace, toilet and sink.

[. . .]

In this way, Santa Maria Nuova increasingly functioned as a general medical resource for the entire Florentine community, defining its primary mission in specifically medical terms. In other words, whereas it had been founded to serve the poor, with special emphasis on the sick, by the early sixteenth century it was serving the sick, with special emphasis on the poor. In pursuit of this mission, it had developed close ties with the organized and licensed medical profession in Florence. The care it offered was supervised by physicians and surgeons drawn from the city's elite. . . . Furthermore, by the middle of the sixteenth century, the medical profession itself was beginning to use the hospital as a centre for medical training; the College of Doctors recommended that graduates in medicine from the universities of Pisa and Siena practise in the hospital before attempting their licensing examination and required those who failed to extend their clinical training. By the beginning of the seventeenth century, Santa Maria Nuova housed a full-fledged school of surgery, later expanded to include formal training in lithotomy, ophthalmology, and medical botany and pharmacy.

Like Santa Maria Nuova, the other three Florentine hospitals for the sick poor also developed over the course of the later fourteenth and fifteenth centuries a specialized medical organization that relied on the services of the medical profession. Just as important, they were apparently very selective in the patients they admitted, as is clear from 'the books of the sick' and the 'books of the dead' that survive in the archives of the hospitals of San Paolo and Santa Maria Nuova; these remarkable documents contain detailed information concerning hospital patients from the late fifteenth century on, including names, dates of admission and death or discharge, admission and bed numbers (in the case of male patients), and occasionally ages, occupations, and diagnoses. These data reveal a striking and consistent pattern. First, they testify to an unexpectedly low mortality. Over the decade between 1503 and 1512, for example, the average death-rate in Santa Maria Nuova was 10.5 per cent of the several thousand male patients received each year, and between 1518 and 1522 it averaged only 8.6 per cent. . . . Furthermore, the length of stay of the average male patient was unexpectedly short: about eight days for those who died in San Paolo and ten for those who left, and twenty-one days for those who died in Santa Maria Nuova. Among the dead males in both hospitals (and the sick in San Paolo), the great majority had been there twenty days or fewer.

These figures raise as many questions as they answer. Not all of the discharged patients can be regarded as cured; some were doubtless only improved or left the hospital for other reasons. None the less, the figures suggest that these hospitals functioned largely or exclusively as hospitals for the acutely rather than the chronically ill, and that the latter were excluded in the course of the diagnostic examination that according to the statutes preceded each admission. . . . This does not mean that the hospital accepted only mild or curable cases. The books of the dead contain many references to patients who were carried in without signs of life . . ., expired under examination before even being assigned to a bed, or died during their first day in hospital. But it does imply that hospital administrators had made a conscious decision to concentrate their beds and their resources on patients who could be expected to die or recover in short order, making room for yet other sick poor.

This hypothesis is confirmed by what information we possess about the patients' illnesses. These were rarely noted in admissions and death records, with the exception of a single year, 1567-8, in which the infirmarer[17] of San Paolo recorded diagnoses for nearly all the male patients admitted to his ward. During that time, the majority (220 out of almost 400 for whom diagnoses survive) had fevers of various sorts, 'fever' being a common term for a number of acute infections. The next largest group (about sixty patients) complained of skin diseases, ulcers and boils. A further twenty-three were admitted for accidental injuries, wounds, fractures and bites, while at least fifteen suffered from syphilis. The illnesses of the rest were miscellaneous, including haemorrhoids, exhaustion, cataracts, dysentery, smallpox, typhus and constipation. Only very infrequently did the infirmarer indicate chronic conditions, such as phthisis,[18] old age and dropsy;[19] the sole exception was syphilis, which manifested itself in acute episodes. It is of course difficult to interpret these diagnostic categories and to identify in our terms the diseases to which they refer. It seems clear, however, that the vast majority of patients admitted to San Paolo in the mid-sixteenth century suffered from acute diseases or conditions.

[17] In medieval hospitals, the administrator in charge of the infirmary.
[18] A wasting disease of the lungs.
[19] Accumulation of watery fluid in the body.

The policy seems to have been somewhat different for female patients, as far as it is possible to judge from the erratic and rudimentary women's records of Santa Maria Nuova. The female ward had seventy beds, compared to the hundred in the male ward. Correspondingly fewer women seem to have been admitted, and their death-rate appears to have been somewhat higher. Furthermore, the women who died in the hospital seem to have had a longer average length of stay – fifty-three days in 1518–19, as opposed to twenty-one for the men – and although the majority of them, like the men, left quickly, a significantly greater proportion stayed for periods of several months or, in a few cases, several years. This suggests that the women's ward was far more crowded than the men's, and that the women's hospital may have had a somewhat different policy concerning admissions. Women were disproportionately represented among the city's aged; the municipal books of the dead record twice as many women dying of old age as men. The plight of Florence's many poor widows, together with the general Florentine fixation on women as particularly deserving objects of charity . . . may have pressed the female wards to loosen their admissions criteria and to receive a larger number of women who were old, disabled or chronically ill.

None the less, the figures for both men and women in general belie the notion that all early hospitals were warehouses for old and terminally ill people or focuses of unchecked infection, places from which few returned alive; as the records show, people entered them voluntarily, expecting to get better, and their expectations were usually fulfilled. The effectiveness of the hospitals for the sick arose in large part from their admissions procedures, but it also reflected the nature of their therapeutics. Many acute illnesses are self-limiting and respond well to warmth, rest, nourishing food and simple surgical procedures. These were in fact the treatments of choice in this period, inside the hospitals and outside them. The distinction between care and cure did not exist in Renaissance medicine. Physicians shunned aggressive intervention, which they saw as dangerous to both patient and professional reputation, opting instead for conservative and supportive therapy.

[. . .]

In Renaissance Florence, therefore, the sick poor were not in general targets for isolation and confinement, except to some extent in the special case of plague, and the public and private forms of medical assistance available to them did not have that end in mind. There is no evidence that the communal surgeon acted as an agent of state surveillance . . . or the hospital for the sick as an instrument of 'repression' or 'segregation'. In addition to being genuine expressions of Christian charity, these institutions were certainly tools of social policy, but the problem they aimed to solve was the chronic shortage of labour and rise in wages caused by recurrent epidemics of plague. Their principal intention, visible in clearest form in the choice of public doctors, was to offer free medical treatment of the highest quality possible to a well-defined sub-group of the Florentine poor: productive workers suffering from acute and treatable illnesses such as fractures, eye infections, hernias, fevers and skin diseases. Their goal, far from being one of confinement, was to cure these workers and return them to the labour force in the shortest time possible – a goal doubtless shared by the patients themselves.

6.5
Caring for the sick poor:
St Bartholomew's Hospital, London (1653)

Minutes of the Meeting of the Board of Governors for
St Bartholomew's Hospital, London, 3 January 1653;
St Bartholomew's Hospital Archives, Ha 1/5
[Minute Book, 1647–65], fols 88v–89r.

The governors of St Bartholomew's Hospital were responsible for oversight of the day-to-day administration of the hospital. By virtue of the charter of 1547, the hospital was refounded and placed under the control of the city of London. Originally, twelve unpaid governors officiated, many of them drawn from the highest ranks of city government (the most senior governor was often the Lord Mayor). However, by the middle of the seventeenth century, their number had expanded and included many who had made generous donations to the hospital. Nonetheless, the number actively engaged in the routine of governors' meetings was probably small and limited to those with a special interest in the smooth running of the hospital.

The extract cited here dates from a meeting held on 3 January 1653. This was a politically significant moment in the life of the hospital as it, like all other aspects of life in England following the execution of Charles I (1649) and the creation of a puritan republic, was deeply affected by these events. The puritan fixation with godly reformation is reflected in the high moral tone of the governors' edict.

It being this day informed that the Patients of this hosp[ita]ll which have their dyet allowed unto them in money, come thereby to have their sores and deseases inlarged and their Cures retarded by their ill disposing thereof, some mispending it at Alehowses to the disordering of theire bodyes, and after it is spent are forced to begg to the Great dishonnor of this howse, others bestowing their allowance upon Trash and such things w[hi]ch is worse, and more unwholesome for them than the howse dyett, And others having their money allowance doe out of a covetous disposicon abridge themselves of those things which are necessary and fitt for them, Because they would save their money, though it bee to the impaireing of their healthes and prolonging of their Cures, upon the Consideracone aforesaid and to prevent the like for the future it is thought fit and ordered That noe Patient whatsoev[e]r shalbee p[e]rmitted to receive any dyet money But shalbee satisfied with the howse allowance in victualls Except such of the Doctors Patients as are ffevourish or otherwise diseased soe as they cannot eat the howse allowance without preiudice to their Cures. And alsoe such of the Chirurgions Patients as are dismembred. And it is further ordered That such such [sic] sick p[er]sons shall not dispose their moneyes themselves But shall receave Brothes[,] Cawdells[20] or other things suitable and fit for their Condicon from the Sister of such ward they are in, who is hereby appointed from tyme to tyme to provide the same. And the dyet money of such Patients as are thought fit to bee allowed itt; whether they have the halfe or whole dyett, shalbee paid by the steward to the sister for dischargeing her disbursements in p[ro]videing p[ro]visions as aforesaid.

---

[20] A thin gruel, mixed with wine or ale, and sweetened and spiced, which was frequently given to sick people.

6.6

The establishment of the county hospital at Winchester (1736)

'An Account of the Establishment of the County Hospital at
Winchester' in John Woodward, *To Do the Sick No Harm:
A Study of the British Voluntary Hospital System to 1875*
(London and Boston, Routledge & Kegan Paul, 1974),
appendix 2, pp. 149–52.

During the course of the eighteenth century, numerous new voluntary hospitals were founded throughout England. These were based on popular subscription, the largest donors being granted the right and privilege to present poorer patients to the hospital for admission. Winchester was one of the first of these new provincial hospitals and was the brain-child of Alured Clarke (1696–1742), a prominent Whig churchman, who drew up its rules and raison d'être (below). Immediately prior to his death in 1741, he was made dean of Exeter and was responsible for the foundation of the Devon and Exeter Hospital, which was modelled on Winchester.

1. It is the only certain way of relieving the Poor-Sick; who are frequently neglected and over-looked at their own Homes; because Physicians and Surgeons can neither give their attendance, nor dispense their Medicines with any convenience at more places than One, and because their concerns are of too private a nature to engage the attention of any but the very Few Who make it their business to inquire after Them.
2. It is the most safe and eligible manner of doing it; because the care and neatness, as well as the simplicity and regularity of Diet, with which the Poor are kept in an Hospital, do all contribute much sooner to their Recovery, than their own way of living; and are often more effectual than Physic in the Cure of Several of the most inveterate Distempers.
3. The Expence of relieving a great number of Sick Persons in an Hospital, bears no proportion to that of assisting them at their separate Homes: And the Widow's Mite entrusted with Those who can dispose of it to the utmost advantage, will go farther towards answering the Ends of Charity, than a Sum of Money bestowed at random

on such as are incompetent judges of the use of it, or of the proper manner of laying it out.

4. It opens a Channel for private Charities which has been long wanted, and enables persons to lay them out to certain advantage; because Every One has it in his power from the moment he subscribes, to recommend a Patient, and by that means, may be assured, that his Bounty cannot be misapplied: Whereas almost all private Charities have hitherto been wasted, and rendered ineffectual thro' indolence, or want of knowing how to direct the expence; or by the various sorts of Mismanagement, which are in some measure unavoidable, and which are too well known, and too heavily felt, to need any particular explanation.

5. It is incapable of being so far abused or misapplied, as to make Any One repent of their Bounty; which will appear to Those Who consider that, tho' the greatest part of the income should really be perverted, there would still be more good done by it, than by a larger Sum in any other manner. For a thousand persons will be relieved here at a less expence, than would be required for an hundred in the ordinary way of giving Alms.

6. It is a Charity that is subject to no Imposture, but what must be discovered by the Physicians and Surgeons.

7. It prevents most of the Evils that are common to the Poor, by administring a present support in the time of Sickness; and does in some measure supply all their Wants more effectually than Money; for Money itself cannot provide that instant Relief which is here always at hand, and gives the Poor (in the case of Accidents, to which they are more subject) a considerable advantage over their Betters: The Supplies, that are immediately wanted, are here granted in kind without any delay. Advice and Medicines are to the Sick, what Food is to the Hungry, and Clothes to the Naked.

8. It provides for the relief and comfort of Multitudes who are unable to be at the expence of Advice or Physick, but are not distinguished by the name of The Poor, because They do not come under the care of a Parish or a Workhouse; and yet are the principal objects of this Charity, and most of all entitled to the regards of the Public; since They are in present want; and are of the diligent and industrious, that is, of the useful and valuable part of all Society.

9. It multiplies every Good that can be done to the Poor in any other way, by easing whole Families of the burden of attending and providing for their sick Relations; so that the Miserable are relieved and comforted, and their Families are at liberty to earn their own Support at the same time.

164

10. It preserves Them from the ill usage of ignorant Quacks and Impostors Who too often take advantage of their Necessities; and not only insensibly drain them of the little Money Them have under pretence of selling cheap Medicines; but frequently destroy their Health for want of Honesty or Skill.

11. It is of infinite Use to All Other persons as well as the Poor, by furnishing the Physicians and Surgeons with more experience in one Year, than They could have in ten without it.

12. It is a most certain means of increasing the number of the People; as well as of saving a multitude of Hands, who are often lost for want of timely assistance: And it deserves to be remembered, that a third part of what every labouring Man earns, is so much clear gains to the Public.

13. It encourages Parishes (when They are relieved of the great burden of supporting the Sick) to provide better for the maintenance of Orphans and Aged Persons. And it is certain, that the number of both these sorts must gradually decrease, by a provident care of the Sick; Who will be enabled for the most part to educate their Children, as well as to provide beforehand for their own Support against the Extremities of Old Age.

14. It reduces the number of Vagrants by depriving them of one of their most plausible Reasons for begging from door to door, under the specious pretence of sick Relations or Friends for whom They are concerned: So that they who are Idle and able to work, will be obliged to have recourse to some Employment, and make themselves serviceable Members of the Community, when they are not supplied in the usual manner from the public and private Charities, which are too often distributed without any due regard to the different Necessities of the Poor.

15. It must have the strongest tendency to promote a Spirit of Religion and Virtue amongst the Common People; which by degrees may recover them out of that profligate State of Life which is the general complaint of these Times, and of the utmost consequence to the Well-being of the whole Kingdom. The most certain method of recovering Men from their evil Courses, is to remove them out of the way of bad examples for so long a time as is necessary to beget contrary Habits. And it may be reasonably presumed that great numbers of the Poor will be insensibly reclaimed by the exact regularity of Manners, which is maintained in an Hospital as well as by the frequency of such Reflections as are naturally suggested in the House of Mourning. They are provided here with the use of the best Books, and have daily opportunities of being instructed by Those,

whose Duty it is to attend upon this very thing. And as an Hospital is supplied with Patients from all parts, it must needs be, that a Spirit of Religion and Gratitude will be gradually spread throughout a whole Country. For We can never hope to secure their Affections, soften their Passions, reform their Manners, and possess them with a sense of their Duty to God and Their Superiors so effectually as by this feeling way to Instruction.

16. It is the most comprehensive of all Charities; because there is scarce any One Species of doing good which is not promoted by it. For the Sick are visited and relieved; the Stranger is taken in; the Ignorant instructed; the Bad reclaimed; present Wants are supplied, and future ones prevented; and (by easing Families of the burden of supporting their sick Friends) it is also a Means of feeding the Hungry, clothing the Naked, cherishing the industrious Poor, and preserving a multitude of useful Members to the Public Etc. Etc.

These are the Benefits which without any shadow of doubt are peculiar to this Charity, and are of great consequence to All and Singular; to the Rich as well as the Poor; and to the public as well as the private Estate of Men. Any One of them should be sufficient to convince Us of its use, and All of them together must warm Men into proper resolutions of encouraging and supporting a Charity, which is the Glory of other Countries and has long been the Reproach of Our Own.

6.7

The medicalisation of the hospital in Enlightenment Edinburgh, 1750–1800: the case of Janet Williamson (1772)

Guenter B. Risse, *Mending Bodies, Saving Souls: A History of Hospitals* (Oxford, Oxford University Press, 1999), pp. 231–51.

The Edinburgh Royal Infirmary was founded in 1729, one of the first of many voluntary hospitals founded in Britain in the eighteenth century. Increasingly, during this period, the hospital became the site of clinical instruction. In the case of Edinburgh, its most famous exponent was William Cullen (1710–90), whose neurophysiological theories constitute one of the most important innovations in medicine in this period. After studying at Glasgow and Edinburgh, he rose through the ranks of the Scottish medical profession and was finally rewarded with a chair in medicine at Edinburgh University in 1766. During this period, he became well acquainted with all the leading figures of the Scottish Enlightenment and, through his own reputation, helped to establish the university as one of the most important centers of medical education in eighteenth-century Europe.

At the heart of Cullen's new medical theory lay the idea that the key to the functioning of the human body lay in the nervous system. He also set out to reclassify diseases according to new criteria based on his novel neurophysiological theories. Most infectious diseases were classified in the category of *Pyrexiae* or febrile diseases, which might assume various forms. One such was *synochus*, an inflammatory fever accompanied by delirium, which he diagnosed in the case of the patient, Janet Williamson, in 1772.

On Sunday morning, December 13, 1772, a young woman, Janet Williamson, came to the gates of the Royal Infirmary of Edinburgh 'desirous of accommodation in the house,' perhaps accompanied by a relative or neighbor. Tired, restless, and aching all over, she had been battling severe headaches and a fever for about a week. 'Fevers' were notorious, especially during Edinburgh's wet winters. Now Janet also felt an 'oppression' in her chest, in spite of the fact that someone had bled her three days earlier to ease the symptoms. Directed by the porter, she must have proceeded to the hospital's waiting room. . . . Why would a young woman such as Janet seek admission to the hospital, especially on the 'Scotch Sabbath?' . . .

Unlike other British voluntary establishments, the Infirmary admitted sick persons every day. Aged 19 and single, Janet Williamson was listed in the Infirmary's General Register of Patients as a servant. . . .

[. . .]

To screen applicants properly, the hospital needed to ascertain the 'deserving' nature of the poor who applied for admission. For this purpose, unless there was an emergency, the Infirmary required a letter of recommendation from known Edinburgh citizens or pastors from other Scottish parishes. . . .

For Janet and other potential patients, therefore, the first task was to find a current subscriber provided with valid letters, not always an easy proposition. Persons like Janet were usually lower-class individuals who had been judged by their superiors worthy of charitable support

167

because they demonstrated self-reliance and a willingness to work instead of being idle. . . . From a mercantilist standpoint, Janet was considered an investment, because of illness now in need of assistance lest she slide into total poverty, degradation, and thus become another burden to society. Her employers among Edinburgh's middle and upper classes were expected to provide the necessary help for ensuring Janet's recovery so that she could return to be a productive worker in her community.

[. . .]

Janet's sponsor could not be identified in the General Register – perhaps an omission by an overworked medical clerk. On the other hand, she may simply have carried a certificate attesting to her employment status if her master contributed regularly to the hospital's Servants' Fund. With the participation of Edinburgh's Presbytery, this special endowment had been created during the 1750s, and annual fund drives on 'Infirmary Sunday' kept the treasury alive. . . .

[. . .]

Back at the Admissions Room, Janet must have been interviewed after waiting patiently for some time. The hospital's physician-in-ordinary on call usually questioned newcomers before his noon rounds. By now, in medicalizing institutions such as the Edinburgh Infirmary, religious admission rituals had been replaced by bureaucratic and medical ones. Having successfully passed the social filter because of her status as a deserving servant, Janet now needed to pass the clinical test of eligibility. Her history was important for the physicians deciding whether she would be admitted. These encounters could be frustrating and deceptive, as prospective patients tried hard to tell doctors the 'right' stories about their sufferings to ensure admission. Physicians, in turn, were on the lookout for symptoms or signs that clearly marked particular diseases, and the applicants went out of their way to provide them. . . .

The clinical test thus served as a second important screening device to separate those who, in the eyes of the admitting professionals, would probably benefit from institutional care, as opposed to the hopelessly sick or those who feigned illness, who 'had been long accustomed to lodge in hospitals and expected to meet with good entertainment and to pass the winter with us'. For this purpose, the admitting physicians needed to determine whether the presumed ailment was 'proper', meaning not only that it was suitable for hospital management but also that, with adequate treatment, the patient had a good chance to recover.

This policy implied that, as a general rule, individuals suffering from acute, self-limited, and benign diseases were admitted. . . .

[. . .]

Perhaps unknown to Janet, her arrival coincided with an accelerated admission of fever cases to the Infirmary's teaching ward, open during the university's academic year from November 1 until April 30. The physician then in charge of this unit was William Cullen (1710–1790), professor of the theory of medicine at the University of Edinburgh. Perhaps the most accomplished and most famous English-speaking clinician of his time, Cullen was soon to assume the presidency of the local Royal College of Physicians. He not only managed the 24-bed teaching ward (divided into male and female sections), he was also responsible for a biweekly course of clinical lectures in which he discussed the clinical management of his cases. Since the subject of fevers was traditionally taught at the peak of its appearance during January, Cullen could often be found in the Admissions Room, personally interrogating potential teaching candidates and dictating his findings to a clerk. In December 1772, the word was out that the professor wanted more fever cases for his ward. Four women suffering from this condition had already been hospitalized, but Cullen always aimed at presenting a number of typical cases to his students. By meeting his pedagogical criteria, Janet became the fifth such person within three weeks admitted to the teaching ward.

After the interrogation was completed and the decision to admit Janet reached . . . [she] finally went up to the female teaching ward, a 12-bed chamber, 50 by 26 feet long and located in the west wing, now virtually a fever ward, where she would have been greeted by the other inmates. . . .

[. . .]

Janet Williamson was probably visited the day after her arrival by William Cullen. . . . Followed by a 'train' of assistant physicians and students, university professors such as Cullen made their entrance at a predetermined hour – usually noon – eagerly awaited or dreaded by the patients, who greeted the procession in silence. . . . Bodily postures and discharges, as well as the gross appearance of the tongue, were always checked and carefully noted [and] [b]odily functions such as pulse, respiration, appetite, digestion, motion, and excretion were also routinely recorded. At times, the patient's complaints prompted the use of special diagnostic tests, including urethral inspections with probes and catheters. Tubes were employed to check the throat and printed cards

169

to determine visual acuity. When appropriate, a description of sputum, feces, blood, and urine was appended to the clinical chart, relating the physical characteristics and quantities of such discharges.

... Janet had no appetite and was constipated; her skin was described as hot. Cullen counted her pulse with his famous hourglass – a fast 120 and full. ...

[. . .]

... Janet's clinical history and febrile symptoms suggested a diagnosis of synochus.[21] ... Cullen chose to begin a traditional 'antiphlogistic' (antifebrile) regimen consisting of a low diet, emetics, purgatives, and bloodletting to 'starve a fever'. For him and other attending physicians, dietary prescriptions constituted the first line of therapy. During daily rounds, detailed food instructions were issued, with orders for drugs and other procedures. ...

[. . .]

Besides receiving rest and regular food, Infirmary patients were subjected to treatments with physical methods and drugs. 'Nothing is more evident,' wrote Cullen, 'than that bloodletting is one of the most powerful mean of diminishing the activity of the whole body, especially of the sanguiferous system.' Indeed, the withdrawal of blood retained its importance in spite of the significant shifts in medical theory since ancient times. Cullen justified bloodletting because it could lessen the tension and spasms occurring in a febrile body. He had recast the traditional therapeutic strategies designed to restore humoral balances, with the focus now on adjusting bodily excitement through either nervous stimulation or sedation. Among the agents considered stimulants were meat, wine, exercise, fresh air, warm baths, and tonic drugs; the depressant regimen included rest, a vegetarian diet, bloodletting, purging, and antispasmodic and sedative medicines.

To the trained eye, the sudden removal of four to eight ounces of blood seemed indeed to improve several cardinal symptoms accompanying fevers. Pulse rates fell, body temperatures declined, pain sensations lessened, the reddish color of the skin paled, and the patients were overtaken by a feeling of relaxation, even faintness, and sleep. Although temporary, such physiological responses suggested to eighteenth-century practitioners that bloodletting was still a useful measure in all inflammatory states and the keystone of their antiphlogistic regimen. Thus, during her first two days in the infirmary, Janet

---

[21] A continuous or uninterrupted fever.

was bled eight ounces and also given a saline enema. Cullen also ordered ipecac powder,[22] his favorite fast-acting emetic, designed to cleanse the weak stomachs of all fever patients. In a sense, these were traditional measures that most individuals employed under similar circumstances at home. Janet's reaction went unrecorded.

When patients experienced a very high fever and were delirious, infirmary physicians often also ordered fomentations with flannel cloths dipped in hot water, believing that they produced a relaxing and soothing effect. In Janet's case, the nurse fomented her legs and feet hourly while she was delirious, not only to quiet her down but also to allow other patients in the teaching ward to get their night's rest. When her condition worsened, and she began complaining of chest pains and a persistent cough – both signs of a respiratory infection – an expectorant, a mucilaginous[23] mixture, was added to the regimen.

To complicate matters, the surgical clerk found it impossible to locate a good vein in Janet's arm or hands to draw the blood. Therefore, he was forced to obtain blood from a foot and recorded that her symptoms were somewhat relieved. . . .

[. . .]

Cullen ordered a second withdrawal of eight ounces of blood from his patient on the evening of her third day. The measure apparently provided more relief of Janet's symptoms. The emetic, too, was finally having an effect, making her throw up several times, as well as causing her to pass several stools. Janet's pulse was still around 120 but softer and regular. Night delirium and sweats continued. Fever patients were ordered to remove their soaked clothing periodically for washing, but if no additional shirts were available, they lay naked under the sheets. Concerned about her recent respiratory symptoms, Cullen now also ordered the creation of a blister on Janet's back between the shoulder blades, not however for the reason that humoral therapeutics suggested such a course, namely to remove harmful substances from the body. Rather, in Cullen's neurophysiological theory, blisters stimulated the body and nervous system and thus neutralized the action of fever-producing substances. . . .

[. . .]

On the sixth day of her hospitalization, Janet reached a critical stage in her illness, a subject traditionally debated by practitioners. The fever

[22] A drug made from the root of the ipecacuanha plant, native to South America, and widely used for its purgative and emetic properties.
[23] Viscous or gum-like.

seemed to abate and her cough was less frequent, but partial deafness was still a problem and the blister had failed to rise. For the first time, however, the patient was able to take some food. Cullen prescribed a powder of golden root or *virga aurea*, a bitter, astringent remedy designed to counteract systemic debility. To the delight of her attending physicians, she seemed to tolerate this bitter powder. Then, on December 22, Janet became quite nauseated, forcing Cullen to discontinue the medication without telling her that she was experiencing a side effect of the remedy. A day later, she was clearly on the mend, sleeping a good deal and free of delirium, with a lower pulse and more appetite.

At this point, Janet may have been switched to the Infirmary's middle diet consisting of cooked meat and vegetables. Fomentation of her feet and legs continued as did the administration of an expectorant mixture after her cough became more productive. Following Christmas Day, Janet slowly improved, her pulse now 80. However, part of her arm at the elbow had begun to hurt and swell, a feared complication of an earlier venesection attempt. . . .

[. . .]

Finally, on New Year's Eve, Janet's status was officially changed to that of a convalescent, and she was placed on a full diet.

Part seven

New models of the body, 1600–1800

7.1

William Harvey and the discovery of the circulation of the blood

Andrew Cunningham, 'William Harvey: The Discovery of the
Circulation of the Blood' in Roy Porter (ed.), *Man Masters
Nature: 25 Centuries of Science* (London, BBC Books, 1987),
pp. 68–76.

William Harvey (1578–1657) studied philosophy at Cambridge before
going to Padua, at the time one of the most important centres of medical learning in Europe, where he studied medicine and anatomy. On
his return to England he established a successful medical practice,
became a member of the London College of Physicians, and served as
physician to both James I (1603–25) and Charles I (1625–49). He is best
known for his anatomical investigations into the function of the heart,
which led him to discover the circulation of the blood. Here, the historian Andrew Cunningham challenges the traditional view of Harvey
as a pioneer of scientific modernity and suggests that we should seek
to understand him instead as an Aristotelian anatomist reviving an
ancient medical project.

In the midst of [his] very busy life as a practising doctor, Harvey did
something very unusual: he found time and space to undertake an enormous programme of research at his own expense. For fifty years,
mostly at home, and with no institutional support, Harvey passionately
and doggedly pursued anatomical research of the kind he had learnt

from Fabricius:[1] and when he began he was probably the only person in England to be doing anatomical research at all. One can see from this how impressed he must have been by that research programme. It was the Aristotelian programme of research into 'the animal', the only anatomical research tradition to which he had been fully exposed.

His teacher, Fabricius, had been the first person to revive, in its fullness, the Aristotelian form of research into 'the animal'; Harvey was the second. This is what made his work unique. For he thus had a different set of questions and a different viewpoint from all his contemporary anatomists. And it is this which was to lead him, unexpectedly, to discover the circulation of the blood. But the topics on which he began research in the early 1600s were not concerned with the blood, let alone its movement. They were the same as or similar to those of Aristotle and Fabricius: the generation of animals; respiration; the local motion of animals. One of his topics, however, was on the central organ of the body. It was, in Harvey's own words, on 'the motion, pulse, action, use and utilities of the heart and arteries'. Why should Harvey have chosen such a project? He later wrote that he was actually willing to publish on this topic because when Fabricius 'learnedly and accurately delineated . . . each part almost of animals, he left only the heart unattempted'; yet his reason for choosing it in the first place lay in the fact that it was a typically Aristotelian object of inquiry: according to Aristotle's characterisation of the animal body, the heart was the most important organ. As Harvey later put it, 'the heart of animals is the foundation of life, the ruler of each of them, of the microcosm it is the sun from which all *vegetatio* derives, all vigour and strength emanates'. '*Vegetatio*' means the growth, maintenance and reproduction of the animal (i.e. everything except sensation, motion and thought): it refers to all those aspects of life which animals have in common with plants. Indeed, the true object of all Harvey's anatomical inquiries here, as it had been of Aristotle's and Fabricius' before him, is the agency controlling this aspect of the life of the animal: what they all referred to as 'the vegetative soul'. In this sense the heart is the centre, source, principle, and origin of the life of the animal, and that is why Harvey set out to study it and its vessels.

[. . .]

[W]hat he was investigating was not 'man' but 'the animal'. That is to say, the account he was trying to give of what the heart is for – what role it plays in the life of 'the animal', and why it is necessary for that life –

---

[1] For Harvey's teacher, Hieronymus Fabricius (Girolamo Fabrizi d'Acquapendente), Professor of Anatomy at Padua from 1565 to 1613, see above extract 3.6.

174

had to be true of *all* hearts in *all* animals. It had to be true of hearts which have fewer chambers than the human one; it had to be true of the hearts of animals with cold blood as well as those with warm. Most important of all . . . it had to be true of the hearts of animals without a lung as well as those with. But, as Harvey found very early on in his research, 'whatever earlier people have said about systole and diastole[2] – about the [alternating] motion of the heart and arteries – all these things they have related while eyeing the lung!' Harvey, however, was going to look at the heart and arteries *without* considering the lung. He had a novel object of study: it is the heart (the whole of it) plus the arteries. No-one since Aristotle had investigated this particular set of things.

Thus at the very moment that he took up this set of organs to explore, Harvey was out on his own. His only predecessors in such inquiry were Aristotle and Fabricius, and eventually he was reduced to criticising even them. . . .

[. . .]

It is not currently possible to reconstruct the precise sequence of experiments which led Harvey to discover the circulation of the blood, for the book he published in 1628 about the discovery was a carefully worked-out argument, not a laboratory notebook. He called his book *An Anatomical Exercise on the Motion of the Heart and Blood in Animals*, and wrote and published it in Latin. But we can listen here to the breathless way he describes the moment when it occurred to him that the blood circulated. Harvey has been arguing that the blood must pass from the right side of the heart to the left via the lungs (the so-called 'lesser' circulation):

> Truly when I had often and seriously considered with myself and long turned over in my mind how great the quantity of blood was – evident partly from the dissection of living animals for experiment's sake, and from the opening up of blood-vessels and from many ways of investigating, partly from the symmetry and magnitude of the ventricles of the heart and of the vessels which go into it and out from it . . . partly from the beautiful and careful construction of the valves and fibres, and from the rest of the fabric of the heart, and likewise from many other things – viz., the abundance of blood passed through was so great, and the transmission was done in so short a time, that I realised that the fluid from the ingested food could not supply it: and indeed that we should have the veins empty, quite exhausted, and the arteries on the other hand burst with too much intrusion of blood, unless the blood did pass back again by some way out of the arteries into the veins, and return to the right ventricle of the heart.

[2] The expansion and contraction of the heart.

> I began to think myself whether it had a sort of motion as if in a circle, which afterwards I found to be true, and that the blood was thrust forth and driven out from the heart through the arteries into the flesh of the body and all the parts, by the beating of the left ventricle of the heart . . . and that it returns through the veins into the vena cava, and to the right ear of the heart . . .

What settled it all for Harvey, it seems, was the presence of little 'doors' (membranous flaps) in the veins: such things do not occur in the arteries, so what purpose could there be for them in the veins? Fabricius had actually discovered these 'little doors',[3] but had thought their purpose was to slow the outward flow of the nutritive blood. Faced with his new dilemma about the route of blood, Harvey investigated them anew and discovered that they allowed only one-way flow – that they were *valves*. Their role had to be to prevent the blood, returning through the veins to the heart, from slipping back.

   Thus did Harvey discover the circulation of the blood. But he had not been trying to discover whether the blood circulated, nor had he initially even been trying to confirm a hunch that it circulated. Harvey was engaged in a quite different enterprise, with its own goals and purposes. This was one reason why the idea that blood circulated dawned on him only slowly and reluctantly. But there was another reason too. Harvey was a willing follower of Aristotle in his whole approach. Aristotle the philosopher and investigator of 'the animal', provided Harvey with his method, his logical tools, his topic, his goals. Indeed Harvey conducted his anatomy in a philosophical spirit: like a good philosopher he was looking for *causes*, trying to give accounts which explained why 'the things themselves' are as they are. The problem that arose from Harvey's devotion to Aristotle was that Harvey could not be totally happy with his new discovery, because he could not find out the most important thing about it: he could not discovery *why* – for what purpose – the blood circulated. For a philosophical anatomist, as Harvey was, this was the greatest disappointment: he had to settle for 'speculating' and 'likely reasons'.

[. . .]

Harvey's discovery of the circulation of the blood was an accidental by-product of his attempt to revive and reinstate in seventeenth-century England the anatomical enterprise that Aristotle had conducted in Athens twenty centuries before. This greatest of modern discoveries about the body was made by a man trying to do anatomy like an ancient

---

[3] See extract 3.6 above.

Greek philosopher. Only an Aristotelian anatomist could have thrown up the particular set of phenomena which required the hypothesis of the circulation of the blood to explain them: and only an Aristotelian anatomist did. . . .

All this may seem a bit strange. For we would instinctively expect this great discovery to have been a product of a deliberate attempt to release men's minds from their bondage to the teachings of the 'ancients', and in particular from the teachings of Aristotle. Given that this discovery was made in seventeenth-century England, we would also expect it to be associated with the 'mechanistic' way of thinking. . . . 'Mechanistic' explanations of natural phenomena are ones which seek to explain events primarily in terms of the motion of the smallest particles of inert matter: it is the approach of which we are the heirs, and which underlies our modern science. We are so imbued with this way of thinking, that the temptation is for us to reconstruct this discovery so that it accords with a mechanistic view, by (for instance) stressing the one instance of measurement that Harvey uses in his argument, and the analogy he makes between the action of the heart and that of a pump. And, because it seems so obvious to us that the blood circulates – it seems to us that it was a fact just waiting to be discovered – we would expect Harvey to have been the final person in a tradition of people *looking for* evidence and proof of the circulation. But all this would be wrong. For Harvey, the body did not act like a machine in any way: it was alive, and all its activities and functions were those of life. For him the beat of the heart was a vital, not a mechanical, phenomenon, and the blood itself was alive.

In his own day Harvey's approach, though only newly brought back into practice, was very old-fashioned. He looked to Aristotle as his primary authority, and had no time at all for such people of his own day as Descartes, who were promoting the 'mechanical philosophy'. Indeed, Harvey's anatomical practice was as old-fashioned as his politics. Throughout his life he was a loyal supporter of the monarchy, never wavering even in the darkest days of the Civil War and Commonwealth.[4] He dedicated his book announcing the discovery to the King, his patron and employer, Charles I. It was not just a matter of flattery that Harvey's opening words there describe the king in his kingdom as being like the heart in the body: 'Most serene King', he wrote, 'the heart of animals is the foundation of life, the ruler of each of them, of the microcosm. It is the sun from which all *vegetatio* derives, all vigour and strength

[4] The English Civil Wars of 1642–46 and 1648 saw the defeat of the royalist cause and the execution of Charles I in 1649. For the next eleven years, the Commonwealth of England was ruled as a republic until the restoration of Charles' eldest son, Charles II, in 1660.

emanates. The king is equally the foundation of his kingdoms, and of his own microcosm he is the sun, of the State he is the heart from which all power emanates, every favour originates'. It is clear that when, as a loyal Aristotelian, Harvey first chose to study the heart in the animal, he was also, as a loyal monarchist, choosing to study it as the king of the animal body.

7.2

The mechanical body: Descartes on digestion

René Descartes, *Treatise of Man*, ed. and trans. Thomas Steele Hall (Cambridge, Mass., Harvard University Press, 1972), pp. 5–8, 113.

René Descartes (1596–1650) is one of the seminal figures in early modern philosophy. Born in France, in 1629 he moved to the Netherlands where he lived for the next twenty years. In 1649, he was invited to Sweden by Queen Christina and died there in the following year. His major achievement in philosophy was to reject the traditional scholastic approach to the subject, which dominated university teaching in the period, and to replace it with a mechanistic approach to life and the natural world. In his *Treatise of Man* (first published posthumously in 1662), he set out to describe the functions of an imaginary machine capable of performing all the activities of a living body, including digestion, breathing and vision. By demonstrating that all these activities might be reduced to one principle – matter in motion – Descartes claimed to have shown that the vital functions of all animals were ultimately reducible to the same cause.

First, then, the food is digested in the stomach of this machine by the force of certain liquids which, gliding among the food particles, separate, shake, and heat them just as common water does the particles of quicklime. . . .

Know too that the agitation that the food particles receive in being heated, together with the agitation of the stomach and bowels that contain them, and the arrangement of the fibers of which the bowels are composed, cause these particles – in the measure that they are digested – to descend little by little toward the conduit through which the coarsest of them must go out. [Know] too that the subtlest and most agitated particles meanwhile encounter here and there an infinity of little holes through which they flow into the branches of a large vein that carries them toward the liver . . . nothing but the smallness of the holes serving to separate these from the coarser particles; just as, when one shakes meal in a sack, all the purest part runs out, and only the smallness of the holes through which it passes prevents the bran from following after.

[. . .]

I desire you to consider, further, that all the functions that I have attributed to this machine, such as [a] the digestion of food; [b] the beating of the heart and arteries; [c] the nourishment and growth of the members; [d] respiration; [e] waking and sleeping; [f] the reception by the external sense organs of light, sounds, smells, tastes, heat, and all other such qualities; [g] the imprinting of the ideas of these qualities in the organ of common sense and imagination; [h] the retention or imprint of these ideas in the memory; [i] the internal movements of the appetites and passions; and finally[j], the external movements of all the members that so properly follow both the actions of objects presented to the senses and the passions and impressions which are entailed in the memory – I desire you to consider, I say, that these functions imitate those of a real man as perfectly as possible and that they follow naturally in this machine entirely from the disposition of the organs – no more nor less than do the movements of a clock or other automaton, from the arrangement of its counterweights and wheels. Wherefore it is not necessary, on their account, to conceive of any vegetative or sensitive soul or any other principle of movement and life than its blood and its spirits, agitated by the heat of the fire which burns continually in its heart and which is of no other nature than all those fires that occur in inanimate bodies.

7.3

Debating the medical benefits of the new anatomy: Girolamo Sbaraglia versus Marcello Malpighi

Howard B. Adelmann, *Marcello Malpighi and the Evolution of Embryology* (5 vols, Ithaca, Cornell University Press, 1966), vol. 1, pp. 559–62, 570–1, 575.

Girolamo Sbaraglia held the chair in medicine at Bologna from 1664 to 1704, and was also a member of the city's College of Physicians. During this period, he staunchly opposed the anatomical investigations of a group of innovative physicians working in Italy, citing as one of his reasons the failure of these new approaches to impinge upon medical practice. His objections first appeared in a letter, published in 1689, which was targeted at one of the group's leaders, Marcello Malpighi (1628–94). The clash was both personal and professional. Malpighi himself was one of the most important anatomists and physiologists of the seventeenth century. As a professor at Bologna, he devoted himself to the painstaking investigation of human and animal bodies, often using the recently invented microscope as a new tool in his studies. His reply to Sbaraglia was published posthumously.

The original text of Sbaraglia's letter is in Latin; here, we have used the English translation of Adelmann, which is in fact an abridgement of the original (i). Malpighi wrote in Italian. Again, we have used Adelmann's abridged translation, which we have occasionally expanded (ii). Additional translated material appears in square brackets. Both texts originally appeared in Malpighi's *Opera posthuma* (London, A. and J. Churchill, 1697), pp. 84–91, 99–187.

(i)

In the present century there are very many who desire to cure, but very few properly prepared to do so successfully. All with one voice agree that no stone should be left unturned in endeavoring to protect and strengthen the health of mankind, for without health our enjoyment of life and living is embittered. But men boast of this aim more than they seek after it, and they derive a barren pleasure from proceeding not where they ought to go but where the rest are going; nor do they recognize that the better things do not please many people.

... There are three things that the physicians of our time have received with great approval: finer anatomy, plant anatomy, and comparative anatomy. When I have demonstrated that these three kinds of anatomy contribute little or nothing to the sounder practice of medicine, it will immediately be evident that, while many eagerly desire to heal, very few have the proper orientation for curing successfully.

This is, morally, a laborious task, because the minds of many are preoccupied; because what is new, though empty, is more attractive to them than what is old, though full; because it is difficult to disprove dubitative[5] statements; and because there is no consensus among the learned as to their observations, for all do not see the same thing, and this is particularly true when things extremely small are being investigated. . . .

First of all, I confidently assert that a knowledge of finer anatomy is useless in warding off disease, and this is attested by men of great authority, of whom Galen is the best example. In several places he has divided anatomy into useful and useless parts. For example, in the third chapter of the second book of *De anatomicis administrationibus* he chides some anatomists for cultivating too diligently that part of it which is of no use whatever to medicine and neglecting the other, which all regard as the principal, highly useful, and necessary one. Yet in Galen's time, because the microscope was not available, the subtleties of today were not being sought after. What would he write today if he saw physicians studying fibrils, networks, miliary glands, and other exceedingly minute particulars? For it is one thing to study anatomy in order to know the most intimate structure of the viscera and another to study it in order to know what therapy should be employed. And this position is supported by the methodists and empiricists of old and also by the famous chemists of our day, Van Helmont, for example.

Examine the various viscera, then, and after acquiring a better knowledge of their structure consider whether any new function has been discovered and whether practical medicine has been enriched. Certainly there are many organs of the body that still retain their old function even after the Moderns have labored hard upon them. Galen regarded the kidneys as instruments for the secretion of the urine; in the past century Bartolommeo Eustachio[6] added canaliculi, of which

---

[5] Doubtful.

[6] The Italian anatomist Eustachio (c. 1500–74) was the author of *Opuscula anatomica* (*Anatomical studies*) (1564), which dealt with the kidney, ear and veins.

Galen did not know the kidney is composed; and modern authors have confirmed their existence and added some glands [the glomeruli] to them. Yet the kidneys are not as a result excluded from the function of secreting; they still secrete urine, and renal therapy has not been improved. The same may be said of the breasts, testes, and liver, where knowledge of the many vessels, the many reservoirs, ducts, glands, and capsules contributes no new uses. . . . Galen taught that the liver separates the bile from the blood, and this is all we know now after so many centuries and so many experiments and lucubrations. Hence, if anatomy is necessary because of the light it sheds upon functions, practice gains nothing from a more thorough anatomy which contributes no different functions.

[. . .]

And as to the diseases of the brain and lung, are there, for example, any better cures today for apoplexy, epilepsy, catalepsy, dizziness, or soporific affections than there were in past centuries? No. Surely Cimmerian[7] darkness still surrounds us everywhere. When the memory is damaged, remedies are still applied to the head, as Galen advises; but who of the most recent anatomists could by the most diligent anatomical dissection demonstrate the seat of this power and the way in which it is excited? Who from his reflections, from the things he has clearly seen innumerable times in animals and in man with the microscope or in any other way could ever, I shall not say throw light on practice, but even search out a path leading toward it, or incite the mind to discover some remedy? The same is true of organs the mechanics of which appear more clearly than they do in the brain. The accurate investigation of the structure of the liver, for example, has not shown the way the bile is separated (this, I believe, is the work of another extremely small, concealed contrivance never to be known, if my conjectures do not deceive me) and consequently has shown no remedies when it fails to be separated. Just as broken, luxated,[8] and corrupted bones are made well by skill, though the structure of bone is not known, so, too, the other parts are probably restored.

[. . .]

What should be studied is not the composition of the parts but the features and causes of diseases that are common and universal. Thus ulcers are cured equally well in one part or another, and the better

---

[7] In ancient Greece the Cimmerii were fabled to live in complete darkness.
[8] Dislocated or put out of joint.

physicians have denied that medicines affect only certain parts of the body. Even when corrosive juices appear in definite places, it is the fluid that should be considered, not the finest structure, which generally requires to be repaired, whatever it may be, and if a particular remedy is required, use, experience, and analogy will suggest it; it will not be deduced from the finest components of the parts.

You may object that according to the Ancients the heart was the sun of the microcosm, the monarch of the body, and that it is now a mill ass, so great is the difference in the function to be assigned to it. . . . I concede the new function, but I do not concede that from this new remedies have been devised for diseases of the heart. The old cures are still in use, and no new cardiac medicines have been added. We should therefore conclude that up to now all these labors have not benefited the practice of medicine.

(ii)

Nature . . . always acts uniformly, and man's sagacity is not so feeble as to be unable to discover a good part of her artifices[.] [So we admire the discoveries of Astronomy]   [And the same we can say about] the machines of our body, which are the basis of medicine, [since they are] made up of cords, filaments, beams, levers, tissues, fluids coursing here and there, cisterns, canals, filters, sieves, and similar mechanisms. Man, examining these parts by means of dissection, philosophy, and mechanics, has learned their structure and use; and, proceeding a priori, he has succeeded in forming models of them, by means of which he demonstrates the causes of these effects and gives the reason for them a priori. From a series of these, aided by ratiocination, and understanding the way Nature operates, he founds physiology, pathology, and then the art of medicine.

[Evidence of this is the] optic *camera*,[9] [in which the mathematician produces all the effects which are observed in the vision both in health and sickness. And he can demonstrate a priori that the effects resulting from the various shapes of the lens, or from the distance or the closeness of the parts, are necessary. Thus, the way we see and the lesions of sight are demonstrated by knowing the man-made machine which is analogous to the eye.] . . . [Respiration, which occurs through the machine of the thorax, is demonstrated by anatomy and mechanics, and a machine similar to the thorax can be made.] . . . Furthermore, for the

[9] Camera obscura.

coction, filtration, precipitation, and dulcification[10] of fluids Nature for the most part employs glands as workshops. As a result, the physician who knows mechanics will readily come to know the trituration[11] that is effected in the stomach by the fleshy fibers and an *aqua fortis* separated by the glands of the stomach from the universal fluid . . . and the filtration occurring in the glands of the kidney. Consequently Reissel[12] could construct a machine to demonstrate all these operations and phenomena. Though the senses cannot reach the finest structure of the porous glands of the viscera and the composition of the menstrua which these glands separate, the intellect instructed in mechanics can nevertheless arrive at them by ratiocination; thus by using distillation and precipitation it recognizes the nature of the salts and minerals composing the menstrua and deduces a priori the structure of these machines and the composition of these fluids by the laws of motion and differences in shape.

[. . .]

If this is so, it is clear that medicine can be founded upon a priori reasoning, that is, upon the knowledge of causes and the mechanical means by which Nature operates both in health and disease; and if we proceed with the knowledge of medicines gained from experiment and mechanics, cure can be effected.

[. . .]

. . . The glandular structure of the pleura and pericardium, which I have described, [throws light upon medical practice, showing the production of watery dropsy. Those parts are made up of holes and riddles[13] so that fluids can accumulate in the cavities which they enclose, that is, the thorax and lower abdomen, to keep the viscera wet and apart, so that they do not collapse on to each other. Every time there is an overproduction of that serum due to a fault either in the holes or in the universal fluid, it cannot dissipate or perspire and it collects in the abdomen, which, as a result, swells. . . . From this knowledge, one can deduce the

---

[10] Sweetening.

[11] The process of reducing to a fine powder by grinding.

[12] Salomon Reissel or Reisel was a counsellor and physician to the Duke of Württemberg. A follower of Descartes, in 1693 he published a description, including illustrations, of a 'Statua Humana Circolatoria' (Human statue showing the circulation), which appeared in *Miscellanea Curiosa, sive Ephemeridum Medico-Physicarum Germanicarum Academiae Naturae Curiosorum*. Allegedly, the hydraulic machine could imitate all the activities of the human body.

[13] A coarse-meshed sieve.

probable cure of this type of dropsy proposed by Nuck,[14] and administer remedies that thicken the blood and narrow the holes of the peritoneum].

7.4

New theories, old cures: the Newtonian medicine of George Cheyne

(i) George Cheyne, *A New Theory of Continual Fevers* (London, G. Strahan & J. Vallange, 1701), pp. 42–3 in Theodore M. Brown, 'Medicine in the Shadow of the *Principia*', *Journal of the History of Ideas*, 48 (1987), pp. 631 5.

(ii) George Cheyne, *An Essay of the True Nature and Due Method of Treating the Gout* (London, G. Strahan & H. Hammond, 1722), pp. 38–9.

(iii) *The Letters of Dr. George Cheyne to the Countess of Huntingdon*, ed. Charles Mullett (San Marino, California, Huntington Library, 1940), pp. 54–6.

George Cheyne (1671–1743) was one of the most popular physicians in eighteenth-century Britain. Born in Scotland, after graduating he went to London where he moved in a circle of Newtonian physicians and was elected a member of the Royal Society. He subsequently left London for Bath where he built a successful practice among the wealthy and fashionable clients of the spa town. From about 1720 he began writing popular medical self-help manuals, which promoted the benefits of temperance and moderation in all aspects of life. Despite the fact that he, himself, was prone to overindulgence, his works gradually took on an evangelical, almost mystical tone.

In the first extract, taken from his *A New Theory of Continual Fevers*, Cheyne was still writing within a strictly Newtonian framework. The book is characterised by a clear mathematical format and outlines a scientific medicine based on the laws of physics and geometry. The

[14] Anton Nuck (1650–92) was Professor of Medicine at the University of Leiden. He was famous for his anatomical investigations on the glands, which he published as *Adenographia curiosa et uteri foeminei anatome nova* (Leyden, 1690).

second extract is taken from his book on gout, a very common illness among his affluent patients. He explained the disease in mechanical terms and recommended Bath water as a cure. He also insisted, however, that gout was linked to moral dissipation and was best treated with a restrained lifestyle. The third passage indicates that Cheyne was still employing the age-old tradition of writing letters of medical advice to his clients. Here, we can see the importance of the personal relationship that existed between a physician and his wealthy clientele.

(i)

. . . [Suppose] an Obstruction or Dilation of the *Glandular* Vessels, It's evident the foresaid concave Cylinder will be thereby diminish'd or increas'd in any given Proportion: Suppose, e.g. the Diameter of the Cylinder so obstructed is to that of the whole, as 1 is to the [square root of] 2; their Orifices will be as 1 to 2. Suppose again, there are twenty Pounds of Blood in a Man, seeing at the Beginning of the Arterial Vessels, (which constitute the Glands) the Velocity is near the same, as proceeding from the same Cause, the Compression of the Heart: Therefore divide 20 into two Parts, which may be (in this Case) as, 1 is to 2 (which done by this general Rule

$$x = \frac{md}{m + h} \quad y = \frac{nd}{m + h} \quad \text{putting } d \text{ for 20 pounds, } x \text{ for the greater,}$$

and y for the lesser proportional part, m to n for their *Ratio*). The parts will be here 6⅔, and 13⅓; which are the proportional Parts of 20 Pounds of Blood, which would naturally pass in the obstruct-Canal, and in the Remainder thereof, which is passable.

(ii)

The fat and oily parts of sulphur, like other fat and unctuous bodies, are the lightest, the most coherent, and the most springy of all bodies. . . . Join all these qualities together, and you have one of the most admirable remedies in the world, for all intentions in the cure of the gout: by its agreeable taste and lightness on the stomach, (especially when wash'd down with any milky vehicle) its tenacity, ropiness and elasticity; the smallness of its parts; their efficacy in destroying the mischief of all saline particles, with their natural warmth, join'd to the activity of its

186

acid salt, (making it a kind of natural soap) it enters the small vessels, where no other diluent,[15] hitherto known, can come; cleanses their insides from the foulness that sticks to them; imbibes and retains all the gouty salts, and carries them out of the body by perspiration; softens, smooths and relaxes the parch'd and stiffen'd fibres; and by leaving some of its oily parts on their surfaces, sheaths and defends them from the points of the salts afterwards introduced.

(iii)

Madam

I hope your ladyship with your amiable company has got safe to your habitation before this can come to hand and that you begin to feel the good effects of your journey and the waters, with the few simple medicines you tried here, as I most earnestly wish; but having had the honour of more particular conversation with your ladyship, and thereby become acquainted with many particulars I was ignorant of before and made a great many observations in your case which will enable me, without hesitation or puzzle, to direct your ladyship in your future conduct, I will impart a few of them by this [letter], first of all assuring your ladyship in the strongest and most serious manner one who expects to give an account of his words and actions to an infallible being can, that if your ladyship observes the few rules I shall mention you will in time get as well as any person in England and that as long as you observe them you are in no more danger than your fine daughter, Lady Betty. You have had an original sharpness in your blood, with obstructed glands in several parts, but are strong, firm, and well formed in your solids. Till this sharpness is entirely conquered you can expect no lasting uninterrupted health. I am satisfied these sharp juices are in a great degree already conquered, but the glands do not perform their office strongly. Your perspiration is weak, your digestion feeble, and your bowels lax. By no other method to me known, nor I think possible to be known, could your ladyship have been preserved from being extremely miserable and quite unhappy or destroyed. Now, your late and former paroxysms have proceeded from two causes: 1. your frequent child bearing, by which you have not been able to continue your powderous and sweetening medicines, and 2. from too early attempts to enlarge and encrease your regimen. This you will never successfully do, but by slow degrees, as the corn grows, and by insensible steps, and never till

[15] Substance that dissolves or makes more fluid.

the juices are entirely sweetened and the glands pervious, that there may be room in the vessels to admit more chyle, else the superfluity will stagnate and corrupt in your stomach and bowels and run into vomiting or purging. I allow this precise quantity is hard to find, and I know no so certain a rule to go by as to take down the *lightest* and *least* a person can be easy under, and strive rather to underdo than overdo, at least at first, for in a very few days nature will most sensibly tell and warn an underdoing. Your ladyship knows well all I can say on this topic. I only by this intend only to keep your ladyship in remembrance: 1. when you are sick, low, or oppressed, you'll never be relieved without a vomit. If an Anderson[16] do it not, 2. take your ethiops[17] for 8 or ten days and carry it off by an Anderson, least it colic or purge you, and then begin it again. It is the only medicine on earth can effectually sweeten your juices, entirely open all the glands, strengthen your appetite, and plump you up at last as all the preparations of mercury infallibly do, of which this is the safest and best. 3. chew a little bark in a morning before dinner and a little rhubarb before supper; in your riding, at least sometimes, you need not fear too keen an appetite. That can never hurt unless indulged. 4. after a vomit or an Anderson, drink a pint of spa water. Since you could bear the bath without hurting, you will much better bear it, but when you are quite well and much alive drop all your medical helps and keep them, like a great coat, for a rainy day. I think, except riding and good hours, these are all the medical helps you can ever want, and I hope in a little time you will get above them. . . .

Your ladyship's most obliged, faithful, and humble ser[van]t,
George Cheyne

Bath, Apr[il] 14, 1736

---

[16] Anderson's pills were a popular early eighteenth-century nostrum.
[17] A metal-based medicament.

7.5

Medical knowledge, patronage and its impact on practice in eighteenth-century England

Nicholas D. Jewson, 'Medical Knowledge and the Patronage System in 18th Century England', *Sociology* 8 (1974), pp. 369–83.

Drawing on the thriving sociological research of the 1970s, Nicholas Jewson accounts for the variety of competing medical theories in the eighteenth century by emphasising the role of social constraints operating on contemporary physicians. In exploring the insecure status of the physician and his dependence on the patronage of wealthy patients, he was able to provide a coherent explanation for the ebb and flow of medical theories in the social conditions of medical practice. Though some have seen this approach as overly simplistic, Jewson's analysis has been highly influential on historians of medicine who have incorporated his ideas in a number of fields, including the importance of patient power in the eighteenth century.

It is the object of this paper to construct a sociological explanation of the origins and nature of medical beliefs in 18th century England. It will be argued that the distinctive characteristics of contemporary theories and therapies were shaped by the constraints acting upon the process of medical innovation generated within the structure of relationships between patients and practitioners. Medical knowledge will be located in the context of this configuration, and thus will be viewed as a form of social interaction between the sick and medical personnel.

[. . .]

. . . The key feature of this relationship will be identified as the dependence of the elite of the medical profession upon the fees and favours of their aristocratic patients. Through the patronage system the sick were able to exercise control over the course of medical innovation. Hence the form and contents of medical theories reflected the assumptions, obsessions, and interests of the most powerful section of the lay public. . . . It will be seen that, in the absence of academic or professional criteria, patients recruited their practitioners by means of personal selection in the context of primary social interaction. Thus physicians were enjoined to adopt the stereo-typed lifestyle of their genteel clients whilst simultaneously advertising their services by means of individual display. This peculiar amalgam of social conformity and personal eccentricity, when translated into intellectual activity, led to the creation of a profusion of competing theories which, despite their mutual hostility, shared a number of implicit paradigmatic assumptions. . . .

[. . .]

Perhaps the most immediately striking feature of 18th century pathology was the general lack of agreement about the causes of illness and the effectiveness of therapies. Medical knowledge consisted of a chaotic diversity of schools of thought, each strenuously seeking to attain ascendancy over the others. Despite the plethora of shifting viewpoints, however, a closer examination reveals that the 18th century systems of pathology were based upon a common set of assumptions about the nature of health and disease. . . .

The medical beliefs of the classical authors enjoyed great authority in 15th and 16th century Europe. However during the revolutionary upheavals in English society of the mid 17th century the ideas of Hippocrates and Galen came under attack from a number of quarters. One particularly powerful influence upon the development of medical knowledge during this period was that of Newtonian physics. The mechanical philosophy enjoyed remarkable prestige in both scientific and non-scientific circles. The elite of the medical profession accordingly sought to import its fashionable notions into their theories. Most of the medical authors who invoked the name of Newton had little but the vaguest comprehension of his theories. Furthermore a number of different interpretations of his ideas were in circulation. Hence the introduction of Newtonianism into medicine did not herald a thoroughgoing reformulation of theories of pathology. Instead it gave a new lease of life to the ancient conceptions of disease which reappeared under a new guise. The basic entities of the humoural system were re-defined in terms of material entities, such as corpuscular flow or excitement of the muscles, but the general conception of the bodily system propounded by Hippocrates and Galen remained the guiding principle of research and practice. Thus, despite criticism of specific aspects of the ancient texts and the appeal to new sources of legitimation, the classical authors remained the standard works read by medical students at the English universities. In short the conceptual foundations of classical medicine were refined and consolidated by the accommodation of a crude Newtonianism.

What were the major features of 18th century theories of pathology? Firstly contemporary concepts of disease did not employ the modern notion of illness as a localized physiological or anatomical event. Instead . . . health was conceptualized in terms of the overall condition of the constitution. Pathology was systemic rather than organic or cellular. Furthermore, although the various theories were frequently in dispute over the precise cause of illness, typically they subscribed to the belief that disease resulted from one underlying state of the body. In other words 18th century pathology was monistic in form, constructed upon a single explanatory principle. . . . Although pathology was reduced to a single grand design, however, any particular case of illness was regarded as the product of individual circumstances and situations. Each man suffered from his own peculiar combination of factors which accounted for his physiological disequilibrium. Although there was only one pathological condition there were innumerable pathological careers. Thus contemporary systems of pathology provided a complete explanatory scheme capable of accounting for each and every ailment afflicting mankind, whilst at the same time institutionalizing an individualistic conception of illness which recognized each case to be a unique configuration of bodily disorders. . . .

[. . .]

It is the thesis of this paper that the distinctive characteristics of 18th century medical knowledge were formed by the constraints placed upon medical innovation within the structure of social relationships between patients and practitioners. . . .

In the first half of the 18th century English society may be described as a complex hierarchy of wealth and prestige converging at the top onto a tiny group of rich and powerful landowners. . . . The political, economic, and cultural hegemony of the nobility and aristocracy was overwhelming. Deference to superiors was part of the unquestioned fabric of social life into which Englishmen were born and raised. The distinctions of status were everywhere proclaimed and respected in the stereotyped rituals of speech, manners, deportment, livery, architecture, taste, and innumerable other cultural symbols. The major horizontal cleavage in this hierarchical system of stratification was that which separated gentlemen from the common people. The precise point of demarcation of the upper class from the rest of the population was not simply defined however. Ideally a gentleman derived his fortune from his landed estates, though he might be engaged in certain other occupations. The distinction seems to have been made in terms of birth, manners, display and social acceptance. It was his effortless and elegant lifestyle that all classes of society recognized as the mark of a gentleman.

Where did medical men fit into this hierarchy? In all the professions a line was decisively drawn between the upper ranks of practitioners who were accorded the status of gentlemen, and those who occupied the lower positions. . . . Physicians . . . attended the upper classes, and had themselves received the education of a gentleman. Physicians eschewed the manual labour of surgery and pharmacy, which they regarded as beneath their professional dignity. A medical degree from one of the English universities was an essential qualification for membership of the Royal College. The costs of this academic training were high, and kept all but the wealthy out of this section of the profession. Professional education at Oxford and Cambridge consisted of a six years' course in a wide range of subjects, followed by a slightly longer period devoted to a literary study of the classical medical authors. Thus above all else an academic background ensured that those entering upon the practice of physic were scholars and gentlemen. By their deportment, manners, and attire physicians assiduously sought to maintain this standing in their professional lives.

[. . .]

However, in spite of their genteel status and pre-eminence among medical practitioners, physicians did not occupy a place of precedence within the ranks of the upper class. A major distinction was drawn between the aristocracy . . . and the gentry, who were sub-divided into Baronets, Knights, Esquires, and gentlemen. In general physicians came near the bottom of this hierarchy. Only landed gentlemen enjoyed the full admiration and honours of 18th century society. Moreover medicine was not the most prestigious or highly rewarded among the professions. Hence a physician's social advancement depended upon his acquisition of sufficient fortune to purchase an estate, or upon his ability to win the favours of a grateful nobleman. Physicians therefore were committed to the preservation of the existing social order in which they already held a substantial professional and public position. At the same time they were dependent upon the rewards of their small group of upper class patients to sustain and improve their social standing. Aristocratic patients were in a position to choose for themselves the most satisfactory or amusing practitioners from among the host of medical men who clamoured for their favours. It was the patient who judged the competence of the physician and the suitability of the therapy. The wealthy and influential threw their support behind whichever practitioner pleased them and withdrew it from those in whom they were disappointed. Thus it was the client who held ultimate power in the consultative relationship.

Through the channels of the patronage system therefore the nobility and gentry held sway over the medical profession. This was but one part of the great system of control exercised by the mighty land owners which extended throughout English society in the 18th century, and which had a profound influence on the pattern of cultural innovation. The rule of property was based upon a system of personal selection and favours among friends and kinsmen which governed the distribution of rewards in all walks of life. The wealthy and powerful thus had command over extensive networks of personal loyalty and obligation. Social order was founded upon these configurations of permanent vertical dependency between patrons and their clients. Success in a medical career, as in other occupations, depended upon the cultivation of close personal ties with members of the upper class. Furthermore this elite had a keen amateur interest in medical matters, as may be seen from the contents of contemporary magazines and journals written for the upper class. Physicians had no choice but to tailor their theories and remedies to meet the expectations and requirements of their genteel clients. Upper class patients were able therefore to direct the development of medical knowledge by shifting their patronage from one group of innovators to another. . . .

[. . .]

One of the most important manifestations of the patient's power over the practitioner was his ability to dictate the very definition of illness itself. In particular the patient's understandable desire to be cured of his symptoms, rather than diagnosed of his disease, had an indelible impact on contemporary theories of nosology[18] and pathology. Medical knowledge revolved around the problems of the prognosis and therapy of symptoms, rather than the diagnosis and analysis of diseases. Symptoms were not regarded as the secondary signs of internal pathological events, but rather as the disease itself. . . . The symptom based nosology of the 18th century was thus a reflection of a patient dominated medical system. One consequence of this situation was that 18th century physicians carefully recorded and interpreted the symptoms of their patients but rarely if ever physically examined them. Physical examination was presaged by the modern concept of disease which consigns symptoms to the role of secondary indicators.

[. . .]

The strategies adopted by practitioners in their relationships with their

---

[18] The systematic classification of diseases into specific categories.

patients influenced the development of medical knowledge in a number of other ways. In order to justify their high fees it was necessary for medical men to present themselves to the sick not merely as aids to natural recovery, but as ones who actively intervened to change the course of nature. The patient had not merely to get better: he had to be cured. Physicians wished to be seen wrestling with the mysterious forces of life and death upon the battleground of the patient's body. They required therefore remedies which made the patient conscious of the curative powers of his practitioner and of the efforts which had been made on his behalf. Here the monistic pathology and its attendant therapies stood the 18th century practitioner in good stead. He was never at a loss to know the cause and cure of his patient's ailments, whilst the blood-curdling array of heroic remedies were nothing if not memorable to those who endured them. The rationality of 18th century therapies becomes more apparent then when seen in the light of the dramatic quality which the practitioner sought to bestow upon his healing arts.

... The ultimate success of a consultation depended upon the patient's personal assessment of the standard of care that he had received. The sick man's evaluation of the performance of his doctor might well be influenced by the state of his mind as well as the condition of his body. Thus failure to cure a physical complaint, or even inability to avert death, need not necessarily have proved injurious to a physician's career. Similarly the mere cessation of symptoms did not guarantee the sick man's approval. Of prime importance was whether or not the patient believed he had benefited in some way from the attendance of his physician. . . .

The divergent interests of upper class patients and their practitioners were reconciled in the speculative systems of pathology. These theories allowed for an endless array of ailments, defined in terms with which the patient could readily identify, whilst enabling the physician to diagnose each and every malady and display limitless ingenuity in concocting cures. In other words the medical systems of the 18th century conformed to the requirements of the aristocracy and gentry, who held ultimate control over medical practitioners, whilst affording the profession considerable autonomy in responding to the demands of their patients.

... The sick did not adopt either academic qualifications or professional status as the primary criteria in the selection of their medical practitioners. Instead they sought their assurance of the therapeutic effectiveness and ethical propriety of medical personnel through the personal relationships they established with their doctors in the network of face to face relationships which made up the patronage system.

Medical men acquired their occupational licence by means of primary social interaction with their patients.

The particularistic nature of the consultative relationship between upper class patients and their practitioners was reflected in the particularistic conceptions of disease current in the 18th century. The sick demanded personal attention from their doctors, and medical men for their part sought to make themselves indispensable to their clients. It has already been suggested that the monistic systems of pathology insured that physicians were never without an explanation and a cure. Equally however, because each patient was held to have his own unique configuration of bodily processes, the physician could lay claim to special insight into the individual features of the sick man's disorder. The medical systems enabled the practitioner to combine diagnostic infallibility with personal service. As a result the patient rather than the disease remained the focus of theory and practice. . . .

Professional advancement in the medical world of the 18th century, then, was achieved by means of individual recruitment, through personal contacts, of a group of regular clients upon whose fees and favours the practitioner relied. To obtain a clientele of this kind it was necessary for a medical man to move in the social circles from which he hoped to draw his fees, for the public were liable to assess the professional suitability of a practitioner by the status of his lifestyle. Hence above all else physicians sought to be 'in society', and to display those exquisite standards of taste, etiquette, and bearing denied the meaner sort. Such cultural artifacts as gorgeous apparel, stylish manners, and witty conversation both symbolized and legitimized their close contact with the upper class. Similarly the Royal College placed great store by attendance at the English universities, acquisition of the Latin tongue, and familiarity with classical culture because these attributes were basic requirements for acceptance into the social circles of the nobility and gentry. In short since the patient assessed the worth of his doctor in face-to-face interaction it was necessary for the physician to adopt the stereotyped manner and intellectual worldview of his upper class clientele. In addition to establishing his credentials as a gentleman, however, the ambitious physician also had to draw attention to his own special talents and skills. His career depended upon convincing a sceptical society of the superiority of his services over those of his peers. Physicians were encouraged therefore to bring themselves before the public eye by every devious method of self advertisement their prolific ingenuity could devise. The successful physician was one who succeeded in becoming part of upper class society whilst simultaneously exploiting its fads and foibles.

The career of the physician consisted therefore of a peculiar amalgam of ingratiation into the social circles of the nobility and gentry by means of conformity to the norms of upper class life, accompanied by individual struggle for recognition by means of personal display and publicity. The social constraints placed upon an actor in such a situation are likely to induce him to adopt that form of social interaction described . . . as fashion. . . .

The successful physician of 18th century England was a man of fashion in more ways than one. The leading Fellows of the Royal College adorned London society in the season, whilst more humble provincial physicians mirrored their activities at the county level. In addition practitioners extended the field of fashion into medical knowledge itself. The rivalries between the proponents of the various medical theories were part of the larger battle for power and prestige in the career system. Such contests were not intended merely for the delectation of other members of the profession, but were directed to an audience of fee-paying patients. Medical investigators were thus constrained to pay homage to the intellectual predilections of the upper class whilst simultaneously presenting their own individual interpretations of approved and traditional theories. As a result the 18th century systems of pathology were caught in a process of continual reformulation and revision, yet never succeeded in severing connection with a common set of assumptions about health and disease. Adherence to established theoretical premises assured social acceptability, whilst superficial novelty stimulated public interest and justified high fees. Thus the structure of the 18th century career system ensured that medical knowledge remained in a state of turmoil and controversy whilst at the same time prevented fundamental innovation in the underlying structure of medical thought.

. . . Both patients and practitioners regarded the activities of research scientists as irrelevant to the overwhelming problems of therapy which were their primary concern. An 18th century practitioner advanced his career by prescribing cures for symptoms rather than by discovering the causes of disease. There were few prospects in entering upon time consuming and laborious experiments which at best promised no more than limited and tentative conclusions. A physician's reputation was made by bold, decisive and immediate action to relieve his patient's suffering. . . . The sick and the dying could not wait whilst scientists discovered the causes of their agonies, and in any case they were more interested in remedies than in explanations. The speculative systems might have been unreliable and contradictory, but they did at least offer treatment and hope. . . .

[. . .]

Social relationships among medical men themselves also seriously inhibited the development of scientific medicine. The social organization of medical personnel constrained practitioners to individually compete for clients by advertising their skills. Consequently medical innovators sought occupational advancement by utilizing their discoveries in private practice, where they were often kept as trade secrets, rather than by sharing them with professional rivals. The free exchange of information among medical practitioners and investigators was impossible as long as clients, rather than professional colleagues, held control over the distribution of rewards in the career system. Thus it was not until the 1820s and 30s that medical journals devoted to the communication of empirical research findings were established on a firm footing, a century and a half after those of the physical sciences. Similarly medical societies were not formed in large numbers until the late 18th and early 19th centuries. Clearly a necessary, if not sufficient, condition for the growth of a scientific community is a network of relationships in which established wisdom can be freely disseminated to all accredited members. . . .

[. . .]

This paper has traced the consequences of social class patronage, the client/physician relationship, and the structure of the contemporary profession for the development of medical knowledge in 18th century England. A two-way network of dependencies existed between the sick and medical personnel. By virtue of their economic and political predominance the gentry and aristocracy held ultimate control over the consultative relationship and the course of medical innovation. Physicians, on the other hand, enjoyed a measure of counter power over their patients, for the promise of physical and mental health held out by the profession was highly sought after by the sick. The systems of nosology and pathology were founded upon concepts of disease with which upper class patients could readily identify, whilst legitimizing the provision of therapy and the collection of fees by practitioners.

7.6

The popularisation of the new medical theories in the eighteenth century: the novels of Laurence Sterne

(i) Laurence Sterne, *A Sentimental Journey and Other Writings*, ed. Tom Keymer (London, Everyman/J. M. Dent, 1994), pp. 95–9.

(ii) Laurence Sterne, *The Life and Opinions of Tristram Shandy, Gentleman*, ed. Ian Campbell Ross (Oxford, Clarendon Press, 1983), pp. 117–19.

By the middle of the eighteenth century, the literary genre of the novel was enjoying widespread commercial success, particularly among the burgeoning middle classes of Georgian England. In particular, novels of 'sentiment', which charted and celebrated the deep feeling of the storyteller for the distress of those less fortunate than themselves, became best-sellers. In their analysis of subtle emotions, novelists increasingly drew on recent physiological debates on the function and diseases of the nerves, which they then made available to a wide audience.

Having spent an itinerant childhood in Ireland and England, Laurence Sterne (1713–68) studied at Jesus College, Cambridge, before embarking on a clerical career in Yorkshire. In our first extract, *A Sentimental Journey through France and Italy*, first published in 1768, Sterne both built on, and satirised, the literary convention of the sentimental novel. The book itself recounts the feelings and emotions of the novel's main character, Yorick, during his travels abroad, in particular his encounter in France with a young woman named Maria, who loses her mind after being abandoned by her lover. Despite the satirical tone of Sterne's language, contemporary readers saw in Maria an icon of sentimental distress and she became an influential model for later romantic female characters. The second extract is from the work that made Sterne's name as an author, *The Life and Opinions of Tristram Shandy*. In the passage here, Sterne satirises the thoughts of Shandy's father on the risks which a badly supervised delivery can cause to a baby's intelligence. By engaging in detail with philosophical and physiological debates about the location of the soul and the anatomy of the nerves, Sterne was here poking fun at the way in which novel medical ideas had become popular topics of conversation among the 'chattering classes' of fashionable society. At the same time, however, he was heavily reliant on his own readers' knowledge of, and familiarity with, these debates if they were fully to appreciate the humour of the discussion.

(i)

I have but a few small pages left of this to croud it into – and half of these must be taken up with the poor Maria my friend, Mr. Shandy, met with near Moulines.

The story he had told of that disorder'd maid affect'd me not a little in the reading; but when I got within the neighbourhood where she lived, it returned so strong into my mind, that I could not resist an impulse which prompted me to go half a league out of the road to the village where her parents dwelt to enquire after her.

'Tis going, I own, like the Knight of the Woeful Countenance,[19] in quest of melancholy adventures – but I know not how it is, but I am never so perfectly conscious of the existence of a soul within me, as when I am entangled in them.

The old mother came to the door, her looks told me the story before she open'd her mouth – She had lost her husband; he had died, she said, of anguish, for the loss of Maria's senses about a month before. – She had feared at first, she added, that it would have plunder'd her poor girl of what little understanding was left – but, on the contrary, it had brought her more to herself – still she could not rest – her poor daughter, she said, crying, was wandering somewhere about the road –

– Why does my pulse beat languid as I write this? and what made La Fleur,[20] whose heart seem'd only to be tuned to joy, to pass the back of his hand twice across his eyes, as the woman stood and told it? I beckon'd to the postilion to turn back into the road.

When we had got within half a league of Moulines, at a little opening in the road leading to a thicket, I discovered poor Maria sitting under a poplar – she was sitting with her elbow in her lap, and her head leaning on one side within her hand – a small brook ran at the foot of the tree.

---

[19] A reference to Don Quixote, the doleful knight whose adventures and suffering form the basis of Cervantes' great novel.

[20] Yorick's travelling companion.

[. . .]

. . . I look'd in Maria's eyes, and saw she was thinking more of her father than of her lover or her little goat; for as she utter'd them the tears trickled down her cheeks.

I sat down close by her; and Maria let me wipe them away as they fell with my handkerchief. – I then steep'd it in my own – and then in hers – and then in mine – and then I wip'd hers again – and as I did it, I felt such undescribable emotions within me, as I am sure could not be accounted for from any combinations of matter and motion.

I am positive I have a soul; nor can all the books with which materialists have pester'd the world ever convince me of the contrary.

[. . .]

There was nothing from which I had painted out for myself so joyous a riot of the affections, as in this journey in the vintage, through this part of France; but pressing through this gate of sorrow to it, my sufferings had totally unfitted me: in every scene of festivity I saw Maria in the back-ground of the piece, sitting pensive under her poplar; and I had got almost to Lyons before I was able to cast a shade across her –

– Dear sensibility! source inexhausted of all that's precious in our joys, or costly in our sorrows! thou chainest thy martyr down upon his bed of straw – and 'tis thou who lifts him up to HEAVEN – eternal fountain of our feelings! – 'tis here I trace thee – and this is thy divinity which stirs within me – not, that in some sad and sickening moments, *"my soul shrinks back upon herself, and startles at destruction"*[21] – mere pomp of words! but that I feel some generous joys and generous cares beyond myself – all comes from thee, great – great SENSORIUM of the world! which vibrates, if a hair of our heads but falls upon the ground,[22] in the remotest desert of thy creation. – Touch'd with thee, Eugenius draws my curtain[23] when I languish – hears my tale of symptoms, and blames the weather for the disorder of his nerves. Thou giv'st a portion of it sometimes to the roughest peasant who traverses the bleakest mountains – he finds the lacerated lamb of another's flock – This moment I beheld him leaning with his head against his crook, with piteous inclination looking down upon it – Oh! had I come one moment sooner! – it bleeds to death – his gentle heart bleeds with it –

[21] The quotation is taken from Joseph Addison's tragedy, *Cato* (1713).
[22] 1 Samuel 14:45.
[23] Sterne, *Tristram Shandy* 1.12.

Peace to thee, generous swain! – I see thou walkest off with anguish – but thy joys shall balance it – for happy is thy cottage – and happy is the sharer of it – and happy are the lambs which sport about you.

(ii)

Now, as it was plain to my father, that all souls were by nature equal, – and that the great difference between the most acute and the most obtuse understanding, – was from no original sharpness or bluntness of one thinking substance above or below another, – but arose merely from the lucky or unlucky organization of the body, in that part where the soul principally took up her residence, – he had made it the subject of his enquiry to find out the identical place.

Now, from the best accounts he had been able to get of this matter, he was satisfied it could not be where *Des Cartes* had fixed it, upon the top of the *pineal* gland of the brain; which, as he philosophised, form'd a cushion for her about the size of a marrow pea; – tho', to speak the truth, as so many nerves did terminate all in that one place, – 'twas no bad conjecture; – and my father had certainly fallen with that great philosopher plumb into the center of the mistake, had it not been for my uncle *Toby*, who rescued him out of it, by a story he told him of a *Wallourn Officer* at the battle of *Landon*, who had one part of his brain shot away by a musket-ball, – and another part of it taken out after by a *French* surgeon; and, after all, recovered, and did his duty very well without it.

If death, said my father, reasoning with himself, is nothing but the separation of the soul from the body; – and if it is true that people can walk about and do their business without brains, – then certes[24] the soul does not inhabit there. Q. E. D.

As for that certain very thin, subtle, and very fragrant juice which *Coglionissimo Borri*, the great *Milaneze* physician, affirms, in a letter to *Bartholine*,[25] to have discovered in the cellulae of the occipital parts of the cerebellum, and which he likewise affirms to be the principal seat of the reasonable soul (for, you must know, in these latter and more enlightened ages, there are two souls in every man living, – the one

---

[24] Assuredly.

[25] Guiseppe Francesco Borri (1627–95) was an Italian alchemist and empiric who wrote a letter to the Danish physician and anatomist Thomas Bartholinus (1616–80) which was subsequently published as *De cerebri ortu et usu medico* (*On the origin of the brain and its medical function*) in 1669. The use of the epithet *coglionissimo* to describe Borri is best translated as 'most complete fool', from the Italian word, *coglione* or testicle.

according to the great *Metheglingius*,[26] being called the *Animus*, the other the *Anima*); – as for this opinion, I say, of *Borri*, – my father could never subscribe to it by any means; the very idea of so noble, so refined, so immaterial, and so exalted a being as the *Anima*, or even the *Animus*,[27] taking up her residence, and sitting dabbling, like a tad-pole, all day long, both summer and winter, in a puddle, – or in a liquid of any kind, how thick or thin soever, he would say, shock'd his imagination; he would scarce give the doctrine a hearing.

What, therefore, seem'd the least liable to objections of any, was, that the chief sensorium, or head-quarters of the soul, and to which place all intelligences were referred, and from whence all her mandates were issued, – was in, or near, the cerebellum, – or rather some-where about the *medulla oblongata*, wherein it was generally agreed by *Dutch* anatomists, that all the minute nerves from all the organs of the seven senses concentered, like streets and winding alleys, into a square.

So far there was nothing singular in my father's opinion, – he had the best of philosophers, of all ages and climates, to go along with him. – But here he took a road of his own, setting up another *Shandean* hypothesis upon these corner-stones they had laid for him; – and which said hypothesis equally stood its ground; whether the subtilty and fine-ness of the soul depended upon the temperature and clearness of the said liquor, or of the finer net-work and texture in the cerebellum itself; which opinion he favoured.

He maintained, that next to the due care to be taken in the act of propagation of each individual, which required all the thought in the world, as it laid the foundation of this incomprehensible contexture in which wit, memory, fancy, eloquence, and what is usually meant by the name of good natural parts, do consist; – that next to this and his Chris-tian-name, which were the two original and most efficacious causes of all; – that the third cause, or rather what logicians call the *Causa sine quâ non*,[28] and without which all that was done was of no manner of sig-nificance, – was the preservation of this delicate and fine-spun web, from the havock which was generally made in it by the violent com-pression and crush which the head was made to undergo, by the non-sensical method of bringing us into the world by that part foremost.

[26] A name made up by the author. Metheglin was a type of mead, and some have suggested as a result that Sterne may be referring to the celebrated English physician, Richard Mead (1673–1754).

[27] *Anima* refers to the principle of life and sense, i.e. the faculty governing vital motion; *animus* is the seat of reason or intelligence.

[28] Literally, 'the cause without which nothing'; i.e. the indispensable first cause.

Part eight
Women and medicine in early modern Europe

8.1
Female complaints: the flux

Barbara Duden, *The Woman Beneath the Skin: A Doctor's Patients in Eighteenth-Century Germany*, trans. Thomas Dunlap (Cambridge, Mass. and London, Harvard University Press, 1991), pp. 130–5.

Johann Storch (1681–1751) practised medicine in Eisenach, the seat of the independent German duchy of Saxe-Eisenach, and produced numerous books. The most interesting was an eight-volume work on the diseases of women, which was based on the notes he took during his encounters with female patients. It includes the discussion of about 1,800 cases. In analysing Storch's notes, the historian Barbara Duden has tried to recreate how eighteenth-century women made sense of their bodies and its various illnesses. Here, she discusses their use of the term 'flux', which was invoked repeatedly by Storch's female patients. These are cited in a slightly unorthodox manner by Duden. The indented quotes are in fact Duden's paraphrase of Storch; elsewhere, she cites directly from his writings.

The complaint about an inner flux was one of the most frequent reasons why the women turned to the doctor. Just as often they were troubled that the flux may have struck in again. The flux is a strange thing. It described a host of things. 'Flux' is the name for pains a woman felt inside from matter flowing in her body. The women also spoke of 'flux' when something flowed from their bodies. The menses is a 'flux', the 'whites' is a 'flux', and they used the word to describe oozing wounds or open sores on the skin: they 'have a flux' or a 'defluxion' on them. 'Flux' is the term for an illness . . . in which a physiological interpretation on the part of the women finds expression. The word 'flux' combined a subjective experience with a complex meaning. The women suffered from an inner flux, but at the same time they were fearful that this flux inside them could be 'struck in', be driven back, become stuck. They suffered from the flux and from the fear that it might disappear. 'Flux' signified a contradictory echo between inside and outside.

The 'inner flux' caused pains: headaches, ringing in the ears, hardness of hearing, loss of sight, stone blindness, a 'dull or palsying tongue', gout and rheumatism, stomachaches, colics, suffocation of the womb, sharp pain in the legs. These inner fluxes caused aches where they were felt; they were oppressive, constricting, and burdensome, which is why women could not hear, speak, or see, why the quickness of their external movements was paralyzed. The women explain the inner distress in a paradoxical way. They call it a 'flux', but this flux was characterized by the fact that it did *not* move, that it stagnated, or that it abruptly fell upon some inward part. The pain spoke not of an easy flow, but of a laborious and viscous stream, or of a violent assault of the flux.

In September 1730 a thirty-year-old woman complained 'about the sudden attack of a flux, *circa praecordia*,[1] from which she was struck down speechless, indicating with gestures the strong and violent pains . . . she had'. The following day 'she related that she had recovered her speech after taking the second powder'.

Early in the morning one day in December 1722 a 'woman filled with scorbutic blood' urgently sent for Storch 'so that he may help her in a sudden attack of an apoplectic fit'. This woman was so 'struck' that she could not utter a word. After some powders had been administered and the legs warmed, the fit passed within a few hours.

Other women had a flux quite routinely. They might sense the movement of the flowing matter inside themselves for years. In the case of a noble lady this was felt in the following way:

In September 1722 she was assaulted by a 'flux causing cramps and spasms', which she had already felt several times before, the last time violently six years earlier. This time it manifested itself in 'swooning, numbness of the tongue, and in a tingling and prickling in one arm, which moved from the left to the right arm, and then within a short period into the left leg'. In the following weeks she felt the flux first 'tearing' in the leg, then as a boil 'on the thigh'. In January 1723 she sensed a 'flux in the face, while the swollen leg subsided', a 'true sign that the flux was striking inward and a change in the body was impending'. The flux could keep to its 'old place'

---

[1] In her upper abdomen.

for long stretches of time, a condition that was relatively bearable, until acute crises arose whenever the matter started to migrate: in the years that followed it moved into the head, belly, and the limbs.

The outer flux was a mirror image of the inner flux. As women's 'flux of reds or whites', it ensured cleansing and unburdening. The external fluxes included, in addition to the periodic discharges, the 'oozing sores' that the body created for itself in order to discharge matter. In particular the thin segments of the skin, the swollen venous nodes, boils, and abscesses channeled these flows, the evacuation of 'humoral matter', white moisture, pus, and bloody matter. Such a flux, which was uncomfortable, itchy, even painful, was rarely a cause to consult the physician. Unless they came as a sudden hemorrhage, these running flows did not constitute an illness, especially if they were periodic.

A female relative of Storch's 'had a flux on her from her youth, which in the beginning showed itself only as a small rash under the nose . . . Beginning in her thirtieth year, this rash emerged below the breasts, but especially under the left breast . . . This flux occasionally also alternated with a light oozing of the navel. Whenever she felt it in either of these issues, she was well and healthy. But if it did not show itself on the outside she was usually costive and bound . . . In her fortieth year she came down with fits of the stone, and by her fiftieth year she had gathered a considerable accumulation of small and medium stones.

Different meaning clusters can be read from this case. From the viewpoint of evacuations, body regions were seen as similar by the women: the navel, the breasts, and a sore under the nose were the skin locations of a flux. The opposite to an external ooze was something hard, an accumulation of hard matter. Here the women spoke of a paradoxical inversion: the inner flow, if not drained off, engendered a hardening, a petrification; it was actually viscous and clogging. The flux discharged on the outside was a healthy one. The women were alarmed if an accustomed flow was 'striking inward', disappeared from the surface. The 'dried-up' flux caused anxiety. The term 'dry flux' expressed the darker side of the subterranean flux that seeped into the depths of the body and collected there. The experienced link between an externally invisible phenomenon and the real pains felt somewhere else attests a perception that was plagued not so much by what could be seen, touched, and felt as repulsive, as by its disappearance, a harbinger of an inner stagnation. What fueled the fear was not the discomfort of an evacuation, but the perception of the inner space as a space of induration and stoppage. The evil was inside, not outside. An absent flux, an obstructed evacuation of the body, were interpreted as the causes of later ailments. The women were afraid of driving a flow back.

> The wife of a shoemaker, forty years of age, 'has had an oozing and some-times foul-smelling sore under the breast for many years. Having dried up in February 1721, it moved to an untoward place, namely to the genitals, *ad muliebra*'.[2] The pains, especially when passing urine, were so intense that the woman tried to soothe them with cold washes. This bottled up the flux, upsetting the stomach and the guts, causing great anxiety in the stom-ach and the lower body. During the next years whenever the flux, having returned to its old place, dried up, she immediately requested help, 'for fear of dangerous ill effects'. Storch gave her sudorifics and a mustard plaster. She placed the plaster under her breast, it dissolved the skin, and already within an hour 'the flux could be lured out again, and the woman soon felt . . . relief.' This woman died thirteen years later, and the cause of death was this: after she had fallen down the cellar stairs, the flux under the breast subsided and failed to return, whereupon all the matter got stuck in her head.

To the women healing meant getting rid of the viscous and hardening matter inside of them. This attitude complicated a possible healing, since it implied a contradictory, nearly irreconcilable balancing act: get-ting rid of a pain on the outer surface could mean a 'repressing' or 'repelling' inside. The women wanted to get rid of pustules, rashes, scabs, sores, or measles. They asked the physician for prescriptions. But at the same time they were worried that these matters may be driven into the wrong direction. Between the felt internal flux and the visible external flux was the threat of the flux that had been pushed back inside.

> A woman in childbed consulted Storch about her fear that a 'recently expe-rienced pustule had been driven back inside'.

> Another woman in childbed had much vexation and distemper, since her unexpected early delivery indicated to all relatives that she must have begun 'congressus' prematurely. Because of this worry she developed a feverish rash, and not just the rash itself alarmed her, but also 'her imag-ining that the spots were being pushed inside'.

> A fourteen-year-old girl wanted to work in a noble household as a maid-servant. Anxious lest a red rash in the face thwart her plans, she drove it out by inducing salivation with a mercurial salve, 'without any preparation and purgation'. As a result she was 'now complaining of stopping in the breast and heavy limbs'. The treatment was aimed at luring the rash out.

---

[2] The female sexual parts.

In Storch's eyes, and no doubt also in the eyes of the women, the art of healing lay in supporting the external flow of impure, dirty, pustular matter until the body had been sufficiently cleansed. Storch believed that the home remedies used by the women were frequently harmful in this endeavor:

> A seventeen-year-old girl had been suffering for some time with wild fits and cramps. And whenever that happened her menses were stopped up. Storch reports: 'As I was inquiring about some cause or another, she remembered that some time ago she had a blistery flux on one hand, which she had cured with a plaster and in part had driven back with cold water while washing lace'.

Here a flux in the hand had been driven back; while the hand had been healed externally, the waste matter caused cramps inside. The girl and the physician made a connection between the healed hand and these cramps.

> A 'delicate, choleric woman' came to Eisenach, consulted the physician, and complained of 'persistent cold feet and legs, shortness of breath, and hot flashes'. On a later occasion 'she disclosed that she had had an oozing flux between the toes after confinement. She had cured it by sprinkling it with white lead powder, and she suspected that this flux had been driven back and was now manifesting itself inside. I agreed with her.'

> A woman was suffering from gout. She washed the painful limbs with well water and found relief thereby. But then she felt an 'oppressed breast' and 'noticed by herself that she had driven the gout pains back in with this washing.'

In his reflections and prescriptions the doctor picked up the women's concern, their fear of driving a flux back inside. He strove to prevent what, in medical terms, he called a 'repelling' of the flux. His aim was to support the flows gently, to guide them, and, if necessary, to lure them to the outside. To that end he used in particular blister plasters, *vesicatoria*,[3] and fontanels. A blister-raising plaster – of mustard, Spanish fly, or some such substance – helped above all to divert the flow, to redirect it, by attracting and drawing it out from a distance. It was applied to distant parts of the body and created a stimulus by causing pain. The fontanel (literally, 'small fountain') was an artificial wound that was kept open by a wide wick made of hair, a seton, to allow the continuous drainage of fluids.

> A woman clothseller, who was exposed to cold weather at the market and to dampness in the cellar while serving beer, suffered for years from an

---

[3] Ointments or plasters for raising blisters on the skin.

errant flow. Finally, after 'she had gotten through another attack', Storch advised her to let a fontanel be placed on her leg in order to prevent the flux from being driven back so often.

Fontanels and *vesicatorium* were answers to a flux that was causing torment inside, remedies prescribed by the doctor and administered by the surgeons or barber-surgeons. The surgeon induced on the skin no more than what the body itself should be doing and in many cases was doing. Fontanels and blister-plasters resembled the lichen, the so-called weeping exzema: 'Once a flux had taken up its permanent seat ... patience is the best remedy, since its presence preserves the body from debilitating attacks and takes the place of a fontanel'. The poorer women in Storch's practice complained about the natural sore. Aristo-cratic ladies were concerned with one more issue that could become dry: 'on the 21st', Storch noted in the case of one patient, 'I had to ... examine an old fontanel on her arm, which had much scar tissue and slough around it. Despite all precautions it was closing up and causing her a defluxion in the eyes and a stoppage of the nose'. The afflicted eyes did not improve until the old fontanel had been replaced by a new one on the foot. The remedy worked so well that the patient urgently requested to have an issue made on her other leg as well. Even an abscess, into which an artificial object was placed after it had been lanced in order to keep it open, became thus a kind of natural fontanel.

> A woman who had long suffered from a breast abscess, and whose wound had finally closed, was given the following advice by Storch: 'should she again be troubled by the stirrings of old fluxes, she should have them drawn off through a fontanel placed on one leg. But this abscess alone had cleansed her so thoroughly that she remained healthy for several years thereafter'.

Finally, one woman experiences such great floods of blood that she was nearly spent. Still she declined to take the prescribed remedies because 'she has come to believe that it is a flux which had been withdrawn into the body'.

8.2
Popular and learned theories of conception in early modern Britain

Angus McLaren, 'The Pleasures of Procreation: Traditional and Biomedical Theories of Conception' in W. F. Bynum and R. Porter (eds), *William Hunter and the Eighteenth-Century Medical World* (Cambridge, Cambridge University Press, 1985), pp. 332–40.

Angus McLaren has written extensively on the history of sexuality, fertility and contraception in Britain. In this extract, he discusses how new anatomical and physiological investigations into generation in the early modern period affected and transformed traditional and widely-accepted perceptions of sexuality, in particular the fundamental role of female pleasure in conception.

The variety of sources one can draw on to illustrate the continued vitality of Galenic ideas provides support for [the idea] . . . that until the seventeenth century there existed in England a common culture of procreational knowledge in which women's sexual pleasure was seen by both laymen and doctors as necessary for fecundity. In the seventeenth century this common culture was undermined. What one finds happening is that a new 'high' culture of scientific embryology emerged that severed the traditional linking of pleasure and procreation. What had been the common culture became the 'low' culture. As indicated by the reprintings of traditional works such as *Aristotle's Masterpiece*,[4] the older interpretations did not disappear, but they were increasingly viewed by the educated and respectable as aspects of the mind-set of the lewd and vulgar.

From the late sixteenth century onward, medical scientists who adopted the experimental method were faced with the problem of reconciling their new observations with the models of procreation set out by Aristotle, Hippocrates and Galen. The first discoveries were incorporated in the old model, but as enough contradictory evidence was accumulated it became necessary to construct a new paradigm. The dominant view of embryological development up until the sixteenth

---

[4] *Aristotle's master-piece* was an anonymous advice book on sex and sexuality that bore little relation to the actual work of Aristotle. It was first published in the late seventeenth century and, despite numerous changes and additions, remained enormously popular throughout the eighteenth century. It appeared in more editions than any other medical text.

century has been called epigenetic. That is, the idea was that all parts of the new creation developed sequentially. The weakness of the theory was that it did not satisfactorily explain how such a complicated process as the creation of life took place. A rival theory to that of epigenesis was that of preformation. . . .

[. . .]

. . . [P]reformation theories budded in the 1670s and blossomed in the first half of the eighteenth century. They presented an image of a monoparental embryo in which conception implied simply an enlargement of what was already there. There was no 'creation' *per se*. . . .

[. . .]

For our purposes what is most interesting is how the theories related to the role of the sexes. One finds that the animalculists[5] presented women as being little more than passive recipients of the male gift and returned them to their Aristotelian role of breeding machines. The ovist line of argument would appear at first glance to have been more 'feminist' inasmuch as it credited the mother with carrying preformed beings. In fact the ovists also portrayed the woman as playing a far more passive role than that attributed to her by the defenders of the old semence or two-seed theory. Previously it had been argued that the woman had to be aroused and delighted for conception to occur. Now it was stated that her active involvement was minimal. The sperm was active and the egg almost inert. The egg was presented by scientists as 'shaken' into life by the sperm or allowed by its intervention to 'escape' into the Fallopian tube. William Smellie,[6] for example, wrote: 'The *Ovum* being impregnated, is squeezed from its *Nidus*[7] or husk into the tube by the contraction of the *Fimbria*, and thus disengaged from its attachments to the *Ovarium*, is endowed with a circulating force by the *Animalculum*, which has a *vis vitae*[8] in itself'.

In the latter half of the eighteenth century there was a shift away from preformation theory and back to epigenetic views in large part because of unhappiness with the weaknesses of the former model. But there was no return to the theory of the double semence of two homogeneous

---

[5] Those who supported the view that a tiny being exists in the male semen which then grows into a baby during pregnancy.

[6] The Scot, William Smellie (1697–1763), was a celebrated man-midwife in eighteenth-century London, who published a popular compendium of his art entitled *A treatise on the theory and practice of midwifery* (3 vols, London, 1752–64).

[7] Literally, 'nest' in Latin.

[8] 'Power of life'.

fluids; rather one saw the elaboration of the idea of two distinct sorts of building blocks for the new creation. . . . [W]hat is important to note is that in stressing the idea of different male and female sex roles both preformation theories and the later more sophisticated epigenetic theories undercut the older notion of the necessity of both men and women experiencing sexual pleasure.

The common argument advanced in histories of science is that between the sixteenth and nineteenth centuries scholasticism slowly but surely gave way to empiricism. In analysing progress in embryological thought, however, we find that although a science emerged that was more accurate than Galen's in particulars – for example in demonstrating the differentiation of functions in male and female sexual organs – it did not give rise to a general explanation of procreation any more satisfying than that sketched out two thousand years before. Indeed the new explanation appeared in many ways impoverished inasmuch as it said less and less about the social and cultural aspects of sexuality that ordinary men and women assumed were of utmost importance.

Women's pleasure in sexuality had been traditionally justified on the grounds that their sexual organs were very much like men's. Men had to be aroused to ejaculate and it followed logically enough that women also had to experience pleasure if they were to produce seed. Modern science revealed that this was not so, that men and women were anatomically different, that the ovaries were not 'testicles' producing seed. . . . Theoretically there was no reason why such more accurate and detailed accounts of physiological fact should have led to a denigration of women's right to pleasure, but in fact they did.

The new embryological knowledge of the sperm and the egg – the one active and the other purportedly passive – led to new expectations, or was employed to rationalise new expectations, of differing male and female sexual experiences. . . .

[. . .]

. . . Procope-Couteau[9] asked [in the mid-eighteenth century] if it were not true that many women never felt pleasure in the sexual act. An anonymous author writing in 1789 asserted that pleasure was felt by few women but was in any event not necessary. Fodéré[10] informed his

[9] Michel Procope-Couteau (1684–1753) was Professor of Surgery at Paris and Montpellier and the author of various works including *L'art de faire des garçons, ou nouveau tableau de l'amore conjugal*, published posthumously at Montpellier in 1760.

[10] François Emmanuel Fodéré (1764–1835) was appointed to the chair of legal medicine at Strasbourg in 1814. In addition to writing an influential volume on medical jurisprudence, he wrote on scurvy, medical statistics and public health.

female patients that in place of passion, 'complaisance, tranquility, silence, and secrecy are necessary for a prolific coition'. By the mid-nineteenth century Dr Acton[11] was declaring:

There can be no doubt that sexual feelings in the female is in the majority of cases in abeyance . . . and even if raised (which in many instances it never can be) is very moderate compared with that of the male . . . As a general rule, a modest woman seldom desires any sexual gratification for herself. She submits to her husband, but only to please him and, but for the desire of maternity, would far rather be relieved from his attentions.

But patients apparently did not abandon old theories as quickly as did their doctors. In the 1860s Sims[12] complained that it was still:

. . . the vulgar opinion, and the opinion of many savants that, to ensure conception, sexual intercourse should be performed with a certain degree of completeness, that would give an exhaustive satisfaction to both parties at the same moment. How often do we hear husbands complain of coldness on the part of the wives; and attribute to this the failure to procreate. And sometimes wives are disposed to think, though they never complain, that the fault lies with the hasty ejaculation of the husband.

The new view of women – which held that as far as conception was concerned it was of no importance how indifferent or indeed hostile they might be to the sexual act – did result in one unexpected reform. In cases of rape nineteenth-century courts would no longer assume that the pregnancy of the victim implied her acquiescence. . . .

Thus in the medical literature one moved from the picture of the sexually active woman of the seventeenth century to the passionless creature of the nineteenth. Some have suggested that the rise of evangelical religion was responsible for the new stress on women's chastity, decorum and purity. Others have argued that doctors rather than priests played a key role in counselling moderation – that purity and suspicion of sexuality were exploited by physicians in order to enhance their positions as counsellors and confessors. Still others have suggested that the emergence of a new economic view of the world that lauded thrift, prudence and self-control necessarily negatively influenced sensual enjoyments. And finally some have argued that 'passionlessness'

---

[11] Dr William Acton (1813–75) was a celebrated Victorian gynaecologist and sexologist who wrote at length on medical issues concerned with reproduction, venereal diseases and prostitution.

[12] James Marion Sims (1813–83) was an American surgeon who specialised in gynaecology. After developing new techniques for dealing with vaginal fistulas while practising on slave women in Alabama, he moved to New York where he established the Women's Hospital, a major centre for gynaecological research.

was in part a strategy seized upon by women to protect themselves from male sexual demands, in particular in order to limit pregnancies but more generally as a way of allowing women at least a negative control over sexuality. The purpose of this essay has been to examine the role played in this evolution by medical scientists who were influenced by, but who also obviously influenced, the other participants in the debate over sexuality. The main argument of this work is that the rights of women to sexual pleasure were not enhanced, but eroded as an unexpected consequence of the elaboration of more sophisticated models of reproduction.

8.3

A midwife defends her reputation:
Louise Bourgeois (1627)

Louise Bourgeois, *Récit Veritable de la Naissance de Messeigneurs et Dames les Enfans de France, Fidelle Relation de l'Accouchement, Maladie et Ouverture du Corps de Feu Madame. Rapport de l'Ouverture du Corps de Feu Madame. Remonstrance à Madame Bourcier, touchant son Apologie*, ed. François Rouget (Geneva, Droz, 2000), pp. 99–108, 111–12, 118–19. Translation by Elizabeth Rabone.

Louise Bourgeois (1563–1636) first obtained a licence to practise midwifery in Paris in 1598. Thanks to skilful networking, she was appointed a royal midwife in 1601. Unusually, she published several books, including a textbook on midwifery. In 1627, she attended the delivery of Princess Marie de Bourbon, wife of Gaston d'Orleans and the king's sister-in-law, who died a week after parturition. Following a post mortem, Bourgeois was blamed by the physicians for the death of the princess. She wrote a powerful apology, in which she provided her account of the delivery, questioned the result of the autopsy, and argued for the midwife's competence in matters relating to the female body. Further attacks on her reputation followed, and she was finally forced to end her career at court. The first extract is from Bourgeois' own account. The second is taken from the physicians' response to her, and was very probably written by the royal surgeon Charles Guillemeau (1588–1656).

(i)

A true account of the childbirth, illness and autopsy of the late Princess Marie de Bourbon

I, the undersigned, Louise Bourgeois known as Bourcier, midwife to the Queen Mother and the late Marie de Bourbon, having seen a printed report of the dissection performed on the corpse of the Princess, written by the doctors who attended the Princess during her illness, to justify the treatment they gave her, and to blame me for her death, I believed it was my duty to make the truth known, about both the birth and the illness and to show very clearly that the cause of death was in no way caused by the alleged portion of the placenta.

Throughout the pregnancy, Marie de Bourbon was extremely ill. She often suffered from a high temperature, hot flushes, nosebleeds and a cough in the later months, for which she was bled three times. Before she went into labour she had a high temperature, which did not abate during the birth. The birth itself, thanks be to God, was quite easy, as regards the delivery of both the baby and the placenta, which was whole and healthy. The placenta was seen and examined by Jacques de la Cuisse,[13] a master surgeon with a wide experience of childbirth, and by the attending doctors, Mr. Vautier,[14] Mr Seguin,[15] Mr Le Maistre,[16] Mr Tournaire,[17] Mr Brunier,[18] and Mr Guillemeau,[19] all of whom noticed and acknowledged that the placenta was whole and healthy. I swear on my life that this is true.

For this alleged small portion of the placenta, *so strongly attached to the uterus that it could not be separated from it by hand without difficulty,*[20] is not part of the placenta, but the place to which the mass of flesh commonly known as the afterbirth was attached. This place always stays larger and more prominent than the rest of the inner sur-

[13] A celebrated obstetrician.

[14] François Vautier (1580–1652) was advisor and first physician to the Queen Mother. He later became premier physician to the young Louis XIV.

[15] Pierre Seguin (d. 1648) came from a family of doctors and rose to the pinnacle of his profession, being appointed royal professor of surgery in 1594, and of medicine in 1599. Originally one of the physicians to Louis XIII, he sold his post in order to become first physician to Queen Anne of Austria in 1623.

[16] Rodolphe Le Maistre was physician to Gaston of Orleans.

[17] François Tornaire was physician to Marie de Bourbon Montpensier.

[18] Abel Brunier was physician to Gaston of Orleans.

[19] Charles Guillemeau (1588–1656) served as surgeon to two royal masters from 1601 to 1643, being created first surgeon by Louis XIII in 1627.

[20] Bourgeois here cites the physicians' report, which she is attempting to refute. All further italicised material is from the same source.

face of the uterus until all the matter has been expelled from the uterus, because it is where the blood vessels in the uterus end and where they have been joined with the baby's umbilical vessels. This swelling, which is made of the very same substance as the uterus, was wickedly mistaken for part of the placenta. The placenta is only a soft flesh like clotted blood. It cannot adhere so tightly to the uterus lining and harden in such a way that it has to be cut away with difficulty, and using a razor, as it did with Marie de Bourbon, at the same time as the blood is continuously flowing out of the uterus (as it did in the case of Marie de Bourbon). . . .

[. . .]

. . . You should also have reported whether this portion of alleged placenta (that you had so much difficulty separating with your fingers from the right side of the uterus) was rotten, so that it could have given *gangrene to the left side and the part above the rectum*. In your report you show that you know nothing about a woman's placenta and uterus either before or after she gives birth, no more so than your Mr Galien,[21] who never having been married and hardly ever present at a birth, attempted to teach a midwife using a book, which he wrote for that purpose and made it clear that he had never known the uterus or even the placenta of a pregnant woman.

To further prove to you that what I am telling you is the truth, I will offer to prove it in the Hôtel Dieu[22] on the bodies of the women who die by the dozen in childbirth.[23] And what's more, I will submit to the judgement of the doctors and surgeons, with their knowledge of anatomy (as long as they are not united together in a clique, which is potentially very harmful to medicine), who, without passion but according to their conscience and their knowledge will judge your report and mine. I am quite certain that I shall be absolved of all blame, and that you will be proved to be wrong, and that it will not be the unfortunate uterus falsely accused of gangrene that was the cause of death, but an inflammation of all the internal organs of the lower stomach. *According to your report the whole of the lower stomach was filled with fetid, bloodied matter and the uterus itself was swimming in this matter*. Such a great quantity of matter could only come from the inflamed, and ultimately gangrenous, veins and internal organs inside the stomach from which all the serous fluid in the blood had seeped. This is the opinion

---

[21] Galen.

[22] A hospital for the poor in Paris.

[23] In the original, 'meurent dans la huictaine'; literally, 'die in their eights'.

expressed by Dr Riolan[24] in the presence of the King, the Queen Mother, and Cardinal Richelieu, that the cause of death (which by then could not be prevented) was the gangrene formed in the internal organs of the lower stomach. The Princess's stomach was stretched taut like a drum and as large as if she had not given birth. Dr Riolan judged there to be no tautness in the uterus area, and the other doctors present agreed. I will add that the Princess, from the time she gave birth up to her death, had a flow from the stomach of greenish, almost black, bile, which clearly shows that her entrails were very hot and rotting. Such matter passing through the large intestines caused this deterioration that you notice *on the part of the uterus above the rectum*. It would have been more truthful to say above the large intestine.

If you had been intending to make an honest report, with the good intention of publicising the truth, you would not have omitted comments that should go in a report, nor would you have implied untruths. You should, in the first place, have described the excessively large size of the lower stomach, both before and after death, which is evidence of the gangrene in the lower stomach, which means there is inflammation, which did not form in twenty-four hours. You should also have mentioned the colour and consistency of the organs, which is what changes during illness, and which is how one knows for certain the cause of a death. Either you do not know the natural colour and consistency of organs, to be able to see the change; or it went against your arguments not to admit the inflammation and gangrene in the internal organs. What is the purpose of noting *the largeness and smallness of the ventricle, the liver, the vesicle of bile, the spleen, the kidneys and the bladder* (everyone's bladder is small when it is empty), while saying nothing of their colour and consistency? And not even mentioning the size of the uterus, of which you should have made special mention. *You observed healthy lungs, with no sign of adherence to the ribs, and the brain with no defect.* You should have said whether the lower parts of the stomach were healthy or damaged, which you didn't dare touch, because your consciences did not permit it. If your intention had been to publicise the truth, you should have been accompanied by other doctors [at the dissection], who were impartial in this matter, or the King's doctors, so that you were not the only participants involved in such an

[24] Jean Riolan the younger (1580–1657), a celebrated physician and the son of an even more renowned medic, Jean Riolan the elder, who died in 1610, and with whom Bourgeois had worked as is evident from book 1 of her *Observations diverses sur la sterilité, perte de fruict, fœcondité, accouchements et maladies des femmes, et enfants nouveaux naiz* (*Several observations on sterility, abortion, fecundity, deliveries and female complaints, and new born children*) (Paris, 1609–26).

important business. I am certain that there are good people, with great knowledge of such matters, who would never have tolerated the allegations about the placenta, which had been tried and found guilty before the dissection in order to blame me entirely for the death. . . .

I am neither so wicked, nor so ignorant of the profession I have been following in this city and at the court for thirty-four years, honourably and loyally, as can be seen from the good results I have achieved and from the books I have written on the subject, which have been reprinted several times and translated into all sorts of languages, and earned the gratitude of the greatest doctors in Europe, who have benefitted from reading my books, that if I had realised that I had left some part of the placenta [in the uterus], then I would have said something to remedy this. Alternatively, if I had still not noticed it (although it is quite easy to see when you inspect the placenta) I would within twenty-four hours have found it by the bleeding, which always happens to women when part of the placenta has not been expelled. . . .

If you allege that the late Princess, on the fourth day of her confinement, expelled some small membranes as fine as a cobweb, which could be a small part of the amniotic or chorion membranes,[25] I will reply with what I am told that Hippocrates (who was very knowledgeable about women's illnesses, as testified by the many books he wrote on the subject) noted in Book Two of the *Epidemics*,[26] that the wife of a tanner, on the fourth day after she successfully gave birth, discharged part of a membrane without any ill effect. This great doctor wanted to record for posterity that this is neither dangerous nor significant.

Never has it been witnessed, or written by any good author, that a small piece of dried, unrotted placenta attached to the uterus was a cause of death. I read in Paul of Aegina's *Surgery*[27] that a doctor should not be surprised if a woman does not discharge the placenta, as some women expel them in pieces or rotted down four or five days after giving birth. I am told that a great surgeon and anatomist, *ab Aquapendente*,[28] is of the same opinion and that he saw several women expel a

[25] Internal and external membranes which surround the foetus.

[26] Bourgeois is referring to Book 2 of the *Epidémies* (*On epidemics*), section II, article 17, where Hippocrates reports that a woman expelled a portion of chorion membrane four days after she gave birth.

[27] Paul of Aegina was an ancient Greek surgeon whose works were first published in Greek in 1528. Book 6 only was translated into French in 1539. In it (section LXXV) he refers to the delivery of the placenta and the difficulties sometimes encountered with this operation. He says it is not a cause for concern if the placenta cannot be removed as it will drop of its own accord after a few days.

[28] For Hieronymus Fabricius (1537–1619), whose works on surgery were first published in Latin in 1617 and French in 1649, see extract 3.6 above.

fragmented or rotten placenta, and survive. You are wrong to attribute the cause of death to this little piece of placenta that you claim to have found. You should rather refer to the continuous high temperature, both before and after the delivery, and the cough, which caused the Princess great distress, and the discharge from the stomach, which happened too soon after the birth. These three illnesses are very dangerous to a woman who has just given birth and you should pay more careful attention to them. But to know about women's illnesses, it is necessary to have worked with midwives and to have been present at births, as your great master and legislator Hippocrates did. He consulted midwives about women's illnesses and relied on their judgement. That is all I have to say at present to defend and justify myself against lies and libels, which are damaging to my reputation, which I submit to the arbitration of the doctors of Paris and others who are fit to pass judgement and impartial, and such as it pleases their Majesties to order.

Paris, the eighth of June, 1627

Louise Bourgeois, known as Bourcier.

(ii)

Remonstrance to Madame Bourcier about her 'Apology' against the report the doctors wrote on the cause of the terrible death of Marie de Bourbon

I admit, Madame Bourcier, that you published your 'Apology' for a very powerful reason. For if you were so unfortunate as to find that in some way you were responsible for the death of our great princess, the most painful death we could inflict on you would not be a severe enough punishment. ... For if you had examined your misconduct on this deplorable subject, you would have published nothing but regrets and tears; and if you had considered in a mature way the doctors' report and the just unhappiness of all good French people at the great loss this death has caused them, you would have spent the rest of your life without speaking, rather than admitting as you do (by thinking of accusing the doctors of carelessness) that this great princess was not as well cared for as she should have been. ...

Consider these things, Madame Bourcier, and be content within the limits of your duties; don't bother yourself any more with taking over [the work of] doctors. For you are neither responsible for their actions nor are you qualified to judge them. The misfortunes which have happened to you too often while you are exercising your profession, and

218

even this latest one which is so deplorable, are testimony enough to your limitations, without you taking the trouble to write it down; content yourself with having shown these limitations to us, to our great pity, and do not publish this abroad. For you could not do that without offending all those of your fellow French people who hold you in any good esteem. Do not glory in the name of midwife or act as one. See what can be drawn from your presumption and from your writings and do not speak so arrogantly against men who are more experienced and more successful than you are in your profession, if you do not want to be blamed by everyone who sees, by the relative success of your affairs and those of whom you are attempting to blame, the exact opposite of what you are saying.

[. . .]

. . . Madame Bourcier says that the Princess gave birth quite easily. A first child is not born without great difficulty, principally to she who was of a delicate disposition, full of courage and determination. She was ill from 4 o'clock in the morning until 10 o'clock, by which time she had strained quite powerfully and this is when the aforementioned Bourcier should have been careful because of the cough, lungs, and continued high temperature that she says the Princess had; it was not enough to say 'be brave your Highness', she should have watched the time and assisted the Princess appropriately and gently. After the Princess had delivered her baby, she spent three quarters of an hour pushing to expel the placenta, but this was extremely difficult. They made her swallow raw eggs, put her fingers in her mouth and push, treating her as roughly as you would treat the wife of a poor ploughman. They pressed on her stomach and uterus, without thinking what the use of so much force could do to such a sensitive, delicate Princess. She had pain on her left side, where the pressure and bruising had been greatest; the debonair yet listless Princess kept her hand there. She was showing where she hurt and referring to the pain she felt. They did not stop bandaging her stomach ever tighter with compresses, without considering the pain she was in. What is more, I was told that several days later a certain trainee put their hand even more roughly into the gangrenous area in an attempt to pull out the remains of the placenta, although he had been told beforehand that it had all been expelled. If this is true, I say that it would not be possible to invent any sort of worse treatment. And so what happened next? Swelling; the area became inflamed. The bandage tightened and compressed and choked the natural heat, in such a way that gangrene set in on the outside and the inside. It should be noted, however, that there was no gangrene at the point where the little piece of placenta was still attached, but there was on the left side, where the patient felt continuous pain. Because the attendant did not notify the doctors in time, they could not bring the appropriate remedy, so the gangrene gradually increased and caused the death of the wonderful Princess. France will mourn for eternity for the gentleness and charity God so perfectly bestowed upon her.

8.4

The clientele of London midwives in the second half of the seventeenth century

Doreen Evenden, 'Mothers and their Midwives in Seventeenth-Century London' in Hilary Marland (ed.), *The Art of Midwifery. Early Modern Midwives in Europe* (London, Routledge, 1993), pp. 9–19.

Early modern midwives were among the most ubiquitous of medical practitioners and have recently become the focus of much research. Historians are now beginning to tap a range of hitherto unexplored archival evidence which has allowed them to reconstruct the practice, careers and relationships with clients enjoyed by midwives. The following extract is based on Doreen Evenden's analysis of the testimonials written for midwives seeking a licence to practise in addition to an anonymous midwife's unpublished book of accounts.

Hundreds of midwives' testimonial certificates provide the best surviving evidence of the ecclesiastical licensing process in seventeenth-century London and information about the midwives' clientele. These documents were presented to church authorities by aspiring midwifery licensees residing in the metropolis of London and its environs. In addition to the ecclesiastical sources, which also include bishops' and archbishops' registers, the records of an anonymous London midwife who went about her work of child delivery in the waning years of the seventeenth and the early part of the eighteenth centuries (1694–1723) supplement the more impersonal church records at several junctures. A careful examination of these records has permitted insights into the work of London midwives with regard to what we have called 'repeat business', the geographical distribution of their practices, the social standing of their clients, and the client and midwife referral 'system'. . . .

[. . .]

The evidence for repeat business is derived from both testimonial certificates provided by satisfied clients and the anonymous midwife's account book. Testimonial documentation in some cases specified the number of children the midwife had already delivered for the referee; for the year 1662 testimonials for all twenty-four successful candidates recorded the number of children they had delivered for each of the women testifying on their behalf. The account book provides information on the number of deliveries per client, thus giving a reasonable indication of the relationships which existed in late Stuart London between a midwife and her clients. It demonstrates that the midwife routinely carried out her work to the satisfaction of many of her clients who continued to use her services throughout their childbearing years.

[. . .]

The testimonial evidence sheds light on the extent of repeat business at only a single point in the ongoing relationship between a midwife and a client: the time of an application for licensing. It could be expected that the reliance of many of these women upon a particular midwife would continue, and thus that the actual extent of repeat business would exceed the figures [revealed by this research]. A general pattern is discernible, confirmed by the account book of the, as yet, unidentified midwife which covers the years 1694 to 1723.[29] During that period, this active midwife attended over 376 clients, more than one-third of whom she delivered several times. . . .

The majority of Mistress X's clients expressed a high level of confidence in her skills by summoning her repeatedly when they were brought to bed, and they freely recommended her services to other family members. Mrs Page, who used her services three times, told her sister about the midwife who then also became a client. Mrs Duple of Blackfriars was delivered by Mistress X six times between 1703 and 1714; her sister became a client in 1704 and 1706. One of our midwife's most fecund clients, Mrs Dangerfield of Whitechapel, first used her services in July 1699. By March 1712 she had called upon the midwife nine times. Dangerfield's trust in and reliance on her midwife's skills undoubtedly influenced her own sister who became a client of Mistress X in 1713. . . .

---

[29] Hereafter referred to by the author as 'Mistress X'.

The women of the socially prominent and wealthy Barnardiston family showed a similar satisfaction with the midwife's abilities. Six Barnardiston women used her services on a regular basis. . . .

Since several of the anonymous midwife's clients were themselves the daughters of women who had been brought to bed by the midwife, there is every possibility that Mistress X was attending women whom she had brought into the world, a remarkable tribute to the level of confidence and personal rapport she enjoyed. For example, Mrs Tabram of Butcher's Hall Lane was delivered by the midwife four times from 1697; 20 years later, our midwife delivered 'Ms. Tabram's daughter' who was living in Chapter House Lane. Altogether at least nine daughters of former clients were brought to bed by the popular midwife. Two clients, Mrs Maret and Mrs Benet, summoned Mistress X when their serving women gave birth. . . .

London midwives did not restrict their practices to the parish in which they lived, a fact which has hitherto eluded students of seventeenth-century London midwifery, leading to the assumption that midwives carried out too few deliveries to gain the experience necessary for competence. . . . [T]he abundant evidence that midwives seeking licences normally provided references from satisfied clients beyond the boundaries of their own parish demonstrates that, even at that point in their professional career, London midwives practised over a large geographical area. Rose Cumber, licensed in [1610], presented sworn testimony from women who resided in [the parishes of] St Swithin and St Andrew Holborn although she herself resided in St Bridgid Fleet Street. Elizabeth Martin of St Giles Cripplegate called on only one client from her home parish in 1626 when she applied for her licence; women from St Antholin, St Dunstan in the West, St Martin in the Fields and St Michael Pater Noster added their testimonies. In 1629, Alice Carnell of St Dunstan in the West was licensed after presenting evidence from clients, none of whom resided in her parish. . . .

The account book of our unidentified London midwife, Mistress X, demonstrates a similar mobility and geographical diversity of practice. Although addresses were not recorded in every case, clients from at least thirty parishes within the city walls claimed her services. But these formed only a part of her practice: in the years covered by her records the busy and popular midwife travelled far beyond the confines of the City. To the east, she journeyed to Leytonstone, Spitalfields and Whitechapel where she attended, among others, Mrs Dangerfield in her numerous confinements; to the north, to the area of Finsbury Fields and the northern reaches of the vast ward of Cripplegate Without; to the west, she delivered women in the Strand, the Haymarket and Drury

Lane. Among her clients on the South Bank was the prosperous Mrs Sims who was brought to bed five times by the peripatetic midwife. Mistress X's practice encompassed not only the City but almost all of suburban London north of the River Thames as well as Southwark. Her sprawling practice is all the more remarkable in view of the backward state of intra-metropolitan communications. At the same time as the anonymous midwife was travelling ill-lit streets to the numerous nighttime confinements which she recorded, one visitor commented that the city was 'a great vast wilderness' in which few were familiar with even a quarter of its streets. In the last year of recorded practice, most of Mistress X's deliveries were in the East End of London or its eastern suburbs, probably close to where the midwife resided. It can be suspected that the shrinking catchment area was a result of ill health or old age. Though there is no way of determining how representative Mistress X was, it is absolutely certain that very few, if any, licensed midwives (of whom more than nine hundred have been uncovered) restricted their practice to a single parish.

There is no evidence that midwives advertised their skills by means of printed advertisements. Word of mouth recommendation by satisfied clients living close to one another apparently played a key role in establishing pockets of women who used the midwife's services, and may explain some of the cases which lay at the geographical periphery of the practice of Mistress X. Mrs Rowden of Drury Lane employed her in March and less than six weeks later a client from nearby Tower Street called on her. On 29 October 1707, Mrs Nicolls of St Martin's Street was delivered; a few days later, on 7 November, Mrs Hampton of the same street called the midwife to her delivery; a month later, Mrs Wood, also of St Martin's Street, was delivered of an infant daughter by Mistress X. Mrs Field and Mrs Hobkins, both of Aldgate Street, were delivered within three days of each other. Also delivered within three days of one another were Mrs Duple's sister (referred by Mrs Duple) and her neighbour, the shoemaker's wife in Swan Yard.

Testimonial evidence suggests that female clients on occasion sought a midwife on the basis of recommendations by women whose husbands were employed in the same craft or trade as that of the prospective father. For example . . . Winnifred Allen of St Andrew Wardrobe enlisted the wives of three tailors from two different parishes when she applied for a licence, and Elizabeth Davis of St Katherine Cree Church supplied the names of three women (one of whom had used her services six times), all of whom were married to men employed in the exclusive goldsmith trade. . . . In the case of Eleanor Stanfro of the parish of St Leonard Shoreditch, where a large number of weavers made their home, parochial and occupational links converged; four of the six testimonial clients from her home parish were married to weavers. Seamen's wives also apparently referred their midwives to other women whose husbands were similarly engaged. All six of Elizabeth Willis's clients, all three of Mary Salmon's, and all four of Sara Griffin's were married to seafaring men.

Out of the fifty-three testimonials which gave occupational designations for clients' husbands in 1663, thirteen or almost 25 per cent demonstrated similar occupations for two or more spouses. Similarly, in the years 1696–1700, out of the forty testimonials which declared occupations, twelve, or 30 per cent, gave the same occupation for at least two of the women's husbands. Although Mistress X seldom recorded occupational information for spouses, among the few instances where she has done so, we have two examples which confirm testimonial evidence of occupational links between clients of individual midwives. In 1704 the midwife 'laid' two shoemakers' wives within five weeks of one another; similarly, in 1715, two tailors' wives were delivered less than five weeks apart, one of whom lived in the Minories and the other at a considerable distance to the west in the Strand.

The existence of other networks between women and their clients can be traced in the testimonials. Mary DesOrmeaux, wife of Daniel, a jeweller of St Giles in the Fields, was a member of the French church in the Savoy (home of the Huguenot congregation) when she applied for a midwifery licence in 1680. All five women who gave sworn testimony on her behalf were French immigrants. . . . It is apparent, and understandably so, that, whenever possible, female immigrants turned to midwives of their own nationality, who spoke the same language and shared the same cultural heritage, to assist them when they were brought to bed. . . .

The authors of two studies of midwifery and gynaecology in the early modern period have both concluded that women turned to male midwives because they believed that male practitioners could offer them better care. If this was the case, women of the upper echelons of seventeenth-century London society could reasonably be expected to be among the first to desert the traditional midwife and seek the services of the male midwife. The evidence, however, points to a different conclusion. Wives of London gentlemen continued to use the services of midwives well into the next century, as both testimonials and the anonymous midwife's account book demonstrate.

Midwives applying for licences frequently included the name of a gentlewoman among those giving sworn testimony on their behalf. . . .

[. . .]

An indication of the continuing loyalty of gentry women to their midwives can be found in testimonial evidence at the end of the century. Of
seventy-five testimonials presented to the vicar general for the City of
London in the years 1690–1700, sixty-five contain occupational and
status designations. Of 198 possible designations, fourteen husbands
were listed as members of the gentry. Thus, 7 per cent of the women
supporting the midwives' applications were from the upper level of
society. The testimonials preserved in the Lambeth Palace archives
were analysed separately for the purposes of comparison. Of the sixty-
two testimonials which survive for the years 1669–1700, fifty included
occupational information. Out of a possible 174 designations, twenty-
three spouses were named as 'gentleman' (over 13 per cent). This
would indicate that midwives who sought licences from the jurisdiction
of the Archbishop of Canterbury, rather than the jurisdiction of the
Bishop of London, not only drew their clientele from a more influential
and affluent sector of society, but that this elevated group continued to
use the services of the midwife.

[. . .]

In seeking referees, midwives quite possibly looked to respectable
members of society, and the evidence from the testimonials is not necessarily representative of their practices as a whole. The practice of
Mistress X, however, reflects the range of clientele listed in testimonials – indeed her accounts suggest higher levels of employment by the
well-to-do. Her account book makes a clear distinction regarding the
status of clients: women from the lower and middle class are designated 'Ms' or 'mistress', while women of the upper ranks of society are
given the more respectful form of address 'madam'. We are, therefore,
able to identify a sizeable segment of her clientele, which was largely
made up of the wives of men of prestige and affluence. Although there
is a very close connection between the size of the fee charged by the
midwife and social designation, there are indications that occasionally
the courtesy title of 'madam' was extended more for social than economic reasons. Madam Andrews of St Bartholomew Lane, for example,
paid less for her deliveries, £1 14s. and £1 16s., than many a 'mistress'
among the midwife's clients.

Our anonymous midwife identified no fewer than twenty of her
clients as 'madam' and in addition delivered a lady. Lady Clarke paid £6
in 1720 when she was delivered of a daughter. These twenty-one
women, several of whom were extremely fertile, accounted for roughly

9 per cent of the busy midwife's practice and provide some support for the argument that midwives were not deserted in favour of male practitioners by women of substance at the turn of the century. On one of the last folios of the casebook, the names of Lady Shaw, Lady Clarke, Arthur Barnardiston (a wealthy merchant), Samuel Barnardiston, John Barnardiston and Lady Barnardiston appear, indicating the elite status of a section of Mistress X's clientele.

At the other end of the social scale, we find evidence that midwives remained faithful to their oath which required that they not discriminate between rich and poor women who were in need of their services. Susan Kempton's testimonial (signed by her vicar) stated that 'she is not only helpfull to the rich and those that can pay her but also to the poore'. Individual parishes frequently assumed responsibility for paying for the delivery of poor women of the parish and also of vagrant women who could not be removed from the parish before they gave birth. . . .

8.5

The making of the man-midwife: the impact of cultural and social change in Georgian England

Adrian Wilson, *The Making of Man-Midwifery: Childbirth in England 1660–1770* (London, UCL Press, 1995), pp. 185–92.

The replacement of female midwives by trained man-midwives in the eighteenth century has been traditionally regarded as one further episode in the gradual improvement of medical practice at the end of the early modern period. Here, the main engines of change are perceived as the circulation of new ideas about nature and the application of a new 'scientific' approach to medicine. Women were the passive recipients of these new trends. In this work, Adrian Wilson challenges this reconstruction and, by exploring how the experience of giving birth was gradually transformed, offers a stimulating reappraisal of this older interpretation, in which he links new fashions in medical practice to broader social and economic changes taking place in women's lives in the eighteenth century.

[H]ow did men come to play the role of midwives? The answer to that question . . . lies in the wider sphere to which childbirth was closely tied: the lives of women. What we must remember is that the traditional role of the midwife was embedded in the collective culture of women. It was the ceremony of childbirth that conferred authority on the mid-wife; the mother's personal choice extended only to the selection of *which* midwife, of those locally available, would deliver her. What gave the ritual itself its immense power was collective female authority, which transcended the whims and wishes of the individual mother: hence the importance of the gossips[30] in the management of childbirth. Mothers, midwives and gossips were bound together by the same web of social bonds that constituted the collective culture of women in general. That culture was made possible by the range of experiences and activities shared by mothers of all social ranks. The basis of this shar-ing was the patriarchal order, that is, the laws and customs that con-ferred upon husbands property in the sexuality, the goods and the labour of their wives. Even the aristocratic wife was subsumed within this order; all women found themselves bound by it. Hence the fact that the relatively humble midwife could assert power over a mother who belonged to the ruling class.

Surely the midwife can only have been displaced from the role if the collective culture of women fragmented. And in fact there are grounds for believing that the old culture did indeed break up during the first half of the eighteenth century. Wealthy mothers began to detach them-selves from their humbler sisters and to construct a new cultural space – most conspicuously in London but also elsewhere. After about 1750 there were two distinct cultures of women: the old, traditional, *oral* cul-ture, characteristic of the lower orders, and a new, fashionable, *literate* culture, the culture of 'the ladies', visible among the aristocracy and the wealthy middle classes.

The two hallmarks of this new female culture were literacy and leisure – of which literacy is far easier to document. In the period 1680 to 1730, women in London acquired writing literacy (visible to the his-torian as the ability to sign their names) to a degree that probably had no historical precedent, and certainly had none in England. Over 50% of London women were able to sign by 1730; the rate had more than dou-bled in 50 years. . . . Still more widespread – although by how much more is difficult to assess – was the ability to read. Not surprisingly, this transformation was reflected in the creation of a new literature, written both *for* women and increasingly *by* women. Almanacs for women

---

[30] Godparents.

appeared as early as the 1680s; in the 1690s the *Athenian Mercury* popularized Newton's new natural philosophy, with women among its audience; and a host of similar initiatives followed in the early eighteenth century. The high point of these developments was of course the novel – a new literary form that emerged in this period and was intimately bound up with women, as readers, as subject-matter, and increasingly as authors. . . .

[. . .]

I suggest that together, literacy and leisure began to break the bonds that had united women in a common culture. As long as the middle-class wife was engaged in manual labour, she shared a certain set of experiences with her fellow women far down the social scale. And so long as female literacy was relatively low, the literate/literary woman was individualized and uncommon – whence the tendency for mid-wives, who were local leaders of women, to be endowed with literacy. But as female literacy expanded, accompanied by an increased degree of leisure, there became possible a new collective culture of women: the culture of 'the ladies', that is, a culture distinct both from that of their husbands and from that of humbler women. . . . By the mid-eighteenth century the educated woman is a far commoner phenomenon, and although she remains constrained by the patriarchal order, isolation is not her main problem. She now belongs to active circles of collective literary involvement, and even the men (Samuel Richardson, Henry Fielding, Samuel Johnson) recognize something of her worth. And as the literary lady made new companions, so she detached herself from the traditional, oral, collective culture – once the collective culture of all women, now that of the lower orders of women. . . .

[. . .]

Nevertheless, the new female culture retained, or constructed, a certain degree of independence from men and . . . it preserved some aspects of the older oral culture. The dilemma facing the eighteenth-century 'lady' was precisely that of maintaining simultaneously a female identity and an identity of gentility. There were many different responses to this challenge; those that are best known and most accessible are of course those of the women writers who now emerged as a major cultural force. It would require a vast research enterprise to reconstruct the corresponding responses among the much wider circle of their readers. Even more interesting would be a study of the complex interplay between the changing reality of women's lives and the equally changing content and form of literature itself, above all, of the novel. Literature simultaneously reflected, deflected and informed the lives of its readers. One indication of this is the highly popular epistolary form. There seems to be a continuum between the epistolary novel (Delariviere Manley, Eliza Haywood, Samuel Richardson), the published correspondence (Mary Delaney), the 'private' letter written with an eye to later publication (as one suspects of many of Mrs Delaney's letters), the personal letter that circulated extensively in manuscript (as happened with some of the letters of Lady Mary Montagu) and, finally, the genuinely private letter, written only for the eyes of a single reader, yet in all probability powerfully influenced in style and in content by published epistolary models. It was precisely this complex connection between life and art that was displayed in the novel, with its conventions of verisimilitude, character, plot, and intimate involvement of the reader. More generally, it was the new female reading public that actually called forth the novel; and the leading male novelists (Richardson, Fielding) were keenly aware of both their female readers and their female authorial colleagues.

[. . .]

Hitherto, childbirth had been the great leveller – in several interlocking ways. It had physically brought together women of different social ranks. It had exposed the aristocratic lady and the cottager's wife to the same risks of illness and even death. With its inevitable blood and pain, it vividly contradicted the phrase 'gentle birth' used to describe the origins of members of the landed classes. And in subordinating the lady to the midwife, it had ceaselessly reminded that lady that she was, for all her pretensions to rank and breeding, a woman like other women; manual labour she might eschew, delegating this to servants, but labour in its other sense, that of childbirth, remained her inescapable lot. As long as women's traditional collective culture remained intact across all social classes, childbirth retained this levelling quality. And surely this was why the man-midwife was so attractive to those wealthy and literate women who by about 1750 had collectively constructed a new female culture. The male practitioner was a midwife who was not a midwife, a childbirth practitioner who stepped into the midwife's shoes and yet differed in all other respects from the traditional female midwife. The midwife, by her very presence – whatever her actual deportment – served as a tangible reminder that ladies were mere women. But the man-midwife offered proof of their superior social status: who but ladies could afford the 10 guineas that William Hunter[31] charged for

---

[31] William Hunter (1718–83) trained under William Cullen at Glasgow before setting up as a private lecturer in anatomy, surgery and obstetrics in London, where he trained some of the leading practitioners of the late eighteenth century.

deliveries? The putative skills of the male practitioner, we may venture, went to support this: whatever the real distribution of skill between male and female practitioners, the ladies doubtless assured themselves that exclusive fees meant exclusive technical abilities. Mentally, therefore, they detached themselves from the dangers of childbirth – a further separation from their less fortunate sisters.

In these terms we can begin to understand the role of 'fashion' in giving momentum to man-midwifery. It has always been alleged that fashion played a crucial part in the making of the man-midwife, but . . . such explanations beg the question as to how this process got started. Set in the context of the new split in women's culture, this ceases to be mysterious. Fashion was in general the symbolic reflection of the new culture of class; in the world of women, for which childbirth was so crucial, fashion dictated the need for the man-midwife. In the same moment as it effected a separation between social ranks, fashion offered a bridge by which those of intermediate or ambiguous status could symbolically climb the ranks and 'ape the quality'. The artisan's wife might not be able to afford a carriage, but every couple of years she could afford a man-midwife. Man-midwifery thus became an area of conspicuous consumption; the new men-midwives cashed in, and the loser was of course the traditional midwife, who saw draining away her most lucrative sphere of practice.

Part nine

The care and cure of the insane in early modern Europe

9.1

Madness in early modern England: the casebooks of Richard Napier

Michael MacDonald, *Mystical Bedlam: Madness, Anxiety, and Healing in Seventeenth-Century England* (Cambridge, Cambridge University Press, 1981), pp. 33–54, 160–4.

The Reverend Richard Napier (1559–1634) was educated at Oxford, where he proceeded B.A. in 1584 and M.A. in 1586. He served as fellow of Exeter College from 1580 to 1590, and in the latter year was appointed rector of Great Linford in Buckinghamshire, a post which he held until his death in 1634. During this period, he also operated as a medical practitioner and astrologer, dispensing advice and cures to thousands of patients from the surrounding area. Fortunately, Napier's casebooks survive and form the basis of the magisterial survey conducted by the historian, Michael MacDonald, into popular and learned perceptions of madness and mental anxiety in early seventeenth-century England.

In the first extract, MacDonald discusses the demography of madness, paying particular attention to the distribution of Napier's patients with respect to gender, age, and marital and social status. In the second, he discusses a particular aspect of the mental anxiety exhibited by Napier's clientele, namely their susceptibility to mopishness and melancholy.

(i)

On one point common wisdom and medical science agreed in the seventeenth century. The likelihood that a man or woman would succumb to madness or melancholy depended upon both physiological predisposition and environmental stress. Some people were more apt to 'take grief' or fear than others, and some circumstances were so oppressive that not even the most stolid soul could remain untroubled. Contemporaries also recognized that the physical differences between the sexes and the bodily changes effected by aging caused men and women to be vulnerable to different afflictions at various stages in their lives. . . .

[. . .]

. . . Medical authorities, emphasizing physiological differences more than social circumstances, remarked that mental disturbances were most common among young males and people who were middle-aged or old. . . . Some social groups, such as indolent aristocrats, bored wives, and scholars, were also believed peculiarly vulnerable to emotional disturbances.

But the early epidemiologists of mental disorder did not demonstrate any consistent link between the natural attributes and social conditions that contributed to psychological suffering and specific kinds of insanity. They succumbed instead to the enthusiastic urge to hoard together the manifold varieties of mental disease they identified into a single heap that included every type of human misery and folly. 'Kingdoms and provinces are melancholy,' [Robert] Burton[1] exclaimed, 'cities and families, all creatures, vegetal, sensible and rational, . . . all sorts, sects, ages, conditions are out of tune . . . For indeed who is not a fool, melancholy, mad? . . . Who is not brain-sick? Folly, melancholy, madness are but one disease; delirium is a common name to all'. No wonder there were few statements about the prevalence of mental affliction that commanded unanimous assent.

[. . .]

The rest of this [extract] examines the demographic characteristics of Richard Napier's mentally disturbed clients and the kinds of communities in which they lived. . . . The only notable correlation between a type of mental affliction and a social variable shows that those who had the fashionable malady melancholy were in better company than the rest of

---

[1] Robert Burton (1577–1640) was the author of the largest and most comprehensive early modern manual of psychology, *The Anatomy of Melancholy* (1st edn, Oxford, 1621), which MacDonald cites here.

Napier's patients, for it was a frequent complaint of aristocrats and gentlefolk. Otherwise, no difference of disease, neither madness nor mopishness nor trouble of mind can be tied to a particular group of clients. The focus [in what follows] will therefore be on the entire pool of mentally disturbed people, and the aim of the discussion will be to identify characteristics special to them by comparing them with Napier's other patients and with the people in the region of his practice. The unit of analysis will be a case of mental disorder, defined for statistical purposes as one or more consultations with Napier for an episode of illness that included symptoms he regarded as mentally abnormal. . . . There were 2,039 cases of mental disorder in Napier's practice by this definition, about 95% of which were experienced by people whom he never again treated for a psychological disorder.

Sex

All over the world today more women suffer from reported psychiatric maladies than men. . . .

. . . The evidence that more than three centuries ago, the women among Napier's clients also suffered from more insanity, sadness, and anxiety than men is perhaps more surprising. He recorded 1,286 cases of mental disorder involving females and 748 cases concerning males. . . . Expressed conventionally as the number of males per 100 females, the sex ratio of Napier's mentally distrubed clients was 58.2, a figure very similar to the ratios reported for modern medical practices in Britain. . . . [A] low sex ratio of mentally disturbed medical patients in a general practice may be caused by several factors, working singly or together. The doctor's medical personality, his character, his specialty, and his biases in diagnosing his patients, or the location of his practice in a demographically odd place may make the sex ratio in the practice peculiar. Socially conditioned habits of medical consultation or physical and social stresses particular to women may also affect the number of female mental patients the physician treats. Did Napier's personal attitudes and habits attract women to his practice? Was his practice in a sexually odd area? Did women consult him medically more readily than men? Did they suffer more physical disease and emotional pressure than men?

Richard Napier was sexually indifferent toward women, openly contemptuous of their intellectual capacities, and strongly disinclined to specialize in female complaints. Nothing in his manner or attitudes can have enticed women to reveal their emotional problems to him. . . .

... [Nor did t]he peculiarities of the 'population at risk', as the epidemiologists call potential medical patients, ... by themselves account for the low sex ratio among Napier's mentally disturbed clients.

Feminine habits of consulting physicians and the greater vulnerability of women to physical and mental stress did affect the sexual balance of the group of tormented people Napier treated. ... Napier spent a large amount of his time ministering to the physical ailments of women. ... Women sought medical treatment more often than men because they were more often ill. In addition to the afflictions men bore, women also suffered from diseases that tormented only their sex. Nutritional deficiencies afflicted young women with anemia. Gynecological ailments, which neither women's cunning nor scientific medicine could cure, caused many to suffer the 'reds' or whites', enduring pain, festering infections, and menstrual disorders until nature and time brought remission – if they did. Childbirth without anesthesia or asepsis was excruciating and dangerous: Difficult and botched deliveries often left women mangled, sterile, or lame – if they survived the infections that appear commonly to have followed dangerous labors. These afflictions were quite familiar in Napier's practice, and they can easily be seen to have contributed to the surplus of mentally disturbed women, for one out of five of them complained to the doctor of a gynecological or obstetrical problem in addition to her psychological distress.

Because women like these were driven to seek medical help more often than men, perhaps they were readier to turn to a physician when they suffered emotionally. ...

The extra burden of disease that women suffered not only led them to consult physicians more often than men did; it also contributed to their superabundance among the mentally tormented in a less direct manner. The protracted agony of many gynecological maladies and the debilitating lassitude of anemia must also have increased the mental stress women were forced to endure. Some doctors did recognize that there was a connection between female diseases and psychological disturbances, and they tried to persuade their fellow practitioners and the literate public that an ailment they called the 'suffocation of the mother'[2] was widespread. They attributed bizarre symptoms, weird perceptions, and grand delusions to this illness and blamed them on the alleged propensity of the uterus to become a vagabond, leaving its

[2] The identification of this disease with the ancient malady, hysteria, was popularised in England at this time in the work of the London physician, Edward Jorden (1569–1632). In 1603, he published a learned treatise on the subject in which he attempted to demonstrate that many of the seemingly supernatural symptoms commonly associated with witchcraft were in fact the product of this physical defect in women.

proper place in the womb and wandering into the upper parts, near the passionate heart. Speculative physiology thus invented a wild explanation for an observation verified by common experience, that women were more vulnerable than men to psychological stress because of illness.

Not all the stress that women suffered was caused by physical illness. . . . 767 of Napier's mentally disturbed clients complained about intolerable dilemmas that corroded their happiness, and many of the people who were tormented by frustrating relationships and upsetting experiences were women. The fact that the sex ratio among these patients (just 52.3) was even lower than the ratios of the mentally disordered and the physically ill suggests that women were also more vulnerable than men to psychologically disturbing social situations. Their individual propensities to anxiety and sadness were enhanced by patriarchal customs and values that limited their ability to remedy disturbing situations, even the catastrophes of family life, the only domain in which the female had any hope at all of influencing events. . . .

Age

Conventional wisdom in Shakespeare's England declared that each stage of life produced its own peculiar affliction of body and soul, and that the vulnerability of men and women to disease and emotional suffering changed as their mental powers waxed and waned with age. Children and ancients sickened and died more often than young people and the middle-aged, and the turbulence of adult life and the bodily decay of old age caused the middle-aged and elderly to suffer more mental disease than other people, according to contemporary writers. Napier's clients, however, found youth much more dangerous emotionally than middle or old age. Almost exactly one-third of his troubled patients were in their twenties. . . . Many of these young people complained to their physician about the anxieties of courtship and marriage and the uncertainties of getting a living and bearing children, problems that accompanied the transition from youthful dependence on parents and masters to full independence as married adults. . . .

The most striking feature of the distribution of ages among Napier's patients, both the physically ill and the mentally distressed, is the rarity of children among them. Paradoxically, seventeenth-century England swarmed with children even though they suffered mortal sicknesses appallingly often. In spite of mortality rates showing that disease slew as many as one-half of the boys and girls under five years old who were born in some cities, about 25% of the population was under ten and from 45% to 50% was under twenty. . . . Because there were many children and because they were more often sick than middle-aged adults, it is surprising that less than 7% of Napier's patients were under ten and less than 20% were not yet twenty. Among psychologically disturbed clients, children were still scarcer: 0.7% were under ten, 7.5% under twenty. Why did parents bring their sick and troubled children for medical treatment so seldom?

Accustomed as they were to see infants and toddlers sicken and die, many parents must have regarded their children's illnesses with gloomy resignation. No expert was needed to diagnose the too familiar diseases that carried away most children, and a physician (or a witch-finder) must have seemed necessary only when the child's illness was unusually sudden or lingering, convulsive or mysterious. That is how many of the illnesses of Napier's youngest patients were described. Nor was there much point in purchasing costly medical treatments for children, because the remedies physicians used were either useless or harmful and often both. Thomas Phaer[3] . . . advised his readers to avoid treating common children's diseases with physic: 'The best and most sure help in this case is not to meddle with any kind of medicines but to let nature work her operations'. . . .

Even today after more than half a century of analysis and speculation about the emotional development of children, there are no reliable figures about how many of them are insane or emotionally disturbed. . . . No other work provides any persuasive information about childhood abnormality that would tell us how many mad or troubled children one might expect to find in a modern medical practice comparable to Napier's. Nevertheless, disturbed children were strikingly rare among his clients, and contemporary attitudes toward children's mental capacities suggest that seventeenth-century parents were less ready than we are to think that their children were psychologically disturbed.

Napier treated only 13 cases of mental disorder involving children under ten, and not all these boys and girls were unmistakably afflicted with maladies of the mind. . . . Opinion of every variety and the practices of legal and religious institutions assumed that children were incapable of reason, and their scarcity among the mentally disturbed may simply be due to the logical consequences of such thinking; because young children were not reasonable, they could hardly suffer from diseases that manifested themselves in unreasonable thoughts and actions. . . .

[3] Thomas Phaer or Phayre (fl. mid-sixteenth century) was a lawyer as well as a doctor of medicine, who published on various subjects including his *Book of children*, cited here.

Seventeenth-century physicians thought that the aged were exceptionally vulnerable to gloom and unhappiness. ... According to Burton's summary of medical opinion, old age was one of the outward natural causes of melancholy, 'which no man living can avoid'. Old age is 'cold and dry and of the same quality as melancholy is, must needs cause it, by diminution of spirits and substance, and increasing of adust[4] humours'. . . . There is, Burton continues, other evidence that the aged suffer more from mental disease:

> After seventy years (as the Psalmist saith)[5] 'all is trouble and sorrow'; and common experience confirms the truth of it in weak and old persons . . . They are overcome with melancholy in an instant, or . . . they dote at last . . . and are not able to manage their estates through common infirmities incident in their age; . . . full of ache, sorrow, and grief, children again, dizzards,[6] they carle[7] many times as they sit, and talk to themselves, they are angry, waspish, displeased with everything . . .

The widespread repetition of such beliefs in proverbs, plays, doctors' writings, and philosophy makes one wonder why old people were not more common among the mentally disturbed in Napier's practice. . . .

The favorite Elizabethan phrase that old age is but a second childhood seems ironically true. The elderly, like little children, were especially likely to perish from their sicknesses, and the sight of old men and women ill and dying must have been very familiar. The barbarous and debilitating medical routines that purged and bled the sick certainly cannot have helped most aged patients, and perhaps their maladies were regarded with the same resignation that parents felt when their infants fell ill. Even in a gerontocratic society ... the plight of old people too weak or poor to work was dire. . . . Some of the old people Napier treated struggled to avoid becoming dependent upon their children by retaining control of their estates, so that their hopeful heirs were forced to attend to their needs and wishes. . . . There were good reasons for old people's reluctance to relinquish control of their property. An elderly man or woman who had not reserved some part of his estate to himself had to rely upon his children's concern and willingness to pay all of his expenses, including the charges to obtain medical treatment. The fact that mortal sickness and mental decay were considered the natural companions of old age may have made the younger persons who controlled the purse reluctant to part with their money. Young

---

[4] Burnt or corrupt.
[5] Psalms 90:10.
[6] Idiots.
[7] Snarl.

people's familiarity with their elders' illnesses and low regard for their mental powers accounts more plausibly for the rarity of the aged in Napier's practice than the alternative speculation that they were proof against the afflictions of the mind.

Marital status

Marriage, according to modern students of mental disorder, is a paradise for husbands and a purgatory for wives. The highest rates of reported psychological illness in England and America are found among married women and single men, the lowest rates among married men and single women. . . . [M]any of Napier's female patients blamed their psychological distress on marital problems, and popular works such as the homily on marriage admitted that women suffered from the tribulations of marriage more than men because they relinquished their liberty when they wed. We would therefore expect that the distribution of marital status among Napier's disturbed patients would closely resemble the patterns found today.

Unfortunately, the astrologer was lax about recording his clients' marital status, and so no statistically significant figures can be tabulated from his notes. Even so, [those which do survive show] that married women are the largest group of patients for whom we have evidence and that if the disturbed clients who were remarried or had children at the time of the consultation are added to those wives, the number of female patients who were probably married swells to 554, 52% of the known marrieds and unmarrieds, 27% of the whole pool of disturbed clients. Husbands, verified and probable, account for only about half as many cases of disorder, 140, or 13%, of those for whom marital status can be determined and 7% of the whole group. There were also more men definitely known to have been single and widowed among the disturbed than there were married men. Even though information is lacking in so many cases, these figures are nevertheless consistent with the hypothesis that marriage had the same dolorous effects on the mental health of women in the seventeenth century as it has today.

Social status

Napier's patients were drawn from the entire range of the social hierarchy. Few were very rich; few were very poor. . . . No historian who is interested in how social status affected the perception and management of mental disorder could ask for better evidence than the diagnostician's own record of the prestige of his clients. These judgments of social standing by a single man are more revealing than pedigrees and lists of occupations, because they were made in the context of assessing the nature of the client's problems. . . .

Napier used three sets of titles to describe his judgment of his patients' status. He scrupulously referred to the aristocracy by their titles or called them Lord or Lady. He called a larger number of his clients Master or Mistress. These people included members of the local gentry, university graduates, fellow clergymen, merchants, and important local craftsmen – the kind of men and women whom the physician regarded as his social equals. He omitted titles of honor from the names of patients who were his social inferiors, calling them Goodman or Goody when he did not know their first names. When one examines the occupations he sometimes recorded for these people it is plain that they comprised a cross section of the farming and artisanal community of the region. Farmers, servants, small craftsmen, and agricultural laborers were most common among these untitled folk. . . .

[. . .]

Although he became familiar with many of the important political and social figures of his day, Napier remained uniquely independent. Unlike many other physicians he did not become a creature of the rich, a servant dependent upon their wealth and favor. He continued to treat people of middling and humble means in large numbers and preferred not to leave his home at Great Linford to attend the nobility personally. . . .

In spite of his greater familiarity with gentlemen and gentlewomen, Napier's practice never became overburdened with noble ladies and courtiers. His fees were comparatively small, typically about 12d. in the early years of the seventeenth century. A consultation with him would have put a laborer out of pocket about one day's wages. The smattering of occupational labels he tagged to his clients show that many servants and humble artisans could pay his charges. . . . Nevertheless, the knowledge that he charged a fee, any fee, must have deterred some of the very poor in the area from seeking his help. . . .

[. . .]

. . . All of this strongly suggests, but (again) does not prove, that Napier's mad and troubled clients represent a faithful cross section of the social composition of the top two-thirds or so of rural society and that throughout the four decades that he practiced medicine his services were available to all save for an indigent minority.

(ii)

The lesser mental disorders ... were distinguished from madness, lunacy, and distraction by the relative infrequency of antic violence and frantic, raging behavior among their victims. The symptoms of melancholy were distinctive enough to show that it was regarded to be a separate type of mental disturbance, although the popularity of the disease encouraged contemporaries to use it to describe virtually any nonviolent emotional disturbance. Napier's usage was comparatively precise. The patients whom he diagnosed as melancholy suffered from deluded fear and sorrow far more often than those who were described simply as troubled in mind. He also recognized another kind of mental disorder less acute than madness and its companions, whose victims he called mopish. Mopish men and women often suffered from the characteristic symptoms of melancholy, especially gloom and solitude. . . . Forty-one of Napier's mopish clients were so glum and withdrawn that . . . they sat sunken in 'dumpish, sullen silence'. . . .

Mopishness nevertheless had distinctive social and psychological signs. It was the social antithesis of melancholy. The dumpish moods of idle gentlefolk frequently earned the classical appellation; the sullen inactivity of husbandmen and artisans merited more often the rude and common word *mopish*. This socially pejorative aura was also reflected in the symptoms Napier associated with mopishness. The idleness of melancholy aristocrats was seldom viewed as a sign of mental illness; it was instead the very mark of gentility, a cause and not a consequence of melancholy. . . .

The truly characteristic psychological evidence of mopishness, however, was a disturbance of the senses. . . . The identification of mopishness with disturbed sense perceptions was not peculiar to Napier. Medical writers seldom used the word *mopish*, but they described an almost identical condition which was called *stupor* or *lethargy* by Galen and his English disciples. A century after Napier's death, William Battie[8] included in his famous treatise on madness a malady called *insensibility*, which he characterized as 'a preternatural defect or total loss of sensation'. That is precisely the meaning of *mopishness* understood by Napier. . . .

The popular usage of the term *mopish* ... can be precisely interpreted in terms of contemporary psychology. The condition it described was a disturbance of the sensitive faculty, rather than the reason. Mopishness was therefore less severe than the maladies that ruined the

---

[8] For Battie, see extract 9.4 below.

reason itself, such as madness and lunacy, because it harmed a lesser faculty, and interfered with wit and will merely by depriving reason of normal perceptions, the raw material of thought. As Napier's records show, this was a very useful diagnostic tool, providing a means with which to separate melancholy from the lesser mental disturbances that made their victims remote and insensible but not sad or anxious. The fact that the concept may be found in popular literature suggests that it was commonly recognized as a type of mental disorder. And yet the popularizers of classical medical psychology largely ignored it in their publications and instead encouraged the tendency to broaden the concept of melancholy to include the symptoms of every mental disturbance except outright lunacy.

... Napier [on the other hand] sought to articulate his patients' maladies into categories that were at once scientifically useful and consistent with popular usage. The physicians encouraged the cult of melancholy. They neglected the empirical distinctions implicit in Napier's methods and popular stereotypes in favor of a vague and confused medical vocabulary. Medical men made few empirically based attempts to improve the nosology[9] of mental disorder before the middle of the eighteenth century. Their preference for the broadest possible application of traditional humoral concepts stemmed in part from the realization that the popularity of melancholy among the educated elite fostered the belief that physicians were the best healers for the maladies of the mind. Doctors were not disinterested taxonomists. They were more concerned to suppress their lay and clerical rivals than to preserve the empirically useful aspects of popular psychology and religious healing.

9.2

Melancholy: a physician's view

Philip Barrough, *The Methode of Phisicke, Conteyning the Causes, Signes, and Cures of Inward Diseases in Mans Body from the Head to the Foote* (London, Thomas Vautroullier, 1583), pp. 35–6.

Philip Barrough (fl. 1560–90), who claimed to have studied surgery for seven years, was granted a licence to practise surgery by the Univer-

---

[9] The study of the classification of disease.

sity of Cambridge in 1559. Thirteen years later, the same body awarded him a licence to practise medicine. His *Method of Phisicke* was a highly popular compendium of traditional Galenic medicine, which first appeared in 1583, and was subsequently reprinted many times in the first half of the seventeenth century. The extract here is taken from chapter 28 of the original edition, entitled 'Of melancholia'.

Melancholie is an alienation of the mind troubling reason, and waxing foolish, so that one is almost beside him selfe. It commeth without a fever, and is chiefly engendered of melancholie occupying the mind, and changing the temperature of it. It is caused thre[e] kind of wayes: for sometime it is caused of the common vice of melancholie, bloud being in all the vaines of the whole body which also hurteth the braine. But oftentimes only the bloud which is in the braine is altered, and the bloud in all the rest of the body is unhurt, and that chaunceth two wayes: for either it is derived from other places, and ascendeth up thither, or els it is engendred in the braine it selfe. Also sometime it is engendred through inflammation, and evil affect about the stomake and sides: and therefore there be thre[e] diversities of melancholiousnes, according to the thre[e] kinds of causes. The most common signes be fearfulnes, sadnes, hatred, and also they that be melancholious, have straunge imaginations, for some think them selves brute beasts, and do counterfaite the voice and noise, some think themselves vessels of earth, or earthen pottes, and therfore they withdrawe themselves from them that they meet, least they should knocke together. Moreover they desire death, and do verie often behight[10] and determine to kill them selves, and some feare that they should be killed. Many of them do alwayes laugh, and many do weep, some thinck themselves inspired with the holie Ghost, and do prophecy uppon thinges to come. But these be the peculiar signes of them that have melancholiousnes caused through consent of the whole body: for in them the state of the body is slender, black, rough and altogether melancholious caused naturally or through certaine thoughtes, or watchinges or eatinges of wicked meats, or through Emeroides, or suppression of menstruis. But they which have *melancholia* caused of vice in the sides, they have rawenes, and much windines, sharp belkinges, burninges, and grevousnes of the sides. Also the sides are plucked upward, & many times are troubled with inflamation, especially about the beginning of the disease. Also there is costivenes of the wombe, litle sleep, troublous and naughty dreames, sweaming of the head, and sound in the eares: Let his dyet be

---

[10] Vow or promise.

such, as doth not engender melancholie. Therefore let him tary in an ayer hote and moist and let them use meanes of good iuyce, that be moist and temperate, and let there bread be well baked & wrought, let there flesh be capons, hennes . . . and such like. Let the sicke use wyne that is white, thinne, and not very old, and let them eschewe wyne that is thick and black, let there excercises be meane, let them ryde or walke by places pleasant and greene, or use sailing on water. Also a bath of sweet water with a moyst dyet let the sicke use often as one of his remedies, sleep is wonderfull good for them, as also moderate carnall copulation. Let them be mer[r]y as much as may be, and heare musicall instruments and singing. But when the whole body abound with melan-cholike bloud, it is best to begin the cure with letting of bloud.

9.3

The hospitalisation of the insane in early modern Germany: Protestant Haina and Catholic Würzburg

H. C. Erik Midelfort, *A History of Madness in Sixteenth-Century Germany* (Stanford, Stanford University Press, 1999), pp. 356–65, 369–84.

The following extract is taken from one of the most recent in-depth studies of the institutional care of the insane in early modern Germany. Using the surviving documentary evidence of admissions' registers, the petitions submitted on behalf of the mentally ill by family, friends and communities, and other contemporary documents, Midelfort has been able to build up a picture detailing the quality and scope of provision in two German hospitals, Haina and Würzburg. The former was a Protestant institution, established on the site of an old monastery after the Reformation by Philipp of Hesse. Würzburg, on the other hand, was a new hospital founded by the Catholic prince-bishop, Julius Echter (1545–1617), a keen proponent of the Catholic or Counter Reformation, in 1576. The town council of Würzburg was pre-dominantly Protestant throughout this period, and Midelfort suggests that the hospital was built by Echter partly in order to encourage support for Catholicism through pious and charitable works.

Protestant Haina

Although Haina became famous in the nineteenth century as a mental hospital, in its origins it had no such specialization. The hospital received the poor mad as it received the poor blind, the poor crippled, and the poor aged. In fact . . . during the sixteenth century, the mad constituted only a tiny proportion of the residents of Haina. After all, there were only nine mentally ill men chained in the vault and only eighteen cages with fifteen inmates and two custodians in 1575, a year when the total number of brethren was close to three hundred. To assume that as few as 8 percent of the hospital's residents were mentally ill, however, is to forget that the vault and cages were intended only for wild and dangerous persons. Many other mentally disabled persons qualified for admission to the hospital because they were unable to support themselves, without necessarily needing to be bound in chains.

To determine how many mentally ill persons there were at Haina, one would need full descriptions of the various patients, inmates, and residents in the hospital, and generally such sources do not exist for the sixteenth century. . . . For Haina . . . however, recently discovered bundles of 'reception rescripts'[11] enable us to draw a crude profile of the hospital population in the second half of the sixteenth century. . . .

[. . .]

These petitions . . . form an unparalleled source for the study of mental disorders among the poor, a group who usually escape the view of even the most diligent researcher. . . . Of the 183 persons for whom a hospital petition survives, 39 were retarded, brain-damaged, or mentally disordered. . . .

If one tries to construct rough categories for these afflicted people, one confronts the often impenetrably vague language of these sixteenth-century documents. [T]he academically trained physician of four hundred years ago could regularly distinguish mental retardation, brain damage, senility, and epilepsy from melancholia, mania, and phrenitis. But the authors of these hospital documents had no interest in medical diagnosis; their only intention was to demonstrate that a person needed care, and no professional diagnosis was necessary for that. . . .

. . . [S]everal of the individual cases cast a bright light into some dark corners of social behavior. . . .

[. . .]

---

[11] Petitions for entry to the hospital.

These cases demonstrate that family members and neighbors were expected to care for their own problems and were to seek aid from the territorial prince only when a person became unmanageable. This was clearly the case with Heinrich Senger of Homberg, who fell into a more and more serious madness. The local pastor, Caspar Arcularius, explained that 'some years ago Senger had behaved strangely both in words and deeds, as if he was a madman'. The neighbors had tried to practice 'Christian love, patience, and sympathy' in tolerating him, but matters had only grown worse. Now in 1593, his reason and human understanding were totally deranged, and he was more than his wife could handle, 'who up to now has cared for him not only with great trouble and effort, but also at the risk of life and limb'. The neighborhood could 'no longer stand to see this miserable specimen, nor could they trust this irrational and senseless person, who might at any hour or moment either kill himself . . . or wound others by hitting, stabbing, burning, etc., and thus produce irreparable damage'. Arcularius concluded that Senger must be admitted to Haina, 'in order that greater misfortune be avoided and that the poor man be helped'. . . . Senger was admitted to the stout cells of Haina.

[. . .]

Another example of gradually strained neighborhood tolerance was the case of Daniel Hoffmann of Stauffenberg. In his case, the burghermaster and council of Stauffenberg wrote in March 1590 to the captain of Giessen, Rudolf Wilhelm Raw, about six miles away, to inform him that Hoffmann was acting as if possessed. He had been found in his barn with a loaded gun and a handful of flax tow (used for starting fires) under his coat. On other occasions, he had thrown knives and other weapons at his wife and children and had tried to stab them; he had also beaten his wife with his fists and had tried to strangle her. The officials of Stauffenberg commanded him to be restrained in a 'blockhouse' or with chains until a more permanent solution could be found. Two weeks later, Hoffmann was confined at Haina, where he would have to stay 'until God might send him some improvement'.

In 1596, a father in Schmalkalden appealed to Landgrave Moritz[12] on behalf of his son. For three years, the boy had been a singer in church and school, but now he was so 'disabled and crazy' that he 'cannot well be tolerated here because of the danger'. He should be admitted to Haina 'until he improves'. The superintendent, Johann Clauer, agreed and ordered the boy confined 'until Almighty God sends him some improvement'.

---

[12] The ruler of the principality of Hesse.

[. . .]

A number of things are striking in these cases of madness and mental disorder. First, the petitioners and the Hessian officials often assumed that improvement of mental condition was possible, although in every case the possibility of cure was ascribed to God alone. The hospital did not initiate any special program of therapy. Second . . . there are surprisingly few instances in which a mad person was thought to be demonically possessed. . . . [O]nly Daniel Hoffman came close, and no one seems to have treated him differently just because he acted 'as if possessed'. . . .

A third noteworthy fact about all of the 39 cases of mental disability in these Hessian hospital records is that the local community was obviously supposed to exhaust its resources before turning to the territorial administration. Even when spouse and neighbors had been driven to despair with their problem, however, they did not apparently attack, punish, ridicule, or demean the afflicted person, or at least they did not openly admit such abuse, if it occurred. They chained or confined the wildly disordered, but only as a last resort and to prevent self-inflicted injury as well as harm to others. There is no evidence that neighbors revered, respected, or were in awe of lunatics and the feebleminded as if they were holy fools or mystical prophets, but the local community was legally required to practice Christian patience and charity.

[. . .]

This much is clear. The Hessian hospital system from its very beginnings housed more than a few mentally disabled residents. By 1600, mental patients were common. With the exception of those who were forcibly detained, we can guess that the mad were as relieved as other residents to find a refuge from the world of famine, poverty, and starvation. In contrast to the mental hospitals that functioned as a repressive prison house of reason, whose seventeenth- and eighteenth-century origins Michel Foucault bathed in a garish light, the sixteenth- and seventeenth-century German hospitals that took their cue from Hesse had their origin in monastic institutions whose watchwords were piety and charity. These ideals are obviously not the ideals of modern mental hospitals, but even with all their moralism, they provided comfort for the helpless in ways so attractive that people clamored to be admitted. These people were not part of an experiment in social discipline or victims of a 'great confinement'.

Catholic Würzburg

From the outset . . . as at Haina . . . mentally disordered patients were mixed indiscriminately among the other patients unless they were thought dangerous. The records do not, however, speak of a separation of the sexes, as in the Hessian high hospitals, but also common place elsewhere. Violent patients were placed in the 'Pilgrim's House' and later in special rooms in the west wing of the spital. . . . Furious deranged patients were always in the minority among the mentally ill, but [Bishop Julius] Echter instructed that the female inmate in charge of the mad should:

[1.] keep the chains and leg-irons, padlocks, and keys to the prison cells in her custody and not allow them to be used or lent or taken else-where without her knowledge; and every time they are needed, she is to provide them;

[2.] be responsible for bowls, cups, mugs and similar eating and drinking utensils, and also for the clothing, alms, and whatever else the mad people need; and faithfully care for these things and keep them clean;

[3.] dispense bread, drink, food, and whatever is daily distributed to them, and not seek her own advantage in these matters at all. What-ever they need for their maintenance, [she should] bring to attention without hesitation and in timely manner before they become sick in their prison;

[4.] adapt herself in every way as much as possible and learn their char-acteristics so that she may not excite them to more nonsense, rage, frenzy, biting, and fury;

[5.] turn them out from time to time, bathe them and dress them in newly washed clothes, clean out the prison and strew it with fresh straw;

[6.] make a little fire for them in winter, when it is rather cold, and take care that no damage results from the fire and that the crazy people in the prisons do not hurt themselves on the hot stoves; and therefore visit them often during the day to observe and see to it that there is no straw, clothing, etc., around the stove;

[7.] absolutely not let them have any belt, garter, knife, or any other thing with which they could harm themselves in any way, and, if she notices that someone has any such thing, bring it to attention at once.

From this document[13] we may underline the following points. It is clear that the female pensioner who had the job of looking after the danger-ously mad might well have had her hands full. She was responsible for the care and safety, the food and cleanliness, the clothing and warmth and comfort of all who were locked up in the hospital's 'prison'. To be sure, the instruction speaks of chains and leg-irons, but the attendant

---

[13] Undated, but probably drafted in the early years of the hospital.

was also to take the individual characteristics of specific patients into account. While conditions were doubtless harsh, she was expected to be a caregiver as well as custodian, bathing her charges and providing for their clothing, fresh straw, and warm ovens when necessary, all with a view to preventing illness. We surely obtain a glimpse here of the situation into which suicidal and dangerous patients were thrown, but we should not conclude that even these persons had to live in hopeless dungeons. . . .

Perhaps the most surprising aspect of the Juliusspital is that patients generally stayed only a short time. Most mental patients, like other patients, arrived for stays of a few weeks or a few months. The governors of the hospital displayed a therapeutic optimism that assumed that only the curable would be admitted, that very few would be granted the status of life-pensioner, and that quick results would therefore have to be registered. With amazing frequency, the records speak of 'cures'. At the remove of four hundred years, it is, of course, impossible for us to tell whether physical or mental improvement was actually visible or whether cures were merely imputed to these troubled persons. Unlike most late medieval German hospitals, however, the Juliusspital was establishing a different ideal of hospital care, one that optimistically intended the treatment and cure of disease and disorder. This ideal is much more visible in the annual records of admissions and dismissals than in the documents like the charter of 1579 or the instruction to the woman inmate in charge of the mad.

[. . .]

In trying to grasp the conditions of real life for the mad, we can go beyond the general principles on which the hospital was based. Fortunately, the admissions books have largely survived from the earliest years of the Juliusspital. . . . The surviving records contain the names and descriptions of over 4,600 persons admitted in the first fifty years of operation.

[. . .]

. . . In its first years, the spital apparently treated no cases of mental disorder, although, as noted, the records are incomplete. . . .

[. . .]

In 1582, the new Würzburg hospital stepped up its activity somewhat, admitting 51 patients for longer or shorter periods. Now we begin to find examples of madness. [Of these] [t]hree were specifically described as mad or mentally disabled. They included one woman

248

admitted because she was suffering from a 'vehement sickness of the head'; the village mayor of Baltheißheim . . . who was 'healthy in body but crazy from time to time in his head'; and a woman of whom it is said (in vague language that recalls the mad of Haina's hospital) that she was admitted 'until God should send a remedy', which He evidently did just eleven months later. . . . Even so, the mad were not a major element in the first few years of the Juliusspital. . . .

As in the Hessian hospitals, however, the numbers of mad increased in the course of time. . . .

. . . [T]he numbers of mad or mentally disabled rose substantially, both in absolute numbers and as a proportion of the total admissions, from 1580 to 1614, but . . . this surge leveled off in the [1620s], at just the time when the hospital began to swell far beyond its original limits. It may be that, as in Hesse, the local population of the prince bishop's lands learned in time to refer their mentally disturbed members to the new hospital. . . .

[The figures] also highlight the fact that here men generally outnumbered women among the mental patients by a ratio of about eight to five, but this was a ratio that fluctuated dramatically over the 50-year period [i.e. from 1580 to 1628] we are examining. Whatever our interpretation of those figures, it would be hard to conclude that women were being treated as mad or labeled as sick and incompetent more frequently than men. . . .

Even more dramatic than the general rise of the mentally ill among the hospital patients in Würzburg during the first thirty-five years was the general rise of 'melancholy' among the mentally ill. . . .

We cannot tell from these records if this dramatic rise of melancholy was owing to the possible increase of melancholy as a diagnostic label at the hospital or to an increasing social tendency to see the melancholy as so troublesome, so disordered, that they needed to be sent away to a hospital, or even to the possible growth of a Galenic optimism that led to the increased referral of the so-called melancholy to the Juliusspital. Some combination of these explanations may well have been at work, but they all testify to . . . the distinct rise of melancholy in the waning decades of the sixteenth century. And here there was an increasing level of concern about melancholy, not only among mad princes and other connoisseurs of the latest fashionable medical treatments, and not just among lawyers eager to deploy a new understanding of the insanity defense, but among ordinary people. This rise of melancholy as a label and as an experience was dramatically evident in Würzburg, but nothing comparable is visible in the Hessian hospital records. This discrepancy suggests that the medical resources and close ties to

Würzburg's medical faculty contributed to the rising popularity of the melancholy diagnosis there. The Hessian high hospitals, by way of contrast, remained more conservatively committed to a vernacular nosology, to the language and medical understanding of ordinary folk.

[. . .]

The hospital also had to deal with a wave of demonic possessions among its mentally disturbed patients. . . .

[. . .]

Repeatedly . . . the Juliusspital recorded striking success with the truly demon-possessed. In 1595, for example, Veronica, the wife of Hans Herbst of Hausen, came in, 'possessed by many demons. She was freed from them by Father Gerhard through exorcisms and other suitable measures'. A similarly mixed therapy helped Kunigundt Schneiderin from Karlburg, 'who was very melancholy and behaved strangely as if she were possessed, as she showed in many [ways]. She was restored [to health] by Father Gerhard with medicine, words of consolation and exorcisms, and was sent back grateful to her children'.

[. . .]

As in Hesse, Würzburg presented a hospital that was clearly a welcome relief from the hard times of the last decades of the sixteenth century. Here the mad were not beaten or abused; they were not forced to work for their suppers, although moderate jobs were found for those who could manage them. They were certainly not part of any 'great confinement', but were rather given whatever medication or therapy seemed professionally indicated. Perhaps because the hospital explicitly sought only curable cases, the rate of cure was extremely high. This is not the place to pursue the later history of the Juliusspital, but it is worth mentioning that when modern teaching clinics were first established in Germany in the 1790s, the Bamberg model that became famous rested in part on the earlier successes of Würzburg's Counter-Reformation sanatorium. There is an irony in the fact that Philipp of Hesse, while moving his territory into the new world of evangelical social institutions, managed to create a hospital system that was medieval in inspiration, whereas Julius Echter von Mespelbrunn, in trying to stem the tide of Protestantism, created a hospital that, at least in its origins and ideas, looked forward with religious and therapeutic optimism.

9.4

New approaches to curing the mad?: William Battie's *A Treatise on Madness* (1758)

William Battie, *A Treatise on Madness* (London, J. Whiston &
B. White, 1758), pp. 1–3, 43–4, 61–2, 68–72, 74–5, 93.

In 1758, William Battie (1703–76), recently appointed as physician to
the newly founded St Luke's Hospital for Lunaticks in London, published *A Treatise on Madness*, in which he sought to present himself
as a medical innovator with regard to the understanding and cure of
the mad. In part, a thinly veiled attack on the therapeutic pessimism
characteristic of the regime to be found in London's only other mental
hospital, Bethlem, it drew the immediate response of the latter's
highly-esteemed physician, John Monro (1715–91). In his *Remarks on
Dr Battie's Treatise on Madness* (London, John Clarke, 1758) Monro
rebutted all Battie's charges and sought to depict his opponent as a
mere pretender to learning on the subject of the mad. The debate
between the two men has traditionally been seen by historians of mad
ness as a straightforward conflict between the 'progressive' Battie and
the inveterate traditionalist Monro. Recent appraisals of the debate,
however, have argued for a more nuanced and balanced assessment of
the merits of the two men and their views on the care and treatment
of the insane.

Madness, though a terrible and at present a very frequent calamity, is
perhaps as little understood as any that ever afflicted mankind. The
names alone usually given to this disorder and its several species, *viz.
Lunacy, Spleen, Melancholy, Hurry of the Spirits*, &c. may convince
any one of the truth of this assertion. . . .

Our defect of knowledge in this matter is, I am afraid, in a great
measure owing to a defect of proper communication: and the difficulties attending the care of Lunaticks have been at least perpetuated by
their being entrusted to Empiricks, or at best to a few select Physicians,
most of whom thought it adviseable to keep the cases as well as the
patients to themselves.[14]

---

[14] Undoubtedly, Battie alludes here to his rival, John Monro, who succeeded his father as
physician to Bedlam in 1752.

[. . .]

But [this] peculiar misfortune . . . want of proper communication, though the chief, is not the only hindrance to our knowledge: for Madness hath moreover shared the fate common to many other distempers of not being precisely defined. Inasmuch as not only several symptoms, which frequently and accidentally accompany it, have been taken into the account as constant, necessary, and essential; but also the supposed cause, which perhaps never existed or certainly never acted with such effect, has been implied in the very names usually given to this distemper. No wonder therefore is it, whilst several disorders, really independent of Madness and of one another, are thus blended together in our bewildered imagination, that a treatment, rationally indicated by any of those disorders, should be injudiciously directed against Madness itself, whether attended with such symptoms or not.

[. . .]

. . . Madness with respect to its cause is distinguishable into two species. The first is solely owing to an internal disorder of the nervous substance: the second is likewise owing to the same nervous substance being indeed in like manner disordered, but disordered *ab extra*;[15] and therefore is chiefly to be attributed to some remote and accidental cause. The first species, until a better name can be found, may be called *Original*, the second may be called *Consequential Madness*.

[. . .]

Original Madness, whether it be haereditary or intermitting, is not removable by any method, which the science of Physick in its present imperfect state is able to suggest.

[. . .]

Madness, which is consequential to other disorders or external causes, altho' it now and then admits of relief by the removal or correction of such disorders or causes; yet in proportion to the force and continued action of such causes, and according to the circumstances of the preceding disorders, it is very often complicated with many other ill effects of those causes and disorders; and, tho' it may not in itself be prejudicial to bodily health, any more than Original Madness, yet by its companions it becomes fatal or greatly detrimental to animal life.

Madness, tho' it may be Consequential at first, frequently becomes habitual and in effect the very same as Madness strictly Original. . . .

---

[15] 'From outside'.

[. . .]

The Regimen in this is perhaps of more importance than in any distemper. It was the saying of a very eminent practitioner in such cases *that management did much more than medicine*; and repeated experience has convinced me that confinement alone is oftentimes sufficient but always so necessary, that without it every method hitherto devised for the cure of Madness would be ineffectual.

Madness then, considered as delusive Sensation unconnected with any other symptom, requires the patient's being removed from all objects that act forcibly upon the nerves, and excite too lively a perception of things, more especially from such objects as are the known causes of his disorder, for the same reason as rest is recommended to bodies fatigued, and the not attempting to walk when the ancles are strained.

The visits therefore of affecting friends as well as enemies, and the impertinent curiosity of those, who think it pastime to converse with Madmen and to play upon their passions, ought strictly to be forbidden.[16]

[. . .]

Every unruly appetite must be checked, every fixed imagination must if possible be diverted. The patient's body and place of residence is carefully to be kept clean: the air he breaths should be dry and free from noisom steams: his food easy of digestion and simple, neither spirituous, nor high seasoned and full of poignancy: his amusements not too engaging nor too long continued, but rendered more agreeable by a well timed variety. Lastly his employment should be about such things as are rather indifferent, and which approach the nearest to an intermediate state (if such there be) between pleasure and anxiety.

[. . .]

Original madness indeed deserves our first attention, as it is the least complicated with any other disorder. But a very little reflection will serve to convince that all our consideration will never enable us to treat this first species of Madness in a rational manner.[17] . . .

[. . .]

Nor does experience, which oftentimes supplies the defect of rational intention in many disorders that are hitherto inexplicable by general

---

[16] In contrast to established practice at Bethlem, Battie outlawed public visiting at St Luke's.

[17] That is, by the application of learned or 'rational' physick.

science and the common laws of Nature, furnish us with any well attested remedy for Original Madness. For, altho' several specifick Medicines have by the merciful direction of Providence been of late successfully applied in some distempers otherwise incurable by art, such as Mercury in the Venereal infection, Opium in pain and watchfulness, the Peruvian Bark in mortification[,] intermittent fevers and many other complaints; and altho' we may have reason to hope that the peculiar antidote of Madness is reserved in Nature's store, and will be brought to light in its appointed time; yet such is our present misfortune, that either this important secret hath been by its inventors withheld from the rest of mankind, or, which is more probable, hath never yet been discovered.

... [But] to our great comfort we shall find that Consequential Madness is frequently manageable by human art. . . .

For altho' delusive Sensation, by whatever external accident it may be occasioned, when considered as a distempered state of the nerves themselves, admits of no rational or specific relief any more than Madness which is not consequential to any known cause; nevertheless the previous disorders and external causes of delusive Sensation are frequently within our reach. And this, as well as any other morbid effect, may in reason be and in fact often is prevented or abated; provided the known cause is taken care of in time, that is before its continued action hath altered the nervous substance to such a degree as to have rendered it essentially or habitually unsound.

[. . .]

When pressure of the brain or nerves is sudden, both these intentions may safely and effectually be answered by the lancet and cupping-glass again and again repeated in proportion to the strength of the patient and the greatness of the pressure; by neutral salts, which gently stimulating the intenstines and sensible parts contained in the abdomen provoke stools and urine. . . . And Revulsion in particular may be successfully attempted by the oily and penetrating steams arising from skins and other soft parts of animals newly slain, by tepid fomentations and cataplasms applied to the head legs and feet, by oily and emollient glysters; which are of very great service not only as they empty the belly, but also and indeed chiefly because they serve as a fomentation to the intestinal tube, and by relaxing the branches of the aorta descendens, which are here distributed in great number, make it more capable of receiving the blood; which will therefore according to the known course of fluid matter be diverted from the head.

[. . .]

We have therefore, as Men, the pleasure to find that Madness is, contrary to the opinion of some unthinking persons, as manageable as many other distempers, which are equally dreadful and obstinate, and yet are not looked upon as incurable: and that such unhappy objects ought by no means to be abandoned, much less shut up in loathsome prisons as criminals or nusances to the society.

Part ten

War and medicine in early modern Europe

10.1

Medicine, surgery and warfare in sixteenth-century Europe: Ambroise Paré

The Apologie and Treatise of Ambroise Paré containing the Voyages made into divers Places with many of His Writings upon Surgery, ed. Geoffrey Keynes (New York, Dover Publications, 1968), pp. 137–8, 28, 140, 147–52, 50-1.

The Frenchman Ambroise Paré (1510–90) was one of the most famous surgeons in sixteenth-century Europe. Born in the province of Maine, Paré was first apprenticed to a barber-surgeon before moving to Paris around 1532–33. Shortly afterwards, he became 'house-surgeon' at the Hôtel Dieu in Paris. He left this post in 1536 to practise as a military surgeon. This change of career, combined with his subsequent publications on surgery, secured his fame. The extracts here are taken from the first English edition, in folio, of Paré's collected works published in London by Thomas Cotes and R. Young in 1634.

(i)

The first discourse wherein wounds made by gunshot are freed from being burnt or cauterized according to Vigoes Methode

In the yeare of our Lord 1536, *Francis* the French King,[1] for his acts in warre and peace stiled the Great, sent a puissant Army beyond the Alpes

---

[1] Francis I, king of France (1515–47). The Valois and Habsburg rulers repeatedly fought for control of the Italian peninsula in the period from 1494 to 1559, not least in the reign of Francis I.

... both that he might releeve *Turin* with victualls, souldiers, and all things needefull, as also to recover the Citties of that Province.... I was in the Kings Army the Chirurgion of Monsieur of *Montejan* Generall of the foote. The Imperialists had taken the straits of *Suze*, the Castle of *Villane*, and all the other passages; so that the Kings army was not able to drive them from their fortifications but by fight. In this conflict there were many wounded on both sides with all sorts of weapons, but cheefely with bullets. I will tell the truth, I was not very expert at that time in matters of Chirurgery; neither was I used to dresse wounds made by Gunshot. Now I had read in *John de Vigo*[2] that wounds made by Gunshot were venenate or poisoned, and that by reason of the Gunpouder; Wherefore for their cure, it was expedient to burne or cauterize them with oyle of Elders scalding hot, with a little Treacle[3] mixed therewith. But for that I gave no great credite neither to the author, nor remedy, because I knew that caustickes could not be powred into wounds, without excessive paine; I, before I would runne a hazard, determined to see whether the Chirurgions, who went with me in the army, used any other manner of dressing to these wounds. I observed and saw that all of them used that Method of dressing which *Vigo* prescribes; and that they filled as full as they could, the wounds made by Gunshot with Tents and pledgets[4] dipped in this scalding Oylo, at the first dressings; which encouraged me to doe the like to those, who came to be dressed of me. It chanced on a time, that by reason of the multitude that were hurt, I wanted this Oyle. Now because there were some few left to be dressed, I was forced, that I might seeme to want nothing, and that I might not leave them undrest, to apply a digestive[5] made of the yolke of an egge, oyle of Roses, and Turpentine. I could not sleepe all that night, for I was troubled in minde, and the dressing of the precedent day, (which I judged unfit) troubled my thoughts; and I feared that the next day I shoulde finde them dead, or at the point of death by the poyson of the wound, whom I had not dressed with the scalding oyle. Therefore I rose early in the morning, I visited my patients, and beyound expectation, I found such as I had dressed with a digestive onely, free from vehemencie of paine to have had good rest, and that their wounds were not inflamed, nor tumifyed;[6] but on the contrary the others that were burnt with the scalding oyle were feaverish, tormented

---

[2] John or Johannes de Vigo (fl. 1500) was an Italian surgeon, whose book on surgery was highly influential in the sixteenth century.

[3] Theriac, a common antidote to poison.

[4] Absorbent materials such as compressed lint used in the dressing of wounds.

[5] A substance which promotes suppuration in a wound.

[6] Swollen.

with much paine, and the parts about their wounds were swolne. When I had many times tryed this in divers others, I thought thus much, that neither I nor any other should ever cauterize any wounded with Gunshot.

(ii)

The voyage of Perpignan, 1542

A little while after Monsieur *de Rohan* tooke me with him poste, to the campe of *Perpignan*; being there, the enemy made a Sally forth, and came and inclosed three peeces of our Artillery, where they were beaten back, to the gates of the Citty; which was not done without hurting and killing many, and amongst the rest *de Brissac*, (who was then chiefe master of the Artillery) received a musket shot upon the shoulder: returning to his Tent, all the others that were hurt followed him, hoping to be drest by the Chirurgions, that ought to dresse them. Being come to his Tent and layd on his bed, the bullet was searched for by three or foure the most expert Chirurgions of the Army, who could not finde it, but sayd it was entred into his body.

In the end hee called for me, to see if I were more skilfull than them, because he had knowne me before in *Piedmount*: by and by I made him rise from his bed, and prayed him to put his body into that posture as it was then when hee received his hurt; which he did taking a javelin betweene his hands as he held the Pike in the skirmish. I put my hand about the wound, and found the bullet in the flesh, making a little tumor under the *Omoplate*:[7]

(iii)

A medicine hindering blistring in burnes, or scalds

One of the Marshall of *Montejan* his Kitchin boyes, fell by chance into a Caldron of Oyle being even almost boyling hot; I being called to dresse him, went to the next Apothecaries to fetch refrigerating medicines commonly used in this case: there was present by chance a certaine old countrey woman, who hearing that I desired medicines for a burne, perswaded mee at the first dressing, that I should lay to raw Onions beaten with a little salt; for so I should hinder the breaking out of blisters or pustules, as shee had found by certaine and frequent experience.

---

[7] Scapula.

Wherefore I thought good to try the force of her Medicine upon this greasy scullion. I the next day found those places of his body whereto the Onions lay, to bee free from blisters, but the other parts which they had not touched, to be all blistered.

It fell out a while after, that a German of *Montejan* his guard had his flasque full of Gunpouder set on fire, whereby his hands and face were grievously burnt: I being called, laid the Onions beaten as I formerly told you, to the middle of his face, and to the rest I laid medicines usually applyed to burnes. At the second dressing I observed the part dressed with the Onions quite free from blisters and excoriation, the other being troubled with both; whereby I gave credit to the Medicine.

(iv)

Where Amputation must be made

It is not sufficient to know that Amputation is necessary; but also you must learne in what place of the dead part, it must bee done, and herein the wisedome and judgement of the Chirurgion is most apparent. Art bids to take hold of the quicke, and to cut off the member in the sound flesh; but the same art wisheth us, to preserve whole that which is sound, as much as in us lies. I will shew thee by a familiar example how thou maist carry thy selfe in these difficulties. Let us suppose that the foote is mortified even to the anckle; here you must attentively marke in what place you must cut it off. For unlesse you take hold of the quicke flesh in the amputation, or if you leave any putrefaction, you profit nothing by amputation, for it will creepe and spread over the rest of the body. It befits Physicke ordained for the preservation of mankind, to defend from the iron or instrument and all manner of injurie, that which enjoyes life and health. Wherefore you shall cut off as little of that which is sound as you possibly can; yet so that you rather cut away that which is quicke, than leave behind any thing that is perished, according to the advice of *Celsus*.[8] Yet oft times the commodity of the action of the rest of the part, and as it were a certaine ornament thereof, changes this counsell. For if you take these two things into your consideration they will induce you in this propounded case and example, to cut off the Legge some five fingers breadth under the knee. For so the patient may more fitly use the rest of his Legge and with lesse trouble, that is, he may the better goe on a woodden Legge; for otherwise, if according to the common rules of Art, you cut it off close to that which

---

[8] For Celsus, see note 27 in Part two.

is perished the patient will be forced with trouble to use three Legges instead of two. . . .

How the section or amputation must be performed

The first care must be of the patients strength, wherefore let him be nourished with meats of good nutriment, easie digestion, and such as generate many spirits. . . . Then let him bee placed, as is fit, and drawing the muscles upwards toward the sound parts, let them be tyed with a straite ligature a little above that place of the member which is to be cut off, with a strong and broad fillet[9] like that which women usually bind up their haire withall; This ligature hath a threefold use; the first is, that it hold the muscles drawne up together with the skin, so that retiring backe presently after the performance of the worke, they may cover the ends of the cut bones, and serve them in stead of boulsters or pillowes when they are healed up, and so suffer with lesse paine the compression in susteining the rest of the body; besides also by this meanes the wounds are the sooner healed and cicatrized; for by how much more flesh or skinne is left upon the ends of the bones, by so much they are the sooner healed and cicatrized. The second is, for that it prohibites the fluxe of blood by pressing and shutting up the veines and arteries. The third is, for that it much dulls the sense of the part by stupefying it; the animall spirits by the straite compression being hindred from passing in by the Nerves: Wherefore when you have made your ligature, cut the flesh even to the bone with a sharpe and well cutting incision knife, or with a crooked knife. . . .

Now you must note, that there usually lyes betweene the bones, a portion of certaine muscles, which you cannot easily cut with a large incision or dismembring knife; wherefore you must carefully divide it and separate it wholly from the bone, with an instrument made neately like a crooked incision knife. I thought good to advertise thee hereof; for if thou shouldest leave any thing besides the bone to bee divided by the saw, you would put the patient to excessive paine in the performance thereof; for soft things such as flesh tendons and membranes, cannot be easily cut with a saw. Therefore when you shall come to the bared bone, all the other parts being wholly cut asunder and divided, you shall nimbly divide it with a little saw about some foote and three inches long, and that as neare to the sound flesh as you can. And then you must smooth the front of the bone which the saw hath made rough.

---

9 A headband.

How to stanch the bleeding when the member is taken off

When you have cut off and taken away the member, let it bleed a little according to the strength of the patient, that so the rest of the part may afterwards be lesse obnoxious to inflammation and other symptomes; Then let the Veines and Arteries be bound up as speedily and streightly as you can; that so the course of the flowing blood may bee stopped and wholly stayed. Which may be done by taking hold of the vessells with your Crowes beake.[10] . . .

The ends of the vessells lying hid in the flesh, must be taken hold of & drawn with this instrument forth of the muscles whereinto they presently after the amputation withdrew themselves, as all parts are still used to withdraw themselves towards their originalls. In performance of this worke, you neede take no great care, if you together with the vessells comprehend some portion of the neighbouring parts, as of the flesh, for hereof will ensue no harme; but the vessells will so bee consolidated with the more ease, than if they being bloodlesse parts should grow together by themselves. To conclude, when you have so drawne them forth, binde them with a strong double thred.

How after the blood is stanched, you must dresse the wounded member

When you have tyed the Vessells, loose your Ligature which you have made above the place of amputation; then draw together the lippes of the wound with foure stitches made acrosse, having taken good hold of the flesh; for thus you shall draw over the bones that part of the skinne and cut muscles drawne upwards before the amputation, and cover them as close as you can, that so the ayre may the lesse come at them, and that so the wound may bee the more speedily agglutinated.[11] . . .

(v)

The Voyage of Hedin, 1553

Charles the Emperor[12] caused the Citty of *Therouenne* to be besieged, where Monsieur the Duke of *Savoy*, was Generall of the whole army: it was taken by assault where there was a great number of our men slaine and prisoners. The King willing to prevent that the enemy should not

[10] A special surgical instrument, which Paré had depicted in the original text.
[11] Stuck together.
[12] The Habsburg Emperor Charles V (1519–55).

also come to beseige the Citty & Castle of *Hedin*, sent *Messieurs* the Duke *Bouillion*, the Duke *Horace*, the Marquesse of *Villars*, a number of Captaines, and about eight hundred souldiers, & during the siege of *Therouenne*, the sayd Lords fortified the sayd Castle of *Hedin*, in such sort that it seemed impregnable. The King sent me to the sayd Lords to helpe them with my Art, if there were any neede. Now soon after the taking of *Therouenne*, we were beseiged with the army. . . . Our souldiers sallied forth upon the enemies, where there was many kild, and slaine with musket shot and swords, as well on the one side, as of the other, and our soldiers did often make sallyes forth upon the ene-mies before their trenches were made; where I had much worke cut out, so that I had no rest night nor day for dressing the wounded. And I will tell this by the way, that we had put many of them in a great Tower, layd upon a little straw, and their pillowes were stones, their coverlets were their cloakes, of those that had any. Whilst the battery was making, as many shot as the Cannons made, the patients sayd they felt paine in their woundes, as if one had given them blowes with a staffe, the one cry'd his head, the other his arme, and so of other parts; divers of their wounds bled afresh yea in greater quantity than first when they were wounded, and then it was I must runne to stay their bleeding. . . . Now through this diabolicall tempest of the Eccho from these thundring Instruments, and by the great and vehement agitation of the collision of the ayre resounding and reverberating in the wounds of the hurt people, divers dyed, and others because they could not rest by reason of the groanes and cryes that they made, night and day; and also for want of good nourishment and other good usage necessary to wounded people. . . . [To eat] they could have had nothing but old Cow beefe, which was taken about *Hedin* for our munition, salted and halfe boyled, insomuch that who would have eate it he must pull it with the force of his teeth, as birds of Prey doe carrion. I will not forget their linnen wherewith they were drest, which was onely rewashed every day, and dryed at the fire, and therefore dry & stubborne like Parchment, I leave you to thinke how their wounds could heale well.

10.2

The cause, diagnosis and treatment of scurvy: James Lind's *A Treatise of the Scurvy* (1753)

Christopher Lloyd (ed.), *The Health of Seamen: Selections from the Works of Dr. James Lind, Sir Gilbert Blane and Dr. Thomas Trotter* (London, Navy Records Society, 1965), pp. 12–21.

Dr James Lind (1716–94) became one of the most prominent figures in nautical medicine in the eighteenth century. After taking his medical degree in Edinburgh, he joined the navy as a surgeon's mate in 1739. By 1747, when he had made his first dietary experiments to prove that lemons and oranges provided the best available cure for scurvy, he had become surgeon of the sixty-gun ship, *Salisbury*. Scurvy had by then become a major problem for merchant ships, as well as navies, due to the much longer journeys undertaken in the eighteenth century. Lind's *Treatise of the scurvy* (1753) was an immediate success and went through three editions and several translations in his lifetime. In 1758, Lind was appointed Senior Physician to the newly opened naval hospital, the Haslar, near Portsmouth, where he remained until his retirement in 1783.

Of the causes of scurvy

I had the opportunity in two Channel cruises, the one of ten weeks, the other of eleven, *ann.* 1746 and 1747 in his Majesty's ship the *Salisbury*, a fourth rate, to see the disease rage with great violence. And here it was remarkable that though I was on board several other long Channel cruises, one of twelve weeks particularly, from the 10 August to the 28 October, yet we had but one scorbutic patient,[13] nor on the other that I remember had we the least scorbutic appearance. But in those who I have mentioned the scurvy began to rage after being a month to six weeks at sea, when the water on board, as I took particular notice, was uncommonly sweet and good, and the state of provisions such as could afford no suspicion of occasioning a general sickness, being the same in quality as in former cruises. And though the scorbutic people were by the generous liberality of that great and good commander, the Hon. Captain George Edgcumbe, daily supplied with fresh provisions, such

---

[13] A patient suffering from scurvy.

as mutton broth and fowls and even meat from his own table, yet at the expiration of ten weeks we brought into Plymouth 80 men out of a complement of 350 more or less afflicted with this disease.

Now it was observable that both these cruises were in the months of April, May and June, when we had, especially in the beginning of them, a continuance of cold, rainy and thick Channel weather, as it is called, whereas in our other cruises we had generally very fine weather, except in winter, when, during the time I was surgeon, the cruises were but short. Nor could I assign any other reason for the frequency of this disease in these two cruises and our exception from it at other times but the influence of the weather; the circumstances of the men, ship and provisions being in all other respects alike. I have more than once remarked that after great rains or a continuance of close, foggy weather, especially after storms with rain, the scorbutic people generally grew worse; but found a mitigation of their symptoms and complaints upon the weather becoming drier and warmer for a few days. And I am certain it will be allowed by all who have had an opportunity of making observations of this disease at sea, or will attentively consider the situation of seamen there, that the principal and main predisposing cause to it is a manifest and obvious quality of the air, viz, its moisture. The effects of this are perceived to be more immediately hurtful and pernicious in certain constitutions; in those who are much weakened by preceding sickness; in those who, from a lazy inactive disposition, neglect to use proper exercise; and in those who indulge a discontented melancholy humour; all which may be reckoned the secondary disposing causes to this foul and fatal mischief.

As the atmosphere at sea may always be supposed to be moister than that of the land, hence there is always a greater disposition to the scorbutic diathesis[14] at sea than in a pure dry land air. But supposing the like constitution of air in both places, the inconveniences which persons suffer in a ship during a damp wet season are infinitely greater than people on land are exposed to; these latter having many ways of guarding against its pernicious effects by warm dry clothes, fires, good lodging etc., whereas sailors are obliged not only to breathe in this air all day, but sleep in it at night, and frequently in wet bed clothes, the ship's hatches being necessarily kept open. And indeed one reason for the frequence of the scurvy in the above cruises was no doubt the often carrying up of the bedding of the ship's company to quarters, where it was sometimes quite wet through and continued so for many days together when, for want of fair weather, there was no opportunity of drying it.

---

[14] A permanent condition of the body rendering it liable to specific diseases.

No persons sensible to the bad effects of sleeping in wet apartments or in damp clothes and almost in the open air without anything sufficiently dry or warm to put on will be surprised at the havock the scurvy made in Lord Anson's[15] crew in passing the Cape Horn, if their situation in such uncommon and tempestuous weather be properly considered.

During such furious storms the spray of the sea raised by the violence of the wind is dispersed over the whole ship, so that the people breathe, as it were, in water for many weeks together. The tumultuous waves, incessantly breaking in upon the decks and wetting those who are upon duty as if they had been ducked in the sea, are also continually sending down great quantities of water below; which makes it the most uncomfortable wet lodging imaginable and from the labouring of the ship it generally leaks down in many places directly upon their beds. There being here no fire or sun to dry or exhale the moisture, and the hatches necessarily kept shut, this moist, stagnating, confined air below becomes most offensive and intolerable. When such weather continues long, attended with sleet and rain as it generally is, we may easily figure to ourselves the condition of the poor men who are obliged to sleep in wet clothes and damp beds, the decks swimming with water below them; and there to remain for four hours at a time, till they are again called up to fresh fatigue and hard labour and again exposed to the washing of the sea and rains. The long continuance of this weather seldom fails to produce the scurvy at sea.

. . . To which it may be added that by observations made on this disease it appears that those who are once infected with it, especially in so deep a degree as that squadron was, are more subject to it afterwards than others. I remember that many of them who returned to England with Lord Anson and afterwards went to sea in other ships were much more liable to scurvy than others.

It will be now proper to inquire into the diet which mariners are necessarily obliged to live upon at sea. And as it appears to be the principal occasional cause of their malady it may be worthwhile to consider sea provisions in their best state, it being found by experience that, notwithstanding the soundness and goodness of both water and provisions, the calamity often rages with great fury and can be removed only by change of diet. Now, if in this case they appear to have so great an influence in forming the distemper, what ill consequences may not reasonably be expected from a much worse state of them, as from putrid

---

[15] Lord Anson (1697–1762) undertook a circumnavigation of the globe in 1740–44. Of 1,955 men who began the voyage, nearly 1,000 had died of scurvy by the time Anson returned to England in 1744.

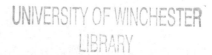

beef, rancid pork, mouldy biscuit and flour, or bad water, which are mis-fortunes commonly at sea? All which must infallibly have bad effects in so putrid a disease.

It must be remarked in general that the sea diet is extremely gross, viscid and hard of digestion. It consists of two articles, viz., the sweet farinaceous substances unfermented, and salted or dried flesh and fish.

But more particularly in our Royal Navy, whose provisions for good-ness and plenty exceed those of any other ships or fleets in the world, every man has an allowance of a pound of biscuit a day, which in the manner it is baked will be found more solid and substantial food than two pounds of ordinary well baked bread at land. And this is a principal article of their diet. But the seabiscuit undergoes little or no fermenta-tion in baking and is consequently of much harder and more difficult digestion than well leavened and properly fermented bread. . . . Well baked bread, which has undergone a sufficient degree of fermentation, is of light and easy digestion, and indeed the most proper nourishment for man, as it is adapted by its acescency[16] to correct a flesh diet; whereas on the contrary sea biscuit, not being thus duly fermented, will in many cases afford too tenacious and viscid chyle,[17] improper for nourishment of the body where the vital digestive faculties are weak-ened and impaired.

The next article in their allowance of what is called fresh provisions is one pound and a half of wheat flour in the week, which is made into pudding with water and a certain proportion of pickled suet. This last does not keep long at sea, so that they have often raisins or currants in its place. But flour and water boiled thus together form a tenacious glutinous paste requiring the utmost strength and integrity of the powers of digestion to subdue and assimilate it into nourishment. We find that weak, inactive, valetudinarian people[18] cannot long bear such food.

There remain two other articles of fresh provisions, of which the allowance to each man is more than they can generally use. The first is ground oats boiled to a consistence with water, commonly called *burgow*. Of this the English sailors eat but little, though in their cir-cumstances it would seem to be wholesome enough, as being the most acescent part of their diet. The other is boiled peas. . . . It is evident that in some cases they must afford gross and improper nourishment.

This is the allowance of fresh provisions, and they have, besides, a proper quantity given them of salt, butter and cheese. The latter of

16 Natural sourness.
17 White, gastric fluid.
18 Weak, sickly people.

which is experienced to differ extremely in its qualities, or in the ease or difficulty with which it is digested, according to its strength, age etc. But the Suffolk cheese will in many instances, instead of assisting digestion, which many other cheese is said to do, prove a load to the stomach itself, as well as the salt butter or sweet oil given sometimes in its place, neither of which indeed correct the qualities of their other foods.

Lastly, of flesh each man has for allowance two pounds of salt beef and two pounds of salt pork per week. But these are found by everyone's experience to be much harder and more difficult to digest than fresh meats. . . . No person can long bear a diet of such salt flesh meats, unless it is corrected by bread, vinegar or vegetables.

[. . .]

For drink the government allows, where it can be procured, good sound small beer;[19] at other times wines, brandy, rum or arrack,[20] according to the produce of the country where ships are stationed. Beer and fermented liquors of any sort will be found the best antiscorbutics and most proper to correct the ill effects of their sea diet and situation, whereas distilled spirits have a most pernicious influence on this disease.

Of the diagnostics or signs of the scurvy

In order to observe greater accuracy in the description of a disease attended with so many and various symptoms, these might have been properly enough ranged under three classes.

The first, containing the most common and constant symptoms, such as may be said to be essential to the nature of the malady.

The second, such as are more casual and accidental, proceeding not so much from the genius of the distemper as from the epidemical constitution of the air, the state or habit of the body, or from the determination of other causes.

And the third, some extraordinary and uncommon symptoms that sometimes, though seldom, have happened in it; and which occur only in the highest and most virulent state of this disease, from the peculiar idiosyncracy of the patient, its combination with other malignant diseases, or from other incidental circumstances.

But for the sake of perspicuity, I choose rather to describe the symptoms in the order in which they generally appear and as peculiar to the

[19] Diluted beer.
[20] Spirit or liquor made from native produce such as coconut and rice.

several stages of the disease, and shall distinguish as I go along those which are more constant or essential from the less frequent or adventitious.

The first indication of the approach of this disease is generally a change of colour in the face from the natural and usual look to a pale and bloated complexion, with a listlessness to action, or an aversion to any sort of exercise. When we examine narrowly the lips or the caruncles[21] of the eyes where the blood vessels lie exposed, they appear of a greenish cast. Meanwhile the person eats and drinks heartily and seems in perfect health, except that his countenance and lazy inactive disposition portend a future scurvy.

This change of colour in the face, although it does not always precede the other symptoms, yet constantly attends them when advanced. Scorbutic people for the most part appear at first of a pale or yellowish hue, which becomes afterwards more darkish or livid.

Their former aversion to motion degenerates soon into an universal lassitude, with a stiffness and feebleness of their knees using exercise, with which they are apt to be much fatigued and upon that occasion subject to breathlessness and panting. . . .

Their gums soon after become itchy, swell and are apt to bleed upon the gentlest friction. Their breath is then offensive, and upon looking into their mouths, the gums appear of an unusual livid redness, are soft and spungy and become afterwards extremely putrid and fungous. ... They are subject not only to bleeding from the gums, but prone to fall into haemorrhages from other parts of the body.

Their skin at this time feels dry, as it does through the whole course of the malady. In many, especially if feverish, it is extremely rough . . . [a]nd when examined it is found covered with several reddish, bluish or rather black and livid spots. . . . These spots are of different sizes . . . [and] are to be seen chiefly on the legs and thighs, often on the arms, breast and trunk of the body, but more rarely on the head and face.

Many have a swelling of their legs . . .[which] gradually advances up the leg and the whole member becomes oedematous.[22] . . .

These are the most constant and essential symptoms of this malady in the progress of its first stage. But a diversity is sometimes observed in the order of their appearance. . . .

[. . .]

In the second stage of this disease they most commonly lose the use of

---

[21] Fleshy excrescences.
[22] Swollen with an oedema.

their limbs, having a contraction of the flexor tendons in the ham, with a swelling and pain in the joint of the knee. Indeed, a stiffness in these tendons and a weakness of the knees appear pretty early in this disease, generally terminating in a contracted and swelled joint. They are subject to frequent languors and when long confined from exercise to a proneness to faint upon the least motion of the body, which are the most peculiar, constant and essential symptoms of this stage.

[...]

They are apt on being moved or exposed to the fresh air suddenly to expire. This happened to one of our people when in the boat going to be landed at Plymouth hospital. It was remarkable he had made shift to get there without any assistance, while many others were obliged to be carried out upon their beds. He had a deep scorbutical colour in his face, with complaints in his breast. He panted for about half a minute, then expired. . . .

It is not easy to conceive a more dismal and diversified scene of misery than what is beheld in the third and last stage of this calamity, it being then that the anomalous and more extraordinary symptoms most commonly occur. It is not unusual at this time for such persons as have had ulcers formerly healed up to have them break out afresh, while on others the skin of their swelled legs often bursts, particularly where soft, painful, livid swellings have been first observed; and these degenerate into such crude, bloody, fungous ulcers as formerly described. Some few at this period (though very rarely) fall into colliquative putrid fevers,[23] attended almost always with petechiae[24], foetid sweats etc., or rather sink under profuse evacuations of rotten blood, by stool and urine, from the lungs, nose, stomach, haemorrhoidal veins etc.; while the disease more frequently in others, by occasioning obstructions and putrefaction in the abdominal viscera, gives rise to jaundice, dropsy and the *affectio hypochondriaca*, or the most confirmed melancholy and despondency of mind, attended with severe nervous rigours; as also to violent colics, obstinate costiveness etc.

Towards the close of this malady the breast is most commonly affected with a violent uneasy straitness and oppression and an extreme dyspnoea,[25] accompanied sometimes with a pain under the sternum, but more frequently in either of the sides, while others without any complaint of pain have their respiration become quickly contracted and laborious, ending in sudden and often unexpected death.

[23] In which the humours become liquified.
[24] Spots.
[25] Difficulty in breathing.

Of the prevention of the scurvy

I shall conclude the precepts relating to the preservation of seamen with showing the best means of obviating many inconveniences which attend long voyages and of removing the several causes productive of this mischief.

The following are the experiments.

On the 20th May, 1747, I took twelve patients in the scurvy on board the *Salisbury* at sea. Their cases were as similar as I could have them. They all in general had putrid gums, the spots and lassitude, with weakness of their knees. They lay together in one place, being a proper apartment for the sick in the fore-hold; and had one diet common to all, viz., water gruel sweetened with sugar in the morning; fresh mutton broth often times for dinner; at other times puddings, boiled biscuit with sugar etc.; and for supper barley, raisins, rice and currants, sago and wine, or the like. Two of these were ordered each a quart of cyder a day. Two others took twenty five gutts[26] of elixir vitriol three times a day upon an empty stomach, using a gargle strongly acidulated with it for their mouths. Two others took two spoonfuls of vinegar three times a day upon an empty stomach, having their gruels and their other food well acidulated with it, as also the gargle for the mouth. Two of the worst patients, with the tendons in the ham rigid (a symptom none the rest had) were put under a course of sea water. Of this they drank half a pint every day and sometimes more or less as it operated by way of gentle physic. Two others had each two oranges and one lemon given them every day. These they eat with greediness at different times upon an empty stomach. They continued but six days under this course, having consumed the quantity that could be spared. The two remaining patients took the bigness of a nutmeg three times a day of an electuary recommended by an hospital surgeon . . . by a decoction of which . . . they were gently purged three or four times during the course.

The consequence was that the most sudden and visible good effects were perceived from the use of the oranges and lemons; one of those who had taken them being at the end of six days fit for duty. The spots were not indeed at that time quite off his body, nor his gums sound; but without any other medicine than a gargarism of elixir of vitriol he became quite healthy before we came into Plymouth, which was on the 16th June. The other was the best recovered of any in his condition, and being now deemed pretty well was appointed nurse to the rest of the sick. . . .

---

[26] Drops.

... I shall here only observe that the result of all my experiments was that oranges and lemons were the most effectual remedies for this distemper at sea. I am apt to think oranges preferable to lemons, though perhaps both given together will be found most serviceable.

10.3

Military medicine in the eighteenth century: John Pringle's *Observations on the Diseases of the Army* (1764)

John Pringle, *Observations on the Diseases of the Army* (London, A. Millar, D. Wilson & T. Payne, 1764 (first edition published 1752)), pp. iii–xiv.

Sir John Pringle (1707–82) matriculated at the University of Edinburgh in 1727. The following year he left to study medicine at the University of Leiden under the famous Herman Boerhaave (1668–1738). Pringle received his M.D. from Leiden in 1730 and four years later he was appointed Professor of Moral Philosophy at Edinburgh, where he also practised medicine. He was appointed physician to the British army by its commander-in-chief, the Earl of Stair, in 1742. In 1745 he was promoted to the post of Physician-General to the army. Pringle saw six years of active service with the British army in the Low Countries before retiring in 1748 to set up a successful medical practice in London. His subsequent publications, which drew largely on his military experiences, advocated hospital reforms and measures to prevent infections.

The diseases of the army, as far as it appears, have been treated of by none of the ancient physicians; nor have we any information about them from the historians, unless when some very uncommon or fatal distemper attended an expedition.

Thus *Xenophon*,[27] in his relation of the famous retreat of the *Greeks*, mentions their being liable to the *fames canina*,[28] to blindness, and to a mortification of the extremities, from the snow, and excessive cold

---

[27] Fourth-century BC Greek historian.
[28] Hunger of a dog.

they were exposed to, on their march. *Pliny*, the Naturalist,[29] is the first who takes notice of the scurvy, which afflicted the *Roman* army, in *Germany*, after it had continued two years in that country; and we likewise find the *Romans* sometimes under a necessity of removing their camps, on account of the bad air of the adjacent marshes. *Plutarch*[30] observes that after a famine *Demetrius* lost *8000* men by a plague. *Livy*[31] informs us of a like distemper that seized both the *Romans* and *Carthaginians* in *Sicily*; and *Diodorus Siculus*[32] describes another plague, attended with a bloody flux, which almost utterly destroyed the latter, at the siege of *Syracuse*; and explains the cause of it in a full and satisfactory manner. But excepting these, and a few more instances, there remains no account of the diseases incident to the armies of the ancients. It may seem strange that *Vegetius*, in his book *De Re Militari*,[33] should write a chapter containing directions how to preserve the health of soldiers; and yet not mention any sickness they were particularly subject to; and that he should speak of the physicians attending the camp, without taking notice of their manner of disposing of the sick, whether in hospitals or otherwise.

The silence of the ancients upon this article is the more to be regreted because as war was their chief study, it might be expected that the orders relating to the care of the sick, were good in proportion to their skill in the other branches of the military art. And indeed as their troops were constantly in the field, and in very different climates, the physicians of those days had it greatly in their power to furnish many useful observations on the nature and causes of camp-diseases, and on the proper methods of treating them.

Nor had this defect been supplied, when I was first employed in the army, by any of the moderns that I knew of, unless by such as had either been little, or not at all employed in the service, at least in military hospitals; and who, on that account, could not be supposed to write better on this head, than that author, who composed a treatise on the Art of War, without having ever seen a campaign. So that after all, this part of medicine, which ought long ago to have been complete, seemed to be still in a manner new: so little is a military life consistent with that state of tranquillity requisite for study and observation.

[29] Pliny the elder, author of the celebrated *Natural History* (c. 23–79).
[30] A contemporary of Pliny, the Greek-born Plutarch was a philosopher and historian whose numerous works were still widely read and taught in eighteenth-century Europe.
[31] Livy or Titus Livius (59 BC–12/17 AD), Roman historian.
[32] Greek historian of the fourth century BC.
[33] Flavius Vegetius Renatus (fl. 383–450) was the author of the only Roman military manual to survive intact.

Perceiving therefore what little assistance I was to expect from books, I began to note down such observations as occurred, in hopes of finding them afterwards useful in practice. And having continued this method to the end of the former war,[34] I then put those materials into order, and with as much clearness and conciseness as I could, endeavoured from my own experience to supply, in some measure, what I thought so much wanting on this subject.

I have divided the work into three parts. In the first, after giving a short account of the air and the diseases more peculiar to the *Low Countries* (so often the seat of our wars) I proceed to give an abridgment of the medical journal, which I had kept of the several campaigns. In this I mention the epidemics and more frequent diseases of our troops, in the order they occurred, the embarkations, marches, encampments, cantonments, winter-quarters, the seasons, the changes of the weather, and, in a word, all the circumstances that seemed to me most likely to affect the health of an army. In this part I have entered little into the description of diseases; much less have I touched upon their cure; reserving both those heads to be considered afterwards. My chief intention here, was to collect materials for tracing the more evident causes of military distempers, in order that whatever depended upon those in command, and was consistent with the service, might be fairly stated, so as to suggest proper measures either for preventing, or for lessening such causes in any future campaign. And I have been the more studious of exactness in this account, as I foresaw that in whatever manner the whole was to be received, this part, at least, would be acceptable, as being a narration of facts, by one who was present and employed all the time. . . .

I have therefore thrown most of the reasoning, that results from the first part, into the second; in which, after dividing and classing the diseases common to a military life, I inquire into the more general causes of them; namely, such as depend upon the air, the diet, and other circumstances usually comprehended under the appellation of the *non-naturals*. And here I have ventured to assign some sources of distempers, very different from the sentiments of other writers upon this subject; and I have also shewn how little instrumental some other causes are in producing sickness, which yet have been thought the most frequent of any. Nor will this liberty, I hope, be condemned, when it is considered what opportunities I have had beyond others to make such remarks; and that, as Natural Knowledge is daily improving, those authors, who write last on subjects connected therewith, are most likely to be in right.

[34] The Seven Years' War (1756–63).

Among the chief causes of sickness and death in an army, the Reader will little expect that I should rank, what is intended for its health and preservation, the Hospitals themselves; and that on account of the bad air, and other inconveniences attending them. However, during the former war, one considerable step was made for their improvement. Till then it had been usual to remove the sick a great way from the camp, whereby many were actually lost before they came under the care of the physicians; or, which was attended with equally bad consequences, if the hospitals were nigh, they were for the greater security frequently shifted, according to the motions of the army. But the *Earl of Stair*,[35] my illustrious patron, being sensible of this hardship . . . proposed to the *Duke de Noailles* . . . that the hospitals on both sides should be considered as sanctuaries for the sick, and mutually protected. This was readily agreed to by the *French* General, who took the first opportunity to shew a particular regard to his engagement. For when our hospital was at *Feckenheim* . . . at a distance from our camp, the *Duke de Noailles* having occasion to send a detachment to another village . . . and apprehending that this might alarm the sick, he sent to acquaint them, that as he knew the *British* hospital was there, he had given express orders to his troops not to disturb them. This agreement was strictly observed, on both sides, all that campaign: and tho' it has been since neglected, it is to be hoped, that on future occasions the contending parties will make it a precedent.

After explaining the general causes of the sickness in armies, I proceed to point out the means of removing some, and rendering others less dangerous. . . .

I conclude the second part with comparing the numbers of the sick at different seasons; in order that the Commander may know, with some degree of certainty, what force he may, at any time, rely upon for service; the effects of short or long campaigns upon the health; the difference between taking the field early, and going late into winter-quarters; with other calculations, founded upon such materials as were furnished by the war. The *data* are perhaps too few to deduce certain consequences from them; but as I have not found any other I could depend upon, I was obliged to make the best use I could of these, which at least will serve for a specimen of what may be done, in this way, upon further experience.

These parts were intended for the information of Officers as well as Physicians. I have endeavoured to relate the facts, and draw my infer-

---

[35] John Dalrymple, 2nd Earl of Stair (1673–1747) was a general and diplomat, who was made field marshall in 1742.

ences in the plainest manner, and with as few scientific terms, as was consistent with the nature of the subject; and I hope with perspicuity enough to be understood by any reader, not unacquainted with the common principles of Natural Knowledge.

But the third part, containing the practice, is designed for those of my own profession only; as it could neither be properly explained, nor prove instructive to others. . . .

I conceive the diseases, to which an army is most subject, to be divisible into two classes; one, comprehending those which are also common in *Britain*; and the other, such as are more peculiar to a different climate, or to the condition of a soldier. Now, as the first have been fully treated of by several learned authors, in the hands of every physician, and also occur in daily practice, I pass them cursorily over; being satisfied with laying down my general method of proceeding, with the difference, if any, to be observed in prescribing in military hospitals.

But, with regard to the other class, including the bilious, and malignant fevers, and the dysentery, as they are distempers less frequent in this country, I thought it proper to treat of them more at length. . . .

[. . .]

In reasoning upon the nature of the bilious fevers, the hospital-fever, and the dysentery, I have frequently had recourse to the *septic principle*; which tho' I think I have sufficiently ascertained in this work, yet to some it may be satisfactory to know, that the corruption of the humours, as the cause of certain diseases, was first hinted at by *Hippocrates*, further taken notice of by *Galen*, and still more fully treated of and applied to medicine in later times; as appears by the Aphorisms of *Sanctorius*,[36] and other noted works of that age. And tho' it was afterwards sunk in the the systems of *Sylvius* and *Willis*,[37] and in that of the mechanic writers, yet it was revived by *Hoffman* and *Boerhaave*;[38] and especially by the latter, who under the article of *alcalis* comprehended all that he thought *septic* or *putrid*. But as my celebrated master had not time to ascertain every part of his doctrine from his own experi-

[36] Sanctorius Sanctorius (1561–1636) was Professor of Medicine at Padua and the author of several important works on medicine.

[37] Franciscus Sylvius (1614–72) was a leading proponent of the iatrochemical and iatromechanical schools of medicine who proposed a new theory of digestion based on the action of acid in the stomach. The Englishman Thomas Willis (1621–75) also adopted various elements of the new chemical and mechanical philosophies in formulating his own, highly influential approach to understanding the function of the human body.

[38] Friedrich Hoffman (1660–1742), Professor of Medicine at Halle, was a thorough-going mechanist, as was the famous Dutch physician Herman Boerhaave (1668–1738), who proposed a hydraulic model of the body.

ence, it was no wonder some mistakes were made, and that the extent of these principles was not fully understood.

Two things induced me to prosecute this subject; the great number of putrid cases that were under my care in the hospitals abroad; and the authority of Lord *Bacon*,[39] who offers good reasons for considering the knowledge of what brings on, and retards putrefaction, as most likely to account for some of the more abstruse operations of nature. My papers on this subject being read at several meetings of the Royal Society, were left in the hands of the Secretary; but finding it necessary to make frequent references to those experiments, I thought it proper to annex them to this work. . . .

10.4
Military and naval medicine in eighteenth-century France

Laurence Brockliss and Colin Jones, *The Medical World of Early Modern France* (Oxford, Clarendon Press, 1997), pp. 689–700.

The improvement of military hygiene and the creation of military hospitals, which gathered pace in the seventeenth century and accelerated further in the eighteenth century, was clearly linked, in France and other European states, to the aggrandising behaviour of the great powers, many of them absolute monarchies, all of which were equipped with large standing armies. It made good economic and political sense for the state to provide extended medical services for its military personnel: it helped trained soldiers to stay battle fit and may have encouraged recruitment in the first instance. In this extract the authors discuss the development of such reforms in eighteenth-century France.

[T]he growth of a standing army, especially in the second quarter of the seventeenth century, obliged the absolute monarchy to confront new problems of control and discipline. One area of the state's concern was to protect the civilian population from the depredations caused by the huge, ill-disciplined, and predatory numbers of military men, deserters,

[39] Francis Bacon (1561–1626), whose *Advancement of learning* and other writings provided the philosophical underpinning for the scientific advances of the seventeenth century.

and demobilized veterans. With traditional welfare arrangements for deserving veterans . . . unable to cope with the scale of the problem, the state resorted to the practices of confinement it was developing in social policy more generally.

The royal edict establishing the Paris Hôpital Général in 1656 had been flanked by an edict ordering disabled soldiers to be despatched to garrisons and stopped from begging in towns. The Hôtel des Invalides established in 1670 was in effect a kind of *hôpital général* for army veterans. Despite its rhetoric of dynastic benevolence, moreover, the establishment was saturated in the mercantilist and populationist concerns of the monarchy. It aimed to confine a potentially dangerous group, keeping them out of harm's way, insulating them from the rest of society, habituating them to productive labour, and maybe even training them in spiritual perfection. . . .

The medical service of the Invalides, which was under the supervision of the war ministry, was noticeably more intense than that of civilian hospitals. Rooms were built deliberately large, airy, well lit, and hygienic, with careful consideration given to water-supply and waste-disposal. There was a separate infirmary for veterans who fell sick and a block for lunatics. The principal physician enjoyed extensive privileges, and the surgical services were strengthened from 1707 by the appointment of a surgeon-major, one of whose tasks was the care of syphilitics, who were kept apart from other inmates. Teaching in surgery was provided from 1718 for apprentice surgeons: the courses became famous throughout Paris in the 1720s when they were taken over by the brilliant surgeon Morand,[40] one of the founders of the Academy of Surgery. The status of the establishment as a medical teaching institution, grounded in the especially profuse supply of cadavers the institution's medical staff were able to secure, was underlined in further legislation in 1728 and 1747.

The Invalides was a pioneer of the medicalized hospital which over the eighteenth century came to be characteristic of health provision within the armed forces. Louis XIV's wars saw the state taking increasing responsibility for the health of troops. . . . Provisional field hospitals were established on campaign; major civilian hospitals were called on to take up any overflow, especially away from the front; and regiments were accorded a standard medical encadrement. . . . In 1708 a network of military hospitals was established, and fixed ratios of medical staffing set.

---

[40] Sauveur-François Morand (1697–1773) was a leading member of a group of Parisian surgeons who acquired international fame for their innovative approach to anatomy and surgery; for the pioneering work of the Academy of Surgery in Paris, see extract 13.2 below.

The hospital network thickened over the course of the century, and it developed in sophistication too. Specialized syphilis institutions operated in Montpellier and Besançon – for serving soldiers sacrificed more freely to Venus than to Mars – and a number of mineral spas were incorporated. The spas at Barèges, Bourbonne-les-Bains, Digne, and Saint-Amand were very specifically aimed at ailing soldiers – notably those with nervous ailments, paralysis, and skin disease. . . .

A particularly striking feature of the military medical establishment was the very high proportion of surgeons within it. Although commanders and aristocratic officers liked the attentions of physicians on their staff for their own health, they viewed the cheap and cheerful services of surgeons and apothecaries as appropriate for the rank and file, especially in times of battle. . . . Though the number of physicians registered only very modest rises [in numbers during the course of the eighteenth century], apothecaries entered the picture for the first time, while the number of surgical posts increased strikingly. Salaries rose too. . . . A sign of growing solidarity and self-esteem in the army medical corps was the adoption of a distinctive uniform for military medical staff: surgeons in 1757, physicians in 1775, and apothecaries in 1786. . . .

The armed forces proved a testing ground for the content of medical and surgical training. Thus although historians conventionally date the 'birth of the clinic' from the 1790s, many of the elements of the approaches associated with that development – teaching practice, an emphasis on bedside medicine, the routine practice of autopsies, and a concern with medical statistics – had all been found in Ancien Régime military hospitals. State regulations in 1747 were the first to mention the need for military hospitals to provide teaching in anatomy (incorporating dissections) by both physicians and surgeons but in fact a number of institutions were already practising this precept. . . . The case for better bedside instruction and surgical training seemed to be highlighted by the wretched experiences of the War of Austrian Succession (1740–8); seven-eighths of individuals who suffered an amputation after the Battle of Fontenoy in 1745, for example, had died of their wounds. In 1769 the chancellor of the Montpellier Medical Faculty, Jean-François Imbert[41] . . . instituted an initiative in clinical teaching at the Montpellier military hospitals which specialized in venereal and skin diseases. State regulation in 1772 required the establishment of training schools . . . in military hospitals, while further measures in 1775 established teaching amphitheatres based within the military hospitals at

---

[41] Jean-François Imbert (1722–85) was chancellor of the Medical Faculty at the University of Montpellier. He also served as the inspector of military hospitals in the Midi.

Metz, Lille, and Strasburg. For the first time in French history, these offered a unified and clinically orientated training in medicine, surgery, and pharmacy, which was targeted at future army health officers. . . . As at the Invalides, medical staff found it easier to get hold of corpses for dissection and teaching purposes than did their counterparts in civilian hospitals. Partly this was due to the fact that military hospitals came directly under the war ministry and were usually not staffed by religious nursing communities, who had rather different ideas about the proprieties of dissection.

The collection and collation of medical statistics too . . . were also developed in military hospitals under the Ancien Régime. . . . Indeed, the new attention to record-keeping within military medicine helped develop the notion of the hospital as a research centre. . . .

[. . .]

A great many of these features of military medicine were replicated, even foreshadowed, in the navy. The concern for social discipline was similar – and similarly mingled with charitable, mercantilist, and populationist motifs. Although there was no naval equivalent of the Invalides, veteran seamen (merchants as well as navy) were catered for by *hôpitaux généraux* in port cities. . . .

. . . The rudiments of a naval health service, foreshadowing the 1708 regulations for the army, were laid down in 1689, fixing levels of medical encadrement, medical supplies for voyages, and hospital provision. Port physicians and surgeons were entrusted with conducting annual lecture courses for local ships' surgeons, though this only ratified what had already started to happen at a local level. In 1722 an official training school for surgeons had been created at Rochefort and similar courses were running in Toulon from 1725 and Brest from 1740. . . . The high number of corpses from the galleys . . . put the institutions in the forefront of the clinical approach. Clinical trials for drugs were conducted within naval as well as military hospitals. Significantly too, the naval medical corps was allowed its own uniform in 1767. . . .

If the health services of the army and navy witnessed innovatory levels of clinical instruction and medical research, they also acted as a laboratory for experimenting with preventive medicine of all kinds. The neo-Hippocratic revival of interest in environmental medicine struck a resonant note in military health circles. Where nursing sisters had shown a commitment to cleanliness whose roots lay in a moral and religious world-view, in military and naval circles the interest in hygiene was more directly linked to the general medical and intellectual *Zeitgeist*, in particular the conviction that illness was not simply a question of sick individuals but that it was located in an environment subject to human intervention and improvement. . . .

The costs of war acted as a perennial stimulant to improvement in this area. High wound mortality, for example, was not just a condemnation of deficient surgical technique, it was an indictment of filthy hospitals and barracks where the sick and wounded died in droves from cross-infection. Military medical regulations introduced towards the end of the War of Austrian Succession in 1747 stressed the role of a healthy environment in the welfare of troops. Triage[42] of hospital inmates into fever-cases, the wounded, and convalescents was increasingly rigorously applied. . . . A greater emphasis on troops' welfare . . . gave the impetus to the wider diffusion of measures of environmental medicine.

Civilian war commissaries . . . situated midway between medical staff and the war ministry, assumed increasingly prominent medical and hygienic responsibilities as the century wore on. Crucial too was the military hospitals' inspectorate introduced in 1718. . . .

The military hospitals' inspectorate proved a bastion of environmental medicine in the armed forces. The brilliant naval physician Pierre-Isaac Poissonnier (1720–98), appointed inspector of navy hospitals in 1769, was highly influential in this domain, and he was aided by his brother Antoine Poissonnier-Desperrières (1723–?1792), an equally able inspector and from 1767 a firm believer in the importance of combating shipboard scurvy *à la Lind* through provision of fresh citrus fruit. In the army, the Paris-trained physician and military bureaucrat Jean Colombier played a similarly pivotal role. . . . In 1772 his *Code de médecine militaire* claimed to be the first work which dealt not only with sickness of the troops but also with the main principles of health and hygiene: 'the cure of most sick individuals', he contended, 'depends almost always as much on regimen as on remedies'. It therefore behoved the government to concern itself as much with the preservation of soldiers' health as the medication of their maladies. Author of a further volume, *Médecine militaire*, in 1778, Colombier became increasingly influential in the health bureaucracy of the war ministry, making major tours of inspection and setting new standards for care and hygiene. The ministry's decision in 1788 to close down many military hospitals and to replace them with regimental infirmaries which would provide a less infectious focus for health care, was largely based on his thinking on disease-prevention.

---

[42] The action of sorting according to type or case.

The medical corps attached to the armed forces was thus attracting individuals of growing stature and broadening intellectual interest. Many of the most brilliant surgical practitioners of the century had had military experience. . . .

The emergence of a military medical press highlighted the broader intellectual impact of the military hospitals' sector and the rising status and self-confidence of the medical services of the armed forces. No fewer than seven newspapers targeted at military medical men were established over the last few decades of the Ancien Régime. Though most were short-lived, they included much high-quality material. . . .

The military imprint on the orthodox medical community was thus considerable and . . . it strongly influenced the civilian hospitals sector. Sick soldiers within military hospitals were the first group of hospital inmates to be utilized systematically as medical guinea-pigs: for scientific motives, but also for profit. This involved on one hand a bed-side observationalism and routine recourse to autopsy, but also a commitment to active testing of economical mass remedies on the collectivity in ways which the normal conventions of private practice ruled out of court. Therapeutic trials – written up and made available in published form for the wider medical community – were predicated, secondly, on a medicine of the site, which aimed at neutralizing hospital space and evacuating it of noxious health threats. *Pace* Foucault,[43] who underestimates . . . the intellectual vitality generated within hospitals in general (and military hospitals in particular) during the Enlightenment, the fundamentals of a creative and investigatory anatomo-clinical medicine were falling into place long before the 1790s.

[43] The French philosopher, Michel Foucault, in a series of influential writings, put forward the view that hospitals, like prisons and other Enlightenment institutions, were used by the French state as a means of imposing greater social control and order on the populace; for an extract from one of his works, see 11.6 below.

Part eleven

Environment, health
and population, 1500–1800

11.1

Air and good health in Renaissance medicine

André du Laurens, *A Discourse of the Preservation of the Sight:*
Of Melancholike Diseases; of Rheumes; and of Old age . . .
Translated out of French into English . . . by Richard Surphlet
(London, Felix Kingston, 1599), pp. 58–60.

André du Laurens or Laurentius (1558–1609) was educated at Avignon,
Paris and Montpellier before becoming Professor of Medicine at the
latter university in 1583. He subsequently became personal physician
to King Henri IV of France. He was best known as the author of works
about anatomy and was a committed Galenist. The volume from
which the following extract is taken is a collection of four discourses
aimed at a non-specialist readership and was first published in France
in 1594. It was subsequently translated into several European languages. This English translation was undertaken by Richard Surphlet
(c. 1560/63–1605/6), a godly preacher and physician, who combined
the two roles on a voyage on behalf of the East India Company. In this
section, du Laurens frames his account within the context of the
Galenic six non-naturals and discusses the impact of the air upon
the sight.

The art which teacheth to heale diseases . . . is ordinarily performed by
three instruments, as Diet, or the manner of living, Chirurgerie, and
Medicine.

The man[n]er of living is alwaies set in the forefront, and hath bin
iudged of the ancient learned to bee the chiefe and most noble part,
because it is most favourable and familiar to nature, not disturbing her

any man[n]er of way, or molesting her in any respect, so, as medicines and manuall operations doe. This man[n]er of living doth not consist onely in meate and drinke, as the common people imagine, but in the ordering of the six things which the Phisitions call not naturall; and these are the ayre, meate and drinke, sleepe and watching, labour and rest, emptines and fulnes, and the passions of the minde.

I will begin my order of diet at the ayre, in as much as no man can want it the least minute, and for that it hath a marveilous force to alter and change our bodies on the sudden. . . . This is the cause why that famous *Hippocrates* did note very well, that of the constitution of the aire doth wholly depend the good and ill disposition of our humours and spirits. . . . It behoveth us for the better preservation of our sight to chuse an ayre which is temperate in his first qualities, as being neither too hot, too cold, too moyst or drie. It is not good to abide in the heate of the Sunne, neither in the beames of the Moone, or in the open aire. The Southerne and Northerne windes are hurtfull to the eyes. Reade that which *Hippocrates* writeth in his third section of Aphorismes. The South winde (saith he) maketh a troubled sight, hardnes of hearing, a heavie head, dull sences, and all the body lazie and lither,[1] because it begetteth grosse spirits. The North winde is very sharpe, and therefore (as saith the same author) it stingeth and pricketh the eyes. The places that are low, waterish, moyst and full of marishes, are altogether contrary to the welfare of the sight. It is better a great deale to dwell in drie places, and such as are somewhat rising. If a man be forced to dwell in moyst places, his helpe is to alter and rectifie the ayre with artificiall fires, made of the wood of Lawrel, Iuniper, Rosemary and Tamariske: or otherwise to very good purpose hee may make the perfume invented of the Arabians, and use it in the chamber where hee keepeth most. Take of the leaves of Eyebright,[2] Fennell, and Margerome of every one an ounce, of Zyloaloe[3] finely powdred a dramme, of Frankinsence three drammes: mingle them altogether, and perfume your chamber often-times therewith.

As concerning the second qualities, a grosse, thicke, and foggie ayre is contrary to the sight, wee must choose such a one as is pure and cleane, purged from all waterish, earthie, nitrous, sulphurous, and other such like mettallike vapours, especially those of quicksilver: the dust, fire, and smoke do wonderfull harme to the eye: and this is the reason why such as have a weake sight should never imtermeddle with Alchimy, for so at once they should consume both their sight and their

---

[1] Sluggish.

[2] Euphrasy: plant used in diseases of the eye, hence its common name as eyebright.

[3] A bitter herbal purgative.

purse: the vapours arising out of standing waters and from dead bodies are very noysome. Neither yet must the ayre bee too lightsome: for an excessive light doth scatter the spirits, and causeth the sight oftentimes to be lost. Wee reade that *Zenophanes* his souldiers having passed the snow, became all of them as it were blind: and *Dionisius* the tyrant of Sicile, did after the same man[n]er put out the eyes of all his prisoners: for having shut them up in a very darke hole, caused them to bee led forth on the sudden into a very bright light, so that they al[l] therby lost their sight.[4]

11.2

Visiting wells and springs in Protestant Scotland

Margo Todd, *The Culture of Protestantism in Early Modern Scotland* (New Haven and London, Yale University Press, 2001), pp. 205–7.

In this work, Margo Todd seeks to recapture the complexity of the social and cultural change which accompanied the Scottish Reformation between about 1560 and 1650. She makes particular use of kirk session records – the proceedings of the regular meetings held in every parish and attended by the minister and a group of lay elders – in which offenders were presented and punished for a variety of offences ranging from sexual immorality to profanation of the Sabbath. From these, she reconstructs the remarkable vitality of many 'profane pastimes' and shows how resort to wells and springs was undertaken as a recreation, as a calendrical celebration and as a source of cure. As indicated here, wherever such activities suggested the attribution of magical powers to the waters or to the saints with which they were associated, the session's response was often severe.

[V]isiting wells and springs . . . shows up very frequently in Scots session minutes. It was a practice probably rooted in pre-Christian veneration of water, which early Christian missionaries incorporated into the Roman version of the faith by blessing the wells and associating them with

[4] Dionysius the elder (c. 430–367 BC) seized power in Syracuse in Sicily in 405. His rule was considered the archetype of cruelty in the ancient world.

Christ or the saints. The magical healing customarily associated with particular wells was simply transferred to their saints, one 'wishing well' (St Cyril's, near Loch Creran in Argyll) even producing enough income from the coins of petitioners to maintain a nearby chapel, where a priest prayed for the pilgrims' wishes to be granted. By one estimate there were more than six hundred such wells in late medieval Scotland. The dates when wells were most frequently visited correspond to the beginnings of each 'raith' or quarter of the ancient Scottish year (May, August, November and February), but the waters were apparently thought to have their fullest power at Beltane, or May Day, and throughout the month of May. Certainly, May was the most convenient and pleasant time to go 'vaguing' in the fields to the wells, with both the weather and the daylight finally emerged from winter gloom and the pressures of the harvest season not yet come. Medieval pilgrimages to wells were joined eventually by fairs and markets, making the events even more festive. After the Reformation, when Sundays became the only days free from work, the sabbaths of May, and especially the first one, nearest Beltane, presented the greatest challenge of the year to sessions intent on enforcing sermon attendance and eliminating ancient superstition. In Perth, it remained a challenge long after the town had supposedly been transformed into a Calvinist enclave.

The session minutes give us tantalising hints of what actually went on at visits to wells. First of all, pilgrimages were made by groups rather than individuals, and particularly by groups of women. They were social events, generally accompanied by music and dancing, communal meals or picnics, and doubtless (in the session's collective mind) lewd and lascivious behaviour. Second, behaviour at the well was ritualised, making use of physical objects in a highly formalised way, to achieve a magical or miraculous end. And the traditional forms and representations were easily interpreted by the session as idolatrous.

The prosecution of several women in May 1618 for going to the well at Huntingtower illumines the nature of the 'idolatry'. The elders charged fourteen women and asked specifically if they had drunk of the well and whether they had left anything there when they left. They answered that they had drunk and had left 'some of them pins or pieces of their headlaces thereat', which the session found 'a point of idolatry in putting the well in God's room'. The elders opined that the women had 'ascribe[d] that to the foresaid well due to God only, as to think to get any help of it and give offerings thereto,' and required the women to be 'humbled on their knees, declare their repentance therefore and promise never to do the like hereafter' and to pay a 6s fine. Clearly the session was anxious to dispel the popular belief that the well had magical power. A few years later, that popular belief led to a charge of witchcraft. Isabell Haldane confessed in 1623 that she had gone to the well of Ruthven and 'returned silent with water to wash' a sick bairn, having 'left part of the bairn's shirt' at the well. The child died after drinking some of Isabell's 'leaf-brew', and since the woman was already in considerable trouble for admitting to consorting with fairies and having second sight, her case was put to inquest. Isabell was convicted and executed.

11.3

An account of the mineral waters of Spa (1733)

Henry Eyre, *An Account of the Mineral Waters of Spa, Commonly called the German Spaw: Being a Collection of Observations from the most Eminent Authors who have wrote on that Subject* (London, J. Roberts, 1733), pp. 14–15, 21–4.

The sale of mineral waters became big business in the eighteenth century and there was an extensive trade in bottled water from many spas, not least from that at Spa, near Liège in modern Belgium. Drinking such bottled waters enabled the consumer to partake of their benefits without the trouble and expense of travel. In this extract, Henry Eyre (fl. c. 1725–c. 1755), a dealer based in London, describes the properties of Spa water, denounces counterfeits, and describes the care which he takes to ensure the best possible supplies for his customers.

The false Notion (which has been most industriously propagated) that the *Spaw Waters* do sparkle much, when poured into a Glass, from a Flask, in which it has been kept, has much favoured the general Abuse of imposing false Waters on the Publick, whereas the true *Spaw Water* has only a very piquant Taste, and in warm Weather will often occasion innumerable Bubbles to settle on the Sides of the Glass, but will not sparkle, when bottled, like the more vitriolick Waters, which are not so well tempered with sulphureous Particles: and are therefore not so smooth on the Palate, but generally leave a disagreeable Harshness, far from being like the agreeable Piquantness (yet Smoothness) of the true *Spaw Water*.

It is not only necessary to avoid these false Waters, but to have particular Regard to the Seasons of filling the *True Spaw Waters*; for to procure these Waters in the utmost Perfection, requires great Exactness, not only in Filling, but Corking, *&c.* . . .

[. . .]

. . . As proper Care will now be taken to import these Waters with all possible Precautions, it may be presumed, that they will soon acquire the Reputation which they have lost: occasioned not only by the false Waters, but by great Part of the true Waters having been filled, by Persons interested in the false Waters, which has occasioned their being filled in bad Seasons, and even in rainy Weather, in order to raise the Reputation of the false Waters, at the Expence of the true. These and other Tricks have been in Practice many Years, and would have continued, had not I met with such extraordinary Encouragement from the Physicians, who are all desirous of having the true *Pouhon* Water,[5] which they know has been very difficult to be got. This induced me to be at the extraordinary Expence of sending two Persons to *Spa*, and keeping them there at my own Charge three Months . . . that I may not only procure the true Water, and filled in the best Seasons . . . but with all possible Cautions, such as providing the best of Corks, having the Tops of the Flasks shaped like Bottles, so that they may be wired down, instead of the usual loose Manner of tying them down with Pack-thread, which the very Air will slacken; and above all to have the Flasks made so strong as to bear Corking the Moment they are filled. If I don't reap the Benefit of this extraordinary Care, I hope the Publick will; by my discouraging the Sale of the false Waters: (an Imposition the most dangerous, as it affects the greatest Blessing of Life, *viz.* Health) for if I do not set a sufficient Mark on them now, I will very soon; and on the Dealers in them likewise, if they continue to sell these false Waters under the Name of the *Spaw Waters*: but I hope to be prevented by this Hint. The Seal of the true *Spaw Water* is according to the annexed Impression.[6] The false *Spaw* is generally sealed with only a Dab of black Wax, without any Impression. . . . [T]o prevent any Imposition on myself or Customers by Changing them, I have ordered all my *Spaw Water* to be sealed at *Spa* with my Seal . . . opposite to the Magistrates Seal. If these Marks do not appear, 'tis certain the Water was not bought at either of my Warehouses.

[5] The Pouhon spring in the town of Spa was the source of what Eyre describes as the 'true Waters'.

[6] At this point in the treatise, Eyre included an image of the seal that he intended to use to authenticate the 'true Waters'.

11.4
The commercialisation of spa waters
in eighteenth-century France

Laurence Brockliss and Colin Jones, *The Medical World of Early
Modern France* (Oxford, Clarendon Press, 1997), pp. 637–8.

In this important book, Brockliss and Jones argue that between about
1500 and 1650 French medicine (especially in the towns) came to be
organised into corporate bodies. Colleges of Physicians, corps of surgeons and associations of apothecaries were granted local legal
monopolies over the provision of health care. These formal structures
largely remained in place up to the French Revolution in 1789. However, the eighteenth century witnessed a huge expansion of commercial cures which transformed the nature of French medicine, on the
one hand offering entrepreneurial medical practitioners opportunities
for great profits and on the other turning patients into consumers. The
development of spas and particularly the growing sales of bottled mineral waters exemplified these developments.

The provision and supply of mineral waters was a further area of health
provision in which practitioners well ensconced within the corporative
medical community were making a commercial reflex. The Enlightenment saw the mineral-water trade pass from ecclesiastics, who had
seen in balneology[7] a sub-branch of the miraculous, into secular hands.
Some ecclesiastics had been rather entrepreneurial: the Cordeliers at
Alise-Sainte-Reine[8] ran massive publicity campaigns for their spa, and
in the first decade of the eighteenth century were said to be shipping
20,000 bottles of their waters to Paris. Yet the eighteenth century saw
such groupings eclipsed. By the eve of the Revolution, counterfeiters
had completely undermined the position of the Cordeliers, for example,
who were responsible for only 3,000 of the 50,000 bottles consumed in
the city. The incorporation of mineral waters into the arsenal of commercial medicines was a triumph – as was so much else – for better
communications and distribution. Travellers to take the waters at Alise-
Sainte-Reine in the 1630s had suffered highway-robbery, death from

[7] The study of the treatment of diseases by medicinal baths, springs and wells.
[8] The waters of this small Burgundian town had long been a site of pilgrimage. The village
was also the site of a community of the Cordeliers, a French branch of the Franciscans.

bandits, and even being eaten by wolves. Now, better and safer roads stimulated travel. Many semi-inaccessible spas in the Pyrenees were opened up by improved communications, often fostered by enthusiastic provincial intendants[9] and by the ministry of war, which utilized spas for convalescing soldiers. On the civilian side, spa waters dissolved social distinctions among the élite, and the sites became the locus of a kind of cross-class sociability which made them honorary outposts of the bourgeois public sphere.

The possibilities for enrichment by the medical and service staff involved with the trade in waters were appreciable: Montpellier-trained physician Théophile de Bordeu[10] pulled out all the stops at court, notably *vis-à-vis* the mercenary Sénac,[11] in order to secure for his father and brother, solid Béarnais physicians both, the inspectorate of local spas, which offered substantial earnings. Local spa supervisors were notoriously mercenary: the intendant at Balaruc in Languedoc, it was said in the 1770s, 'is less concerned with the health of the sick than with a preoccupation to take their money'. He was held to be accelerating throughput at the baths so remorselessly that patients were leaving sicker than when they arrived. Formerly an agricultural labourer, he had become the wealthiest individual in his village. Physicians both worked hand in glove with such figures as the local level, and became involved with the growing bottled-water trade which took off in the Enlightenment, from an extremely low level in 1700. Bordeu combined local patriotism, family fidelity, and empirical therapeutics in stalwartly recommending the Pyrenean *eaux de Barèges*. After 1732 a firm headed by Alleaume[12] and Delage was accorded the monopoly over sales within Paris, and they still held control over the trade in 1760, when more than a dozen different waters were available within the capital from as far afield as the Pyrenees and the Mediterranean coast.

---

[9] Servants of the crown responsible for the oversight of royal government and administration in the regions.

[10] Théophile de Bordeu (1722–76) moved to Paris in the 1750s, where he built up an extensive medical practice. He also published important anatomical research on glandular secretions.

[11] Between 1752 and 1770, Jean-Baptiste Sénac (1693–1770), premier physician to King Louis XV, headed the commission which supervised and vetted all proprietary medicines and mineral waters in France. He used his position to enrich himself spectacularly, taking a fee on every bottle of mineral water brought to Paris and allegedly receiving 100,000 livres a year from this office.

[12] Jacques-Louis Alleaume was a spicer by trade; his son went on to become Dean of the Paris Medical Faculty.

11.5
New approaches to understanding disease: Thomas Sydenham (1624–89)

Thomas Sydenham, *The Whole Works of that Excellent Physician Dr. Thomas Sydenham. Wherein Not only the History and Cures of Acute Diseases are treated of, after a New and Accurate Method; But also the Shortest and Safest Way of Curing most Chronical Diseases. Translated from the Original Latin, by John Pechy, M.D. of the College of Physicians in London* (London, Richard Wellington and Edward Castle, 1696), sigs A1v–A3r.

The work of the English physician, Thomas Sydenham (1624–89), and his conception of disease were enormously influential. A follower of Francis Bacon, he emphasised the importance of observation and the accumulation of data in medical research. Contrary to established opinion, he argued that diseases were specific entities and were not the product of humoral imbalance in the individual patient. A doctor could only derive a true picture of a disease by building up a profile of its characteristic history from the study of a large number of individual case histories. On the one hand, this involved charting the incidence of epidemic diseases from year to year and correlating these with factors like the weather. On the other, it required the collection and collation of a large amount of data in order to establish the characteristic profile of a particular condition. Sydenham published his works in Latin, but seven years after his death these were translated into English by the medical practitioner, John Pechey (1655–1716). Henceforth, he was widely applauded as the 'English Hippocrates'.

But as to the History of Diseases, if any one weighs the Matter carefully, he will soon perceive, that the Writer ought to apply his Mind to many more things than is commonly thought. It will be sufficient to touch upon a few of them at present.

First, It is necessary that all Diseases should be reduced to certain and definite Species, with the same diligence we see it is done by Botanick Writers in their Herbals. For there are found Diseases that are reduced under the same Genius and Name, and as to some Symptoms, are like one another; yet they are different in their Natures, and require a different way of Cure. Every one knows that the Word *Carduus*[13] is extended to a great many Species of Herbs; but he would be thought a very ignorant Herbalist, that should content himself to propose only the general Description of this Plant, whereby it differs from the rest, and in the mean while should neglect the proper and peculiar Signs of every Species, whereby they are distinguished one from another; so it is not sufficient for a Writer to mark only the common Appearances of any Disease: For though the same variety does not happen to all Diseases, yet very many that are treated of by Authors under the same Title, without any distinction of Species, are very unlike, as I hope to make appear plainly in the following Pages, and when they are dibuted[14] into Species, it is most commonly done to serve an Hypothesis built upon the true *Phænomena*; and so such a Discrimination is not so much accommodated to the Nature of the Disease, as to the Humour of the Author, and his Theory of Philosophizing. How much Physick has been obstructed for want of such an exactness in this Matter, many Diseases shew, the Cures whereof had not been now to seek, if Writers in communicating their Experiments and Observations had not took one Disease for another: And this, I suppose, is the reason why the *Materia Medica* is so wonderfully encreased, and to so little purpose.

Moreover, in writing a History of Diseases, every Philosophical Hypothesis that has inveigled the Writers Mind, ought to be set aside, and then the clear and natural *Phænomena* of Diseases, how small soever they are, should be exactly marked, as Painters express the smallest Spots or Moles in the Face: For it can scarce be imagined how many Errors have been occasioned by Hypotheses, when Writers, deceiv'd by false Colours, have assigned such *Phænomena* for Diseases, as are no where to be found but in their own Brains; but they ought to appear, if the Truth of the Hypothesis, which they count certain, were manifest. Moreover, if any Symptom, which exactly suits with the said Hypothesis, really belongs to the Disease they are about to delineate, that they magnifie above measure, as if that were all; but if it do not well agree with their Hypothesis, they either pass it by in silence, or touch it by the bye, unless they can by some Philosophical Subtlety make it serve a turn.

But, *thirdly*, It is necessary in describing any Disease to mention the peculiar and perpetual *Phænomena* apart from those which are accidental and adventitious; such are those which come from the Temper and Age of the Patient, and from the different Methods of Cure; for it often happens, that the Face of the Disease varies according to the var-

[13] Thistle.
[14] Presumably a printer's error in the original for 'distributed'.

ious Processes of Healing, and some Symptoms rather proceed from the Physician than from the Disease, those that labour of the same Disease are treated with different Methods, have various Symptoms; therefore, unless Caution be used, the Judgment about the Symptoms of Diseases will be very uncertain; to say nothing of rare Cases, which do no more properly belong to the History of Diseases, than in the Description of Sage, the biting of the Palmer is to be accounted among the discriminating Signs of that Plant.[15]

Lastly, The Seasons of the Year, which chiefly favour any kind of Diseases, are carefully to be observed. I confess some come at any time; yet others, and not a few, by a certain occult instinct of Nature, follow the Seasons of the Year, as certainly as some Birds and Plants do. I have often indeed wondered, that this Disposition of some Diseases, which is so obvious, has been yet observed but by a few; whereas many have curiously observed under what Planet Plants spring, and Beasts generate. But whatever is the cause of this neglect, I do affirm, that the knowledge of Seasons wherein Diseases are wont to come, is very advantageous for the Physician, both as to the knowledge of the Species of the Disease, and to the manner of extirpating it; and when this Observation is neglected, the Event of either of these is not good.

These things, though they are not all, yet are they the most considerable, which ought to be observed in writing the History of Diseases. The Utility of which History, with respect to practice, exceeds all Estimation, in comparison wherewith the nice Discourses, which nauseously stuff the Books of modern Authors are of no value; for by what more compendions, or other way, can the curative Indications, or the Morbifick Cause, which we are to oppose, be searched for, than by a certain and distinct perception of peculiar Symptoms: Nor is there any Circumstance so small or contemptible, as not to serve for both uses: For though we must grant, that there is some variety upon the account of the temperament of Individuals, and the management of the Cure; yet notwithstanding the order of Nature is so equal in producing Diseases, that the same Symptoms of the same Diseases are most commonly found in divers Bodies; and those which were observed in *Socrates*[16] in his Sickness, are generally the same in any other Man afflicted with the same Disease; as the universal Characters of Plants are the same in all the Individuals of every kind: He, for instance, that has accurately described a Violet, as to its Colour, Taste, Smell, Figure, and the like, will perceive that that Description agrees almost in every thing with all the Violets in the whole World.

[15] A palmer was a pilgrim.
[16] Ancient Greek sage.

11.6

Medical police and the state in eighteenth-century medicine

Michel Foucault, *Power/Knowledge: Selected Interviews and Other Writings 1972-1977*, ed. Colin Gordon (Brighton, The Harvester Press, 1980), pp. 170–2, 175–6.

The controversial works of the French philosopher and historian of ideas, Michel Foucault (1926–84), have proved highly influential in the history of medicine. His studies of asylums, prisons and natural history in the seventeenth and eighteenth centuries were preoccupied with the relationship between the categories by which we analyse and know the world and the operation of power. In the essay cited here, Foucault highlights the way in which the health of a nation's population increasingly became the object of intellectual and political concern during the eighteenth century. Whereas other authors might ascribe this insight to a recognition on the part of the authorities to a specific set of pressing social problems, Foucault interprets the use of the contemporary term, 'medical police', as evidence of the regulatory and authoritarian side of hygiene policies in the Enlightenment.

. . . [O]ne could say that from the heart of the Middle Ages power traditionally exercised two great functions: that of war and peace, which it exercised through the hard-won monopoly of arms, and that of the arbitration of lawsuits and punishments of crimes, which it ensured through its control of judicial functions. *Pax et justitia.*[17] To these functions were added – from the end of the Middle Ages – those of the maintenance of order and the organisation of enrichment. Now in the eighteenth century we find a further function emerging, that of the disposition of society as a milieu of physical well-being, health and optimum longevity. The exercise of these three latter functions – order, enrichment and health – is assured less through a single apparatus than by an ensemble of multiple regulations and institutions which in the eighteenth century take the generic name of 'police'. Down to the end of the *ancien régime*, the term 'police' does not signify, at least not exclusively, the institution of police in the modern sense; 'police' is the ensemble of mechanisms serving to ensure order, the properly chan-

---

[17] A Latin tag meaning 'Peace and Justice'.

nelled growth of wealth and the conditions of preservation of health 'in general'. . . .

. . . [T]he health and physical well-being of populations comes to figure as a political objective which the 'police' of the social body must ensure along with those of economic regulation and the needs of order. The sudden importance assumed by medicine in the eighteenth century originates at the point of intersection of a new, 'analytical' economy of assistance with the emergence of a general 'police' of health. . . . The texts of Th. Rau (the *Medizinische Polizei ordnung* of 1764), and above all the great work of J. P. Frank, *System einer medizinische Polizei*, give this transformation its most coherent expression.[18]

What is the basis for this transformation? Broadly one can say that it has to do with the preservation, upkeep and conservation of the 'labour force'. But no doubt the problem is a wider one. It arguably concerns the economico-political effects of the accumulation of men. The great eighteenth-century demographic upswing in Western Europe, the necessity for co-ordinating and integrating it into the apparatus of production and the urgency of controlling it with finer and more adequate power mechanisms cause 'population', with its numerical variables of space and chronology, longevity and health, to emerge not only as a problem but as an object of surveillance, analysis, intervention, modification etc. The project of a technology of population begins to be sketched: demographic estimates, the calculation of the pyramid of ages, different life expectations and levels of mortality, studies of the reciprocal relations of growth of wealth and growth of population, various measures of incitement to marriage and procreation, the development of forms of education and professional training. Within this set of problems, the 'body' – the body of individuals and the body of populations – appears as the bearer of new variables, not merely as between the scarce and the numerous, the submissive and the restive, rich and poor, healthy and sick, strong and weak, but also as between the more or less utilisable, more or less amenable to profitable investment, those with greater or lesser prospects of survival, death and illness, and with more or less capacity for being usefully trained. The biological traits of a population become relevant factors for economic management, and it becomes necessary to organise around them an apparatus which will ensure not only their subjection but the constant increase of their utility.

---

18 Foucault refers here to the works of two men: *Thoughts on the utility and necessity of a medical police ordinance for a state*, which was published in 1764 by Wolfgang Theodore Rau (1721–72), municipal physician in the German city of Ulm; and *A system of medical police*, published in six volumes between 1779 and 1817 by the Austrian physician, Johann Peter Frank (1745–1821). For an extract from the latter, see below 11.11.

[. . .]

The privilege of hygiene and the function of medicine as an instance of social control

The old notion of the régime, understood at once as a rule of life and a form of preventive medicine, tends to become enlarged into that of the collective 'régime' of a population in general, with the disappearance of the great epidemic tempests, the reduction of the death-rate and the extension of the average life-span and life-expectation for every age group as its triple objective. This programme of hygiene as a régime of health for populations entails a certain number of authoritarian medical interventions and controls.

First of all, control of the urban space in general: it is this space which constitutes perhaps the most dangerous environment for the population. The disposition of various quarters, their humidity and exposure, the ventilation of the city as a whole, its sewage and drainage systems, the siting of abattoirs and cemeteries, the density of population, all these are decisive factors for the mortality and morbidity of the inhabitants. The city with its principal spatial variables appears as a medicalisable object. . . . During the eighteenth century the idea of the pathogenic city inspires a whole mythology and very real states of popular panic (the Charnel House of the Innocents in Paris[19] was one of these high places of fear); it also gave rise to a medical discourse on urban morbidity and the placing under surveillance of a whole range of urban developments, constructions and institutions.

In a more precise and localised fashion, the needs of hygiene demand an authoritarian medical intervention in what are regarded as the privileged breeding-grounds of disease: prisons, ships, harbour installations, the *hôpitaux généraux*[20] where vagabonds, beggars and invalids mingle together, the hospitals themselves, whose medical staffing is usually inadequate, and which aggravate or complicate the diseases of their patients, to say nothing of their diffusing of pathological germs into the outside world. Thus priority areas of medicalisation in the urban environment are isolated and are destined to constitute so many points for the exercise and application of an intensified medical power.

[19] For the health fears generated by the Cemetery of the Holy Innocents in Paris see extract 11.13 below.

[20] Literally 'general hospitals'; these were large institutions established in France in the seventeenth and eighteenth centuries to confine, discipline and care for the poor, sick and indigent.

11.7
Medical statistics and smallpox in the eighteenth century

Andrea A. Rusnock, 'The Weight of Evidence and the Burden of
Authority: Case Histories, Medical Statistics and Smallpox
Inoculation' in Roy Porter (ed.), *Medicine in the Enlightenment*
(Amsterdam and Atlanta, Georgia, Rodolpi, 1995), pp. 289, 292–3.

Traditionally, the decision of Lady Wortley Montagu (1689–1762) to
have her daughter inoculated in London in 1721 is presented as one of
the great turning points in the history of preventative medicine. However, such accounts downplay the huge controversy which sur-
rounded this practice and assume that its efficacy was immediately
noticed and approved. This was far from the case. In this extract,
Andrea Rusnock discusses the campaign mounted by the secretary of
the Royal Society, James Jurin (1684–1750), to gather the evidence
needed to both vindicate and promote the medical virtues of the practice. An important strand in Jurin's approach were his calculations
about the relative risk of dying from natural or inoculated smallpox. In
order to do the sums, he was dependent upon the accumulation of
case histories describing a large number of inoculations, for which he
needed the help of associates in the country.

Statistical evaluation of medical practice is regarded as one of the pillars of modern scientific medicine. Whether through the agency of government commissions, universities or modern hospitals, statistics are
generally the product of bureaucracies, which both legitimate and
obscure the difficulties in collecting and evaluating the numerical data
produced within them. In light of this, it is instructive to examine in
detail an example of the collection of statistics, or more precisely,
numerical figures, in a pre-institutional setting. . . .

The introduction of statistics into medicine, usually located in early
nineteenth-century Paris hospital medicine, has significant roots in
eighteenth-century Britain. . . .

The chief architect of this numerical approach was the physician
James Jurin (1684–1750), who served as secretary to the Royal Society
for the years 1721 to 1727. Educated at Trinity College Cambridge (BA
1705, MA 1709), he briefly studied in Leiden and received his MD from
Cambridge in 1716. He moved to London and wasted little time in

advancing his position both as a physician and a natural philosopher. In 1718 he became a Fellow of the Royal Society, and in 1719, a Fellow of the Royal College of Physicians. . . .

[. . .]

In 1723 Jurin issued an advertisement, initially published in the *Philosophical Transactions* and in his pamphlet, *A Letter to the Learned Caleb Cotesworth*, and reissued in each yearly pamphlet entitled *An Account of the Success of Inoculating the Small Pox for the Year.* . . . The advertisement read as follows:

> All Persons concern'd in the Practice of inoculating the Small Pox, are desir'd to keep a Register of the Names and Ages of every Person inoculated, the place where it is done, the Manner of the Operation, the Days of sickening and of the Eruption, the Sort of small Pox that is produc'd, and the Event.

> They are intreated to send these Accounts, or an Extract from them, comprehending all Persons inoculated from the Beginning, to the end of the present Year, to Dr *Jurin*, Secretary to the Royal Society, some time in *January*, or at farthest *February* next, that so the Result of them may be publish'd early in the spring.

Numerous individuals throughout the British Isles responded to Jurin's request and their letters provide rich details about the actual practice of inoculation and the reception of Jurin's project.

Complete, faithful and accurate case histories were central to Jurin's project, especially in the first year or so when inoculation was an unfamiliar procedure to most people in Britain. . . .

Respondents to Jurin's advertisement ranged socially and geographically. Medical men – apothecaries, surgeons, and physicians – were by far the majority of contributors, but there were also letters from the gentry (for example, Sir Thomas Lyttelton and Lady Catherine Percivall provided detailed accounts of their children's inoculation), from local ministers who vouched for the legitimacy of certain reports, and from a weaver turned medical practitioner. . . .

11.8
Voltaire on smallpox inoculation

Voltaire, *Letters Concerning the English Nation*,
ed. Nicholas Cronk (Oxford and New York,
Oxford University Press, 1994), pp. 44–7.

In his *Letters concerning the English Nation* (first published in English in 1733 and in various slightly different versions in French in 1734), François Marie Arouet, known as Voltaire (1694–1778), used the persona of a French traveller reporting on his observations on England to comment on a wide variety of controversial topics. His eleventh letter discussed inoculation which had been much debated during his visit to England in 1726–28 and which remained controversial, both in England and his native France, at the time of publication. As inoculation had been introduced from the Middle East, Voltaire adopted elements of an orientalist fable to convey his arguments in favour of the practice and to oppose what he saw as superstitious opposition to the practice.

It is inadvertently affirm'd in the Christian Countries of *Europe*, that the *English* are Fools and Madmen. Fools, because they give their Children the Small-Pox to prevent their catching it; and Mad-men, because they wantonly communicate a certain and dreadful Distemper to their Children, merely to prevent an uncertain Evil. The *English*, on the other Side, call the rest of the *Europeans* cowardly and unnatural. Cowardly, because they are afraid of putting their Children to a little Pain; unnatural, because they expose them to die one Time or other of the Small-Pox. But that the Reader may be able to judge, whether the *English* or those who differ from them in opinion, are in the right, here follows the History of the fam'd Inoculation, which is mention'd with so much Dread in *France*.

The *Circassian* Women have, from Time immemorial, communicated the Small-Pox to their Children when not above six Months old. . . .

The Circumstance that introduc'd a Custom in *Circassia*, which appears so singular to others, is nevertheless a Cause common to all Nations, I mean maternal Tenderness and Interest.

The *Circassians* are poor, and their Daughters are beautiful, and indeed 'tis in them they chiefly trade. They furnish with Beauties, the

Seraglios of the *Turkish* Sultan . . . and of all those who are wealthy enough to purchase and maintain such precious Merchandize. . . .

Now it often happen'd, that after a Father and Mother had taken the utmost Care of the Education of their Children, they were frustrated of all their Hopes in an Instant. The Small-Pox getting into the Family, one Daughter died of it, another lost an Eye, a third had a great Nose at her Recovery, and the unhappy Parents were completely ruin'd. Even frequently, when the Small-Pox became epidemical, Trade was suspended for several Years. . . .

A trading Nation is always watchful over its Interests, and grasps at every Discovery that may be of Advantage to its Commerce. The *Circassians* observ'd, that scarce one Person in a Thousand was ever attack'd by a Small-Pox of a violent kind. That some indeed had this Distemper very favourably three of four Times, but never twice so as to prove fatal; in a Word, that no one ever had it in a violent Degree twice in his Life. They observ'd farther, that when the Small-Pox is of the milder Sort, and the Pustles have only a tender, delicate Skin to break thro', they never leave the least Scar in the Face. From these natural Observations they concluded, that in case an Infant of six Months or a Year old, should have a milder Sort of Small-Pox, he wou'd not die of it, would not be mark'd, nor be ever afflicted with it again.

In order therefore to preserve the Life and Beauty of their Children, the only Thing remaining was, to give them the Small-Pox in their infant Years. This they did, by inoculating in the Body of a Child, a Pustle taken from the most regular, and at the same Time the most favourable Sort of Small-Pox that could be procur'd.

The Experiment cou'd not possibly fail. The *Turks*, who are People of good Sense, soon adopted this Custom, insomuch that at this Time there is not a Bassa[21] in *Constantinople*, but communicates the Small-Pox to his Children of both Sexes, immediately upon their being wean'd.

[. . .]

Upon a general Calculation, threescore Persons in every hundred have the Small-Pox. Of these threescore, twenty die of it in the most favourable Season of Life, and as many more wear the disagreeable Remains of it in their Faces so long as they live. Thus, a fifth Part of Mankind either die, or are disfigur'd by this Distemper. But it does not prove fatal to so much as one, among those who are inoculated in

---

[21] The honorific title given to the governor of a province or the general army in the Ottoman empire. Voltaire uses it here to mean 'important official'.

Turkey or in *England*, unless the Patient be infirm, or would have died had not the Experiment been made upon him. Besides, no one is disfigur'd, no one has the Small-Pox a second Time, if the Inoculation was perfect. 'Tis therefore certain, that had the Lady of some *French* Ambassador brought this Secret from *Constantinople* to *Paris*, the Nation would have been for ever oblig'd to her.[22]

11.9
A newspaper account of inoculation for smallpox (1788)

The Times, 25 April 1788, p 3c.

This newspaper report patriotically celebrates the role of English authors and institutions in preventing deaths from smallpox. It describes the debt of the Genevan authorities to the work of Dr John Haygarth (1740–1827), physician to the Chester Infirmary, translated by a local-born physician, Daniel de la Roche (1743–1813), who was practising in Paris at the time. Haygarth was one of a network of religious nonconformists who were eager to promote philanthropic schemes. He collected statistics on population and mortality in Chester and was instrumental in establishing a society designed to promote awareness of the risk of infection from smallpox and the desirability of inoculation. He published an account of the group's work (translated by De la Roche in 1784), as well as a proposal for a national scheme of inoculation in 1793.

Though the articles of news which announce the destruction of mankind, excite most powerfully the reader's curiosity and attention, yet, such as describe the methods by which the lives of our fellow creatures have been preserved, may prove of greater benefit and advantage to the public. In the autumn of 1787, above 600 children were inoculated for the small pox at Geneva, who all, except two, happily recovered from the disease. As the natural small-pox is fatal to one in five, this general inoculation may fairly be computed to have saved 118 lives.

[22] Voltaire refers here to Lady Mary Wortley Montagu (1689–1762), the wife of the British consul in Constantinople, who first observed and commented on this practice and subsequently inoculated one of her own daughters on her return to Britain.

This humane and beneficent transaction was occasioned by a Translation of 'Doctor Haygarth's Account of the Proceedings of a Society for promoting general Inoculation, and preventing the natural Small-pox in Chester, by Doctor de la Roche of Paris, Physician to the Duke of Orleans, and to the Swiss Guards, Fellow of the College of Physicians at Geneva, and of the Royal Society of Physicians at Edinburgh'. – The example of Chester has already been followed with success, by several large towns in England, as Leeds, Liverpool, Newcastle upon Tyne, Whitehaven, Norwich, &c. And it is to be hoped, that the practice of inoculating the poor, as well as the rich, will soon become general through Great Britain; especially when we observe, that the national and benevolent institutions of England, so highly honourable to our national character, and so beneficial to mankind, are imitated by the most enlightened people of Europe!

11.10
Smallpox and inoculation in a provincial town: Luton (1788)

W. Stuart to Sir William Fordyce, 1 March 1788, in *The Gentleman's Magazine* vol. 58 (April, 1788), pp. 283–4.

Founded in 1731, the monthly *Gentleman's Magazine* contained a wide range of articles on literature, art, history, etc., and acted as a forum for the dissemination and discussion of the latest medical and scientific matters. In this issue, the physician and Fellow of the Royal Society, Sir William Fordyce (1736–1802), published a letter written to him by Mr Stuart, the rector of Luton, describing the general inoculation of the parishioners. In an accompanying note, Fordyce explained that he hoped to encourage and facilitate similar actions by placing before the public the details of the procedure. It was also noted that Stuart was the grandson of Lady Wortley Montagu (1689–1762), who had introduced inoculation to England – the family tradition evidently made it a 'good story'.

Sir,
In answer to your letter concerning the success of the inoculation at Luton, I take the liberty of troubling you with the following facts.

Towards the end of last summer, a small-pox of the most malignant kind prevailed at Luton. Notwithstanding every care that human prudence could suggest, as to cleanliness, medicine, and attendance, scarcely more than half of our patients survived this dreadful disease; and though they were kept at some distance from the town, it was found impossible to prevent the infection from spreading. Alarmed at the danger, I endeavoured to overcome the prejudice and fears of the people, and prevail on them to be inoculated. Accordingly, in the course of three days, a surgeon of the neighbourhood communicated the infection to 928 paupers, who were judged incapable of paying for themselves; and soon after to 287 more, mostly at their own charge. Of these 1215, only five died, and those under the age of four months. . . .

Mean time Mr. Kirby and Mr. Chase, the surgeons resident at Luton, inoculated about 700 of the better sort, with an equal success.

[. . .]

On my return to Luton, I mean to recommend annual inoculations at the parish-charge. This may be supported on principles of œconomy, as well as on principles of humanity. The health and safety of the people ought ever to be the supreme object of parochial management. The life of an industrious parent is absolutely invaluable; and he, who thinks it can be rated too high, is no less ignorant of policy, than destitute of feeling.

For nine years that I have held the living of Luton, the average number of small-pox patients is 25. These, at the lowest computation, stand the parish at two guineas each, exclusive of medical assistance. The disease is so apprehended in the country, that the nurses require double pay; and both they and the patients are confined in an airing-house several weeks after the recovery. Should my plan of annual inoculations take place, the expence would not amount to the fifty guineas which are now paid for those who have the small-pox naturally. But, alas! these fifty guineas are but a small part of the real charge and inconvenience produced by this dreadful malady. Its almost constant effect is a permanent augmentation of the parish expenditure. If a labourer dies, his family must be supported. If a mother is lost, the children must be removed to a workhouse, as their father cannot spare time for employments that are merely domestic. In a workhouse they lose innocence, reputation, and that sense of independence which is the surest principle of industry.

I have troubled you with these observations, because I am confident they are applicable to more parishes than mine; and because I am equally confident, that, were inoculation generally practised, it would lessen human misery, save many a useful life, and even promote that œconomy which many think the only object worthy of attention. . . .

11.11
Cleanliness and the state in eighteenth-century Europe

A System of Complete Medical Police: Selections from Johann Peter Frank, ed. Erna Lesky (Baltimore, Maryland, Johns Hopkins University Press, 1976), pp. 183–4, 195.

The Austrian physician, Johann Peter Frank (1745–1821), was educated at Heidelberg and Strasbourg. In 1779 he published the first volume of his monumental *A System of Complete Medical Police*. Five more volumes followed during his life time and two after his death. The size of the work reflected the scale of its ambition which aimed at the regulation of most areas of life and the promotion of hygiene and population growth. It was a great success. Frank was rewarded with numerous university chairs, appointed physician to the Habsburg court and was made director of the main hospital in Vienna. His work on medical police has been seen partly as a culmination of a tradition of writing about such subjects in the central European states, dating back to the mid-seventeenth century, as well as anticipating nineteenth-century public health reforms.

Of the influence of cleanliness on the well-being of the state

In dealing with this important subject of Medical police, I must refer to all that I have said elsewhere about necessary cleanliness of the air, of the various degrees of its spoilage, of the malignant exhalations of bogs, of stagnant waters, of large towns, etc., so that now I can lecture on pertinent matters, without digressions and without having to convince the public that strict supervision in this part of public health care is necessary.

What but an unclean person is in the eyes of well educated persons, the same, and even more so, is an unclean nation when judged by a civilized nation. Although now and again a prejudice penetrates into the ideas which we have of the cleanliness or uncleanliness of a thing, and although the history of so many incredibly dirty yet healthy nations, the

Hottentots, the Greenlanders and others somewhat softens the judgement of a nation's uncleanliness, nevertheless, it is certain that even though an individual person may wallow in mud and slime without detriment because he has been hardened by habit and a completely animal-like way of life, a sociable nation cannot continue with such individuals without the well-being and health of the whole having to suffer enormously, especially in times of epidemics.

It suffices to see how the terrible plague originates mostly in eastern countries, and how terribly quickly it spreads among the unclean Turkish and Greek nations! How on large ships, which after all change their atmosphere every instant, uncleanliness promotes scurvy and malignant putrid fever, how in hospitals and camps the slightest illnesses often deteriorate into the gravest diseases and end in death! . . . On the other hand, look at the Dutch nation, living in the midst of a formerly inaccessible swamp; yet, it is tolerably healthy in the eternal fog only because their cleanliness (of course, pushed to the extreme but appropriate to the unfortunate situation of their low dwelling place) exceeds that of all known nations so much that, as Lord Chesterfield[23] said, the streets in Holland are cleaner than the houses in London. And because this commercial nation clearly knows the power of human diligence against the influence of an unhealthy region! Just look how the solid Cook[24] sailed around the earth several times with so small a loss in human lives only because he enforced punctiliously the strict cleanliness of his ships and his people!

I may assume here that no more detailed proof will be required of me to substantiate the sentence: that uncleanliness is one of the foremost causes of most diseases of people; and that these largely could be healed better by police measures than by physicians, or at least prevented. . . .

But there is such a number of public cleansing institutions that their investigation may easily lead to confusion. Now if I consider the pertinent subjects in the order in which the lectures on institutions of public cleanliness are arranged, with a view to the requirements of the country, the human dwelling, and finally, the citizens themselves and their handicrafts, nothing of importance should be excluded from such a classification. As regards institutions for the country's cleanliness, they comprehend the unhealthy treatment of the soil, the concern for cleansing the atmosphere by utilizing healthy winds, draining swamps and ponds, preventing frequent floods, and consequently also conducting

[23] Philip Dormer Stanhope, 4th earl of Chesterfield (1694–1773), was the oft-quoted author of *Letters to his son*, which Samuel Johnson famously derided for their immorality.

[24] Captain James Cook (1728–79) who first circumnavigated the globe in 1770.

water in secure beds and promoting its flow. .... I ... report here pre-
dominantly on cleanliness in towns and other human societies. For the
towns contain in concentration on a moderately large area all the
causes of uncleanliness which are only very dispersed in the country.
These causes, therefore, deserve the preferential attention of the police
authorities. Here we have to consider the essential cleanliness of the
town's exterior, of its streets, of its public and private buildings, etc.
Among these, the influence of unclean crafts on the health of the
inhabitants, and their own cleanliness, naturally offer themselves for
consideration. ....

[...]

The production and exhibition of foul-smelling cheeses, the exhalations
of herring barrels, of waters from fish and various other smelling wares,
often spoil the air of an entire street, and they should move the police
to at least admonish the grocers and merchants of these foodstuffs not
to exhibit such wares in front of their houses at least and thereby perfume the whole street. A written, or if required, a painted board can
explain to every passerby what is on sale in the house, without making
half the town vomit because of the loathsome stench of piled-up
cheeses, etc., and without poisoning the atmosphere.

11.12
The use of artificial ventilators in hospitals

Stephen Hales, *A Treatise on Ventilators . . . Part Second*
(London, Richard Manby, 1758), pp. 13–21, 25.

The English clergyman and natural philosopher, Stephen Hales
(1677–1761), is perhaps best known today for his work on the physiology of plants. During his own lifetime, however, he was better known
for his work on ventilators designed to remove putrid air from confined
spaces. These were first installed in prisons in order to combat the
dreaded gaol fever, most notably at Newgate in London, and aboard
ships. In this passage, however, their use in the county hospital at Winchester, the first of its kind (see extract 6.6 above), is described. Here,
ventilation is presented not only as preventing epidemics and alleviat-
ing respiratory diseases, but also as beneficial to the recovery of those
hospital patients admitted for wounds and broken limbs.

IT is well known that the foul, putrid Air of Hospitals is a great Disadvantage to the Patients; and this not only consumptively-inclined Persons are sensible of, but also those who, otherwise in good Health, are put into Hospitals for broken Limbs, where they get the Hospital Distemper, which they would not have had in the purer Air of a private House; as do many also whose Disease requires their long Continuance there. Surgeons also observe, that Wounds do not heal so well in such foul putrid Air, as they will do in a purer Air. Whereas, if the Air of Hospitals were changed every Day, Morning and Evening, for a little Time, so as not to have Time to putrify, it is probable that many Patients would recover sooner, and that fewer would die in such purer Air; which would have this further Advantage, to make the Charity of Hospitals more extensively useful, by making Room for a quicker Succession of Patients.

THE first Trial of Ventilators in an Hospital, was made in the County Hospital at *Winchester*; where they are fixed under the Floor, at the farther End of the Ward from the Entrance, yet so as to be worked with great Ease by those in the Ward, by means of a Lever . . . fixed across the Ward between the Beds. . . .

THIS Ward being filled with the Fumes of burning Pitch, they were drawn off, and dispelled by the Ventilators, through Trunks which conveyed them out into the open Air, in nine Minutes, notwithstanding the Length of the Ward is fifty-eight Feet, and its whole Capacity equal to 278 Tuns. When the farther Door was shut of another long Ward, which communicated with this by a long Passage, on working the Ventilators, the Smoke was drawn down the Chimney of that Ward; and with ten Minutes Ventilation the Ward was sensibly sweeter.

[. . .]

. . . The Degrees of Ventilation must . . . be more or less in proportion to the different Temperature of the Air as to Warmth or Coldness, Moisture or Driness, which will be best determined by Experience. The two principal Times of Ventilation should probably be Mornings, and Evenings before the Dew falls; the first to carry off the frowzy[25] Air of the whole preceding Night, the latter to supply the Ward with Store of fresh Air for the Service of the Night. Ventilation will not only be of use to the Patients in many Respects, but will also be very beneficial to the Physicians, Surgeons, Apothecaries, and Nurses, who attend them. During Ventilation, all or some of the Bed-curtains may be drawn, especially in some Diseases, and during the colder Constitution of the Air.

---

[25] Fusty, ill-smelling or stale.

This is what is practised in some Hospitals, when Windows are set open to air them.

[. . .]

SOME are apt to think Ventilators useless in Hospitals, because they can in good warm Weather air the Wards by opening the Windows, and that doubtless much better than by Ventilation; and were there such good kindly Weather all the Year round, then Ventilators would be useless. But since, for the greatest Part of the Year, the external Air is too cold to be admitted in at Windows, because it is a well-known Truth, *viz.* that cold Air admitted into the upper Part of a warm Room, being specifically heavier, falls precipitately down thro' the warmer Air. And this it must doubtless do in the warm Wards of an Hospital, so as to incommode and endanger the Welfare of the Patients; besides that, the Indraft of Air at open Windows will be much greater than what comes in by the more gentle Method of Ventilation. . . . It has been said, that some Hospitals stand in so open and airy a Situation, that they have no Occasion for Ventilators; yet it is well known, that notwithstanding Ships at Sea are in so airy a Situation, that Millions of People have lost their Lives there by the Foulness and Putridness of the Air in Ships; which Inconvenience is effectually prevented by Ventilators, as is now fully proved by repeated Experience in many Ships, which the People on board are so sensible of, that they work the Ventilators with Eagerness.

[. . .]

THIS Ventilation causes the Hospital to be in a manner as sweet as a private House. And it is observed, that fewer by more than one Third die, since the drawing the foul putrid Air out of the Chambers by Ventilation; and it is reasonable to think, that the Danger of so putrid a Distemper as the Smallpox is, will be much greater in a foul putrid, than in a purer Air. The good Effect of this Method, will probably lead to the not keeping the Chambers of the Sick very close in private Houses.

11.13

Public health measures in Paris on the eve of the Revolution: the Cemetery of the Holy Innocents

M. Thouret, *Rapport sur les Exhumations du Cimitière et de L'Eglise des Saincts Innocents; Lu dans la Séance de la Société Royale de Médecine, tenue au Louvre le 3 Mars 1789* (Paris, 1789), p. 5. Translated by Mark Jenner.

In this report to the Royal Society of Medicine the Parisian physician, Michel-Augustin Thouret (1748–1810), describes the closure of the Cemetery of the Holy Innocents in Paris in 1780 as a public health hazard following his investigation into its atmosphere. The whole episode represented a triumph for the Society which had first received a royal charter in 1778. It took a particular interest in combatting and preventing epidemics and in utilising the latest medical and scientific developments such as the analysis of airs in order to promote its aims. Its concern with atmospheric exhalations is strongly evident in this passage.

But it was, above all, with regard to the threats to the salubrity of the air, so much feared on similar occasions, that anxieties became extreme. .... According to the account of a respected physician, the mephitism which emanated from one of the ditches adjoining the Cemetery had infected all the cellars. The terrible effect of this emanation was comparable to the most subtle poisons, to those with which savages impregnate their murderous arrows. The damp-soaked walls which it penetrated could, it was said, transmit the most dreadful afflictions with a single touch.

11.14
Environmental medicine in late Enlightenment Europe

Ludmilla Jordanova, 'Earth Science and Environmental Medicine:
The Synthesis of the Late Enlightenment' in L. J. Jordanova
and Roy Porter (eds), *Images of the Earth: Essays of the
Environmental Sciences* (Chalfont St Giles, British Society for
the History of Science, 1979), pp. 127–9, 132–3, 148–50.

Many scholars have stressed how the Enlightenment expressed a new and greater confidence in the human capacity to understand and mould the natural world through the use of reason. This influential article uses the term 'environmental medicine' to highlight the interconnectedness of medicine and various other branches of natural knowledge at the end of the eighteenth century. Using a comparative and synthetic approach with examples drawn from Europe and North America, Jordanova stresses how the application of these forms of science helped to control and remodel human society. She further suggests that through environmental medicine medical men were able to construct a new public role for their profession.

The connection of events on the earth and in the atmosphere with human ailments was a common theme of the scientific and medical literature of the 1790s. . . .

The environmental sciences – geology, geography, meteorology – were intimately related to the biomedical sciences – physiology, biology, hygiene – as well as to the human and social sciences such as anthropology and epidemiology. . . . [T]he synthetic approach of the late Enlightenment had direct social implications. These consisted in the refinement and elaboration of manipulative techniques of managing individuals and groups by an increasingly self-confident medical profession. . . .

My basic concern is to understand the self-consciously scientific attempts to master the laws of the organism-environment relationship which were expressed in the vast body of literature on the subject at the end of the eighteenth century. It may be convenient to distinguish four facets of this literature: the physical, the physiological, the anthropological, and the social, which display increasingly complex assumptions about the interaction between human beings and their environment.

First, the physical environment, as studied by geology for example, offered direct explanations of how external conditions affected living things. This interest in physical conditions, also seen in climatology, meteorology, topography and geology, is well shown in the extensive published descriptions of travels which proposed to explain the forms of life by reference to the environment. . . .

Second, there was an interest in the physiological details of environmentally caused diseases, seen in the concern with diet, with respiratory problems, and with common diseases believed to be caused by mephitic substances[26] emanating from unhealthy places like marshes and swamps. The medical writing on yellow fever in America during the 1790s was of this kind.

Third, there was an anthropological dimension to environmentalism, which took the form of descriptions and analyses of the lifestyle, health and diseases of other cultures, emphasising variation from one part of the world to another. This was clear in the writings of both lay and medical observers of the time, such as Volney's descriptions of the Near East and of America.[27]

Finally, the social approach analysed the impact of environmental conditions which stemmed not from climate but from civilisation itself. Bills of mortality and the conditions in institutions, factories and slums were used to draw attention to the impact of social and moral environment on human well-being. . . . Hand-in-hand with this went an examination of the role of the medical profession in dealing with socio-medical problems, expressed for example in the writings on medical police which suggested the central role of doctors in maintaining public order.

[. . .]

The concept which, more than any other, suggests the synthesis . . . is that of hygiene. Littré[28] defined it as that part of medicine which deals with the rules for the preservation of health. The term hygiene denoted the concern for the well-being of animals and human beings expressed through the search for principles to ensure health which derived from an understanding of the impact of the environment. Individual and collective habits became objects of great interest to medicine and subject to general social scrutiny.

---

[26] Noxious or pestilential substances that emanated from the earth.

[27] Constantin de Volney (1757–1820), French writer and traveller and the author of *Voyage en Syrie et en Egypte* (Paris, 1787) and *A view of the soil and climate of the United States of America* (London & Philadelphia, 1804; 1st published in French in Paris, 2 vols, 1803).

[28] E. Littré, *Dictionnaire de la langue française* 4 vols (Paris, 1878), ii, p. 2073.

310

. . . According to Hallé,[29] the subject of hygiene . . . had two facets, the social and the individual. The former entailed studying the effect of climate, location, occupation, customs, laws, and government; the latter investigated how the variables of age, sex, temperament, habits, profession, poverty, and travel impinged on human health. The distinction between public and private was a difficult one to draw clearly.

[. . .]

[T]he new sciences of life and those of the environment contained within them theories which opened up the possibility of manipulating and managing the relationship between human beings and their surroundings. The model for this came partly from the experimental control already well established in the physical sciences. But the ethic of management had other more complex origins, especially in political thought. The early eighteenth century, for example, saw the establishment of chairs of *Polizeiwissenschaft*, the science of police, for the instruction of civil servants in the techniques of management. It was in this context that Frank[30] developed the idea of medical police, that is, the administration of the health aspects of the state by those medically trained, especially in public health. . . .

Having acknowledged that the environment was a major determinant of human characteristics, it seemed reasonable to control the variables to produce desirable human features. Among the prime movers in this were the medical profession, a growing and powerful body of middle class men who were intimately involved in the construction and maintenance of the social order. The links of environmental medicine to public policy seem clear enough. . . .

[. . .]

When looked at in this light, the traditional historiography of public health in terms of high minded philanthropy begins to look inadequate. Foucault has already warned us that we must begin to look beneath the surface and see what it concealed, both in the primary sources of the period, with their claims to reform individuals and society, and by implication in the secondary literature, which reproduces the simple 'humanitarianism' of such enterprises. At the very least, one can say from examining the evidence in its historical context that environmental medicine served the interests of the dominant class, for example, in

[29] Jean-Noël Hallé (1754–1822) was a Parisian physician, who was made Professor of Medical Physics and Hygiene after the reorganisation of medical education in 1795, and was the author of an article on hygiene in 1798 published in the *Encyclopédie méthodique, médicine*.

[30] For whom, see above extract 11.11.

suggesting that social or industrial problems had purely individual or domestic causes, and hence solutions. The language and concerns of hygiene suggested the need for a well-ordered, moderate lifestyle, using metaphors of discipline, regulation and self-denial. This synthesis of the environmental and life sciences using the language of the late Enlightenment not only gained in status by its scientific credentials but was also moulded by the reality and needs of everyday life, which shaped people's consciousness of issues such as these, which spanned a range of human activities.

Part twelve

European medicine in the age of colonialism

12.1

Ecological imperialism and the impact of Old World diseases on the Americas and Australasia

Alfred W. Crosby, *Ecological Imperialism. The Biological Expansion of Europe, 900–1900* (Cambridge, Cambridge University Press, 1986), pp. 196–216.

In this work, Crosby argues that Europeans succeeded in colonising the Americas and Australasia because European germs killed off most of the indigenous populations. The author combines history with biological determinism, and reminds the reader that biological factors must be taken into account when explaining European expansion across the globe from the sixteenth century onwards.

Old world germs were entities having size, weight, and mass . . . [requiring] transportation across the oceans, which the *marinheiros*[1] unintentionally supplied. Once ashore and lodged in the bodies of new victims in new lands, their rate of reproduction . . . enabled them to outperform all larger immigrants in rapidity of increase and speed of geographical expansion. Pathogens are among the 'weediest' of organisms. We must examine the colonial histories of Old World pathogens, because their success provides the most spectacular example of the power of the biogeographical realities that underlay the success of European imperialists overseas. It was their germs, not these imperial-

[1] Mariners or sailors.

ists themselves, for all their brutality and callousness, that were chiefly responsible for sweeping aside the indigenes and opening the Neo-Europes to demographic takeover.

[. . .]

The isolation of the indigenes of the Americas and Australia from Old World germs prior to the last few hundred years was nearly absolute. Not only did very few people of any origin cross the great oceans, but those who did must have been healthy or they would have died on the way, taking their pathogens with them. The indigenes were not without their own infections, of course. The Amerindians had at least pinta,[2] yaws,[3] venereal syphilis, hepatitis, encephalitis, polio, some varieties of tuberculosis . . . and intestinal parasites, but they seem to have been without any experience with such Old World maladies as smallpox, measles, diphtheria, trachoma, whooping cough, chicken pox, bubonic plague, malaria, typhoid fever, cholera, yellow fever, dengue fever, scarlet fever, amebic dysentery, influenza, and a number of helminthic infestations.[4] . . .

Indications of the susceptibility of Amerindians and Aborigines to Old World infections appear almost immediately after the intrusion of the whites. In 1492, Columbus kidnapped a number of West Indians to train as interpreters and to show to King Ferdinand and Queen Isabella. Several of them seem to have died on the stormy voyage to Europe, and so Columbus had only seven to display in Spain. . . . When, less than a year later, he returned to American waters, only two of the seven were still alive. In 1495, Columbus, searching for a West Indian commodity that would sell in Europe, sent 550 Amerindian slaves, twelve to thirty-five years of age, more or less, off across the Atlantic. Two hundred died on the difficult voyage; 350 survived to be put to work in Spain. The majority of these soon were also dead 'because the land did not suit them'.

[. . .]

But what killed the Arawacks[5] in 1493 and 1495? Maltreatment? Cold? Hunger? Overwork? Yes, and no doubt about it, but could this be the

---

[2] Disfiguring skin disease of tropical South America closely allied to yaws (below) and syphilis.

[3] Yaws or frambœsia was a contagious disease characterised by raspberry-like tubercles on the skin. It was endemic in the black African populations transported to the Caribbean and the Americas.

[4] Infections caused by intestinal worms.

[5] One of the indigenous peoples of the Caribbean.

entire answer? Columbus certainly did not want to kill his interpreters, and slavers and slaveholders have no interest whatever in the outright slaughter of their property. All or almost all of these victims seem to have been young adults, usually the most resilient members of our species – except in the case of unfamiliar infections. The hale and hearty immune system of one's prime years of life, when challenged by unprecedented invaders, can overreact and smother normal body functions with inflammation and edema. The most likely candidates for the role of exterminator of the first Amerindians in Europe were those that killed so many other Arawacks in the decades immediately following: Old World pathogens.

We shall now turn to the colonies. . . . Let us restrict ourselves to the peregrinations of one Old World pathogen in the colonies, the most spectacular one, the virus of smallpox. Smallpox, an infection that usually spreads from victim to victim by breath, was one of the most communicable of diseases and one of the very deadliest. It was an old human infection in the Old World, but it was rarely of crucial importance in Europe until it flared up in the sixteenth century. For the next 250 to 300 years – until the advent of vaccination – it was just that, of crucial importance, reaching its apogee in the 1700s, when it accounted for 10 to 15 percent of all deaths in some of the western European nations early in the century. Characteristically, 80 percent of its victims were under ten years of age, and 70 percent under two years of age. In Europe, it was the worst of the childhood diseases. Most adults, especially in the cities and ports, had had it and were immune. In the colonies, it struck indigenes young and old and was the worst of all diseases.

Smallpox first crossed the seams of Pangaea[6] – specifically to the island of Española – at the end of 1518 or the beginning of 1519, and for the next four centuries it played as essential a role in the advance of white imperialism overseas as gunpowder – perhaps a more important role, because the indigenes did turn the musket and then rifle against the intruders, but smallpox very rarely fought on the side of the indigenes. The intruders were usually immune to it, as they were to other Old World childhood diseases, most of which were new beyond the oceans. The malady quickly exterminated a third or half of the Arawacks on Española, and almost immediately leaped the straits to Puerto Rico and the other Greater Antilles, accomplishing the same devastation there. It crossed from Cuba to Mexico, and joined Cortés's

---

[6] The name given by geographers to the original super-continent that first began to split apart some two million years ago.

forces[7] in the person of a sick black soldier, one of the few of the invaders not immune to the infection. The disease exterminated a large fraction of the Aztecs and cleared a path for the aliens to the heart of Tenochtitlán[8] and to the founding of New Spain. Racing ahead of the *conquistadores*, it soon appeared in Peru, killing a large proportion of the subjects of the Inca, killing the Inca himself and the successor he had chosen. Civil war and chaos followed, and then Francesco Pizarro[9] arrived. The miraculous triumphs of that *conquistador*, and of Cortés, whom he so successfully emulated, are in large part the triumphs of the virus of smallpox.

[. . .]

Smallpox is a disease with seven-league boots. Its effects are terrifying: the fever and pain; the swift appearance of pustules that sometimes destroy the skin and transform the victim into a gory horror; the astounding death rates, up to one-fourth, one-half, or more with the worst strains. The healthy flee, leaving the ill behind to face certain death, and often taking the disease along with them. The incubation period for smallpox is ten to fourteen days, long enough for the ephemerally healthy carrier to flee for long distances on foot, by canoe, or, later, on horseback to people who know nothing of the threat he represents, and there to infect them and inspire others newly charged with the virus to flee to infect new innocents. . . .

The death rates could be very high. In 1729, two churchmen, Miguel Ximénez and a priest named Cattaneo, started out from Buenos Aires for the missions in Paraguay accompanied by 340 Guaraní. Eight days up the Río de la Plata, smallpox appeared among the latter. All but forty contracted the infection, and for two months the disease raged, at the end of which 121 were convalescing and 179 were dead. The Jesuits, a group more given to numerical precision than most, reckoned that 50,000 had died in the Paraguayan missions in the 1718 smallpox, 30,000 in the Guaraní villages in 1734, and 12,000 in 1765. . . .

[. . .]

The medical history of Australia begins with smallpox, or something very muck like it. The First Fleet arrived in Sydney harbor in 1788, and for some time thereafter the problems of infections among either the

---

[7] The conquest of the Aztecs was accomplished by Hernan Cortés (1485–1547) in less than four years (1519–23).

[8] Capital city of the Aztecs, near modern-day Mexico City.

[9] Francisco de Pizarro (d. 1541) was responsible for the conquest of the old Inca empire between 1530 and 1535. In the latter year, he founded the new Spanish city of Lima.

thousand colonists or the Aborigines were minor. Scurvy was causing trouble among the settlers, but even so they produced fifty-nine babies by February of 1790. The Aborigines were a healthy lot, at least so far as the English could see. Then, in April of 1789, the English began finding on beaches and rocks around the harbor the bodies of dead Aborigines. The cause was a mystery until a family of natives with active cases of smallpox came into the settlement. In February, an Aborigine who had recovered from the disease told the whites that fully half his fellows in the general vicinity of Sydney had died and that many of the others had fled, carrying the infection with them. The sick left behind rarely lived long, perishing for want of food and water. . . .

[. . .]

The disease spread far up and down the coast and inland, raging on for an undetermined period, raking back and forth through the native pop ulations. . . . For scores of years after, old Aborigines with the pocks and scars of the disease kept turning up here and there in the deep hinterlands of New South Wales, Victoria, and South Australia. The pandemic may even have reached the northeast and western coasts of the continent. There was nothing to stop it so long as there were fresh Aborigines to infect. . . . It may have killed . . . one-third of their population, leaving only the tribes in the northwest quarter of the continent untouched.

[. . .]

The exchange of infectious diseases – that is, of germs, of living things having geographical points of origin just like visible creatures – between the Old World and its American and Australasian colonies has been wondrously one-sided, as one-sided and one-way as the exchanges of people, weeds, and animals. Australasia, as far as science can tell us, has exported not one of its human diseases to the outside world, presuming that it has any uniquely its own. The Americas do have their own distinctive pathogens, those of at least Carrion's disease and Chagas' disease.[10] Oddly, these very unpleasant and sometimes fatal diseases do not travel well and have never established themselves in the Old World. Venereal syphilis may be the New World's only important disease export, and it has, for all its notoriety, never stopped population growth in the Old World. . . . Europe was magnanimous in the

---

[10] Carrion's disease or Oroya fever was endemic in the Western Andes. It produces serious blood poisoning and eruptions on the skin. Chagas' disease, or American trypanosomiasis, is transmitted by tiny insects. In its acute form it induces fever, inflammation of the heart walls and often death, and in its chronic form enlargement of the heart followed ultimately by death.

317

quantity and quality of the torments it sent across the seams of Pangaea. In contrast, its colonies, epidemiologically impecunious to begin with, were hesitant to export even the pathogens they did have. The unevenness of the exchange ... operated to the overwhelming advantage of the European invaders, and to the crushing disadvantage of the peoples whose ancestral homes were on the losing side of the seams of Pangaea.

12.2

Health and the promotion of colonialism: Thomas Hariot (1588)

Thomas Hariot, *A Briefe and True Report of the New-found Land of Virginia ... Directed to the Adventurers, Favourers, and Welwillers of the Action, for the Inhabiting and Planting there* (London, 1588), sigs F2v–F4r.

Thomas Hariot or Harriot (1560–1621), mathematician and astronomer, was mathematical tutor to Sir Walter Ralegh (1552–1618) and served as surveyor on Ralegh's expedition to Virginia (Roanoke Island) in 1585. In his *A briefe and true report*, he enumerated the products of the land and extolled the possibilities for trade in the new colony. A work of propaganda, it did not prevent the failure of Raleigh's first colonial enterprise.

[A]ll which I have before spoken of, have bin discovered & experimented not far from the sea coast where was our abode & most of our travailing: yet somtimes as we made our iourneies farther into the maine and countrey; we found the soyle to bee fatter; the trees greater and to growe thinner; the grounde more firme and deeper mould; more and larger champions;[11] finer grasse and as good as ever we saw any in England; in some places rockie and farre more high and hillie ground; more plentie of their fruites; more abundance of beastes; the more inhabited with people, and of greater pollicie & larger dominions, with greater townes and houses.

Why may wee not then looke for in good hope from the inner parts of more and greater plentie, as well of other things, as of those which wee

11 Level, open countryside or fields.

have alreadie discovered? Unto the Spaniardes happened the like in discovering the maine[12] of the West Indies. The maine also of this countrey of *Virginia*, extending some wayes so many hundreds of leagues, as otherwise then by the relation of the inhabitants wee have most certaine knowledge of, where yet no Christian Prince hath any possession or dealing, cannot but yeeld many kinds of excellent commodities, which we in our discoverie have not yet seene.

[. . .]

Whereby also the excellent temperature of the ayre there at all seasons, much warmer then in England, and never so violently hot, as sometimes is under & between the Tropikes, or nere them; cannot bee unknowne unto you without farther relation.

For the holsomnesse thereof I neede to say but thus much: that for all the want of provision, as first of English victuall; excepting for twentie daies, wee lived only by drinking water and by the victuall of the countrey, of which some sorts were very straunge unto us, and might have bene thought to have altered our temperatures in such sort as to have brought us into some greevous and dangerous diseases: secondly the want of English meanes, for the taking of beastes, fishe, and foule, which by the helpe only of the inhabitants and their meanes, coulde not bee so suddenly and easily provided for us, nor in so great numbers & quantities, nor of that choise as otherwise might have bene to our better satisfaction and contentment. Some want also wee had of clothes. Furthermore, in all our travailes which were most speciall and often in the time of winter, our lodging was in the open aire upon the grounde. And yet I say for all this, there were but foure of our whole company (being one hundred and eight) that died all the yeere and that but at the latter ende thereof and upon none of the aforesaide causes. For all foure especially three were feeble, weake, and sickly persons before ever they came thither, and those that knewe them much marveyled that they lived so long beeing in that case, or had adventured to travaile.

Seeing therefore the ayre there is so temperate and holsome, the soyle so fertile and yeelding such commodities as I have before mentioned, the voyage also thither to and fro beeing sufficiently experimented, to bee perfourmed thrise a yeere with ease and at any season thereof: And the dealing of *Sir Wa[l]ter Raleigh* so liberall in large giving and graunting lande there, as is alreadie knowen, with many helpes and furtherances els: (The least that hee hath graunted hath beene five hundred acres to a man onely for the adventure of his

---

[12] The mainland.

person): I hope there remaine no cause wherby the action should be misliked.

If that those which shall thither travaile to inhabite and plant bee but reasonably provided for the first yere as those are which were transported the last, and beeing there doe use but that diligence and care as is requisite, and as they may with ease: There is no doubt but for the time following they may have victuals that is excellent good and plentie enough; some more Englishe sortes of cattaile also hereafter, as some have bene before, and are there yet remaining, may and shall bee God willing thither transported: So likewise our kinde of fruites, rootes, and hearbes may bee there planted and sowed, as some have bene alreadie, and prove wel. And in short time also they may raise of those sortes of commodities which I have spoken of as shall both enrich themselves, as also others that shall deale with them.

12.3
Medicine and acclimatisation

Karen Ordahl Kupperman, 'Fear of Hot Climates in the Anglo-American Colonial Experience', *William and Mary Quarterly* 41 (1984), pp. 213–40.

Kupperman's article discusses how medical theory and popular lay beliefs related climate to people's humoral constitutions. She sets out to show how English settlers acclimatised or seasoned their bodies to the new climates of the West Indies and the American South, and she describes how they subsequently adapted their lifestyles to counter the dangers which they believed were posed by hot climates.

English people contemplating transplantation to the southern parts of North America and to the West Indies in the sixteenth and seventeenth centuries expressed profound anxiety over the effect hot climates would have on them. Heat and the environment it engendered were expected to be alien and even hostile to men and women from England's temperate climate. This article is a study of the interaction between perception and reality, particularly of the way in which evidence was interpreted to sustain the preconceptions English colonists brought with them. The settlers' health fared badly in both the southern mainland colonies and the West Indies. This fact confirmed their expectations and contributed important evidence that hardened generalized anxieties into medical dogma by the eighteenth century. The link between weather and disease then became axiomatic. In 1598 George Wateson, drawing on his experience as a merchant in Spain, wrote 'the first working textbook of tropical diseases', which warned of the diseases engendered by 'intemperate Climats'. From that time through the colonial period, excessive heat was seen as the major reason for southern sickliness.

Early modern science taught that human beings and their native physical environment normally existed in a state of ecological harmony. That is, the human constitution was responsive to and shaped by climate, air, and diet. It followed that men and women who had been bred in England were unsuited to environments that were radically different, such as those of the southern regions of the New World, with their heats and damps and different dietary regimens. Consequently, those who ventured to such places, stayed there, and ate the indigenous foods risked sickness in the short run and a drastic change in physiology and psychology in the long run as their bodies responded to the new environment.

[. . .]

Change in the balance of the humors may have been what was meant by the use of the word *seasoning* to describe the acclimatization of an English person, a process commonly lasting about two years and thought necessary even in southern New England. It was generally believed that the adjustment involved paling and thinning of the blood. . . .

[. . .]

The sun and its heat figured prominently in early English thinking about colonization, and in a profoundly ambivalent way. Fear of hot climates was balanced by the belief that the sun was the source of riches. Despite the widespread conviction that English people would sicken and possibly die in hot climates, the majority of those interested in America went or were sent to the southern regions instead of [temperate] New England or Newfoundland. Early modern science taught that there was a direct trade off between heat and abundance. The sun had a complex relationship with the earth, not only providing warmth but also drawing substances up out of the earth and water. Its purifying power resulted from its attracting poisonous vapours.

[. . .]

The sun's action was also thought to nurture gold, silver, and precious stones within the earth and draw them to the surface. . . . Valuable metals and gems would be found in abundance only in very hot areas.

321

. . . Colonists marveled at how swiftly crops came to fruition, leading to claims of 'incredible usurie' in increase as well as multiple harvests every year. From New England to the West Indies, the great heat of the summer was seen as the source of American abundance.

[. . .]

The sun was thought to be especially dangerous for people not used to laboring in its heat. English writers were preoccupied with the question of how a human body changes when introduced into a hot climate. . . .

[. . .]

. . . Scientists and settlers knew that the function of the sweating mechanism is to conduct heat from the interior of the body to the outside, but they worried about the result of the process because they believed that 'great sweating' left the 'inner parts', particularly the stomach, cold and debilitated. They attributed loss of appetite in hot regions to weakness in the stomach. . . . As a remedy, colonists in the tropics, supported by the best science of the time, turned to drinking 'strong spirits' and eating hot peppers to warm their insides. . . .

[. . .]

Some people believed that the extreme swings typical of America's climate rendered it especially unhealthy. These could be felt in a variety of ways. Newcomers to the West Indies were confronted by the most immediate contrast to their accustomed environment. Mainland settlers were struck by the difference between the great heat of summer and the winter's cold. In all colonies, going to bed sweating with the heat and waking up cold in the night was thought to be the source of many 'epidemical distempers'.

. . . Since the body was struggling to create a new balance of the humors, the traditional approaches of bleeding and purging were still recommended. These had to be used with care, however, especially when natural processes were speeded up. . . .

Colonists sought cures among the products of their new homes. From colony after colony came pleas for physicians to experiment with the herbs and chemicals the settlers were finding. . . . For example, Peter de Osma wrote from Peru to thank Nicholas Monardes, the Seville physician who experimented with New World plants and published a medical treatise about them.[13] He said the doctors in Peru were

---

[13] Nicolas Monardes (c. 1493–1588) was a Spanish physician based in Seville. He popularised the new drugs in his *Dos libros. El uno que trata de todas las cosas que traen de*

'nothyng curious'. William Strachey[14] similarly complained that doctors in Virginia did not understand the ills of the country. Early English colonists on Tobago attributed sickness to lack of knowledge of the medicinal and nutritional qualities of plants native to the island. . . .

Another way of coping was to learn from the Indians and from inhabitants of other hot countries. Colonists acknowledged a large debt to Indian medical practice, emphasizing that to use the products of America without Indian guidance was very risky. . . .

[. . .]

Hot climates, then, were perceived as dangerous, especially for people used to England's moderation. Emigrating to the southern parts of America meant taking great risks, in fact gambling one's health against the possibility of amassing riches. This gamble took place on the national as well as the personal level. A high proportion of those who went or were sent by entrepreneurs lost the wager, but high death rates, because they were seen as a necessary result of transplantation, did not diminish enthusiasm for an English presence in the Caribbean and the southern mainland of North America. . . .

[. . .]

Despite all the dangers and the alien environment [then], English people went to the rich southern mainland of North America and the West Indies in overwhelmingly larger numbers in the seventeenth century than to northern regions that were considered to be more like England. For promoters, planters, and medical men in the colonies, adaptation and survival therefore became major concerns, especially the problem of easing newcomers through the seasoning. Experience demonstrated that the young and strong weathered the traumas of adaptation better than those who were sickly on arrival. . . . Regulation of the rhythm of work and emigration also helped. . . . Virginia settlers early perceived that if new colonists were to arrive in the fall, they would have several months to become acclimatized before they had to face the heat and disease that prevailed during the summer months of hard work. They repeatedly urged this strategy on the Virginia Company, which turned a deaf ear. . . .

nuestras Indias occidentales (*Two books. One which deals with all the things that are brought from our western Indies*) published in three parts in Seville between 1565 and 1574. An English translation appeared in 1577.

[14] William Strachey (1572–1621) was secretary of the council in Virginia (1610–11) and the author of *The history of travaile into Virginia Britannia*, which was not published until 1849.

Colonists were urged to change their eating habits because orderly diet would make them resistant to the ill effects of extreme weather. . . .

[. . .]

Though . . . [the] winter's cold was easier to deal with than extreme heat, southern colonists could do much to control their personal micro-environments through manipulation of housing and clothing. . . .

Eighteenth-century reports make clear that colonists had learned to build their houses to maximise coolness. . . . Chesapeake houses were built around a central hall that drew in breezes; sometimes they were raised to allow free movement of air underneath. Kitchens and other rooms devoted to heat-producing functions were separated from the main house in small buildings, and summerhouses made cool retreats. Underground rooms allowed planters to keep butter and other perishables longer. Common planters' houses as well as those of the great landowners were constructed to allow a free flow of air through them. . . .

Clothing was the most easily manipulated element of the personal environment. Colonists were quick to adapt the clothing of slaves and lesser servants to warm conditions. Servants' dress on Barbados consisted of linen shirts and drawers for men and petticoats for women. The linen garments of the slaves were of canvas, and the materials for Europeans were finer depending on status. . . .

[. . .]

By the eighteenth century, adaptation had made life in the South more comfortable, and the largely native-born composition of the population reduced the role of seasoning as a killer. And yet, inhabitants of the southern mainland and the West Indies continued to think of their regions as less healthy, less apt to produce robust people because of high heat and humidity. . . .

[. . .]

Eighteenth-century physicians knew that fevers were the leading cause of death in the southern mainland as well as the West Indies, but they saw fevers as the direct product of hot weather, especially when combined with high humidity. . . .

Doctors, like laymen, continued to believe that the human body was drastically changed by moving from a cold to a hot climate. The link between heat and disease for these physicians, as for their seventeenth-century counterparts, was changes in bodily humors produced by exposure to 'intemperate climes'. Prickly heat and the leg ulcers that afflicted many were seen as attempts by the blood to throw off 'fiery' and 'acrid' elements, and to excrete them through the skin. Therefore, bathing in cold water or any attempt to control the eruptions was thought to cause more harm to the body by forcing the harmful excretions inward again.

Constant perspiration continued to be seen as a major cause of disease. It led to laxity of the muscle fibers and, because of a sympathetic connection between the skin and the stomach, to weakness in digestion. . . .

[. . .]

Though [eighteenth-century] theories were more complicated, a seventeenth-century reader would have been comfortable with them, based as they were on the same assumptions about human beings in relation to the environment that had informed earlier thinking. Medical thinking based on experiential data from the colonies transformed the vague and unformed beliefs of the late sixteenth and early seventeenth centuries into the certainties of the eighteenth. Evidence from the colonies, interpreted through the lens of the physicians' assumptions about the human body, allowed medical environmentalism to become dogma. The apparently empirical bond between heat and fever, proven experimentally by the colonies, cemented the role of climate in disease in eighteenth-century thinking.

Fear of hot climates was accommodated by the eighteenth century. Southern colonists accepted the danger and discomfort. . . . Most were uneasy about the risks of living in an intemperately hot place, and scientists sought to understand and mitigate the worst effects of heat, but routines of life went on in the face of the danger. . . .

The southern part of America no longer seemed alien. . . . The vast majority of the population, especially on the mainland, were native-born and therefore did not see the flora and fauna as exotic. The colonists were not really colonists; they were Americans by birth: hot and unhealthy though the land might be, it was their home.

12.4

The introduction of European medicine
to New Spain

Guenter B. Risse, 'Medicine in New Spain' in Ronald L. Numbers
(ed.), *Medicine in the New World: New Spain, New France, and
New England* (Knoxville, University of Tennessee Press, 1987),
pp. 29–45.

In this essay, Guenter Risse discusses how Spanish medical institutions and practices were imported to New Spain. The formal structures of Spanish medicine are apparent in New Spain: regulation and inspection by the *protomédico*, and a replication of the training of an elite cadre of physicians in the new University of Mexico. However, as Risse points out, the influence of these two bodies was slight, and it was the hospitals and the *curanderos* of New Spain who made most impact on the health of the American Indians and the Spanish poor who comprised the majority of the colony's population.

Protomedicato

The regulation of medical practice in New Spain followed closely along lines established in the mother country. In 1525, shortly after the conquest of the Aztec empire, the municipal council of Mexico City appointed a barber-surgeon, Francisco de Soto, to act as *protomédico*, concerning himself with the regulation of medical practice and the precarious health of the city's inhabitants. In 1527 the licentiate Pedro López assumed that position, and from then on a succession of *protomédicos* demanded that all practitioners 'explain by what right they practiced'. As in Spain, the reasons for this insistence are not hard to find. A number of irregular healers, both locals and foreigners, streamed into Mexico City, killing, in the eyes of the municipal council or *cabildo*, more people than they cured.

[. . .]

The last decades of the sixteenth century witnessed the arrival in New Spain of a few more university-trained physicians and surgeons and a number of Romance surgeons. Yet the system of inspections continued unabated, perhaps in part because it provided a welcome source of payoffs for participating functionaries. In response to developments in

326

Spain, the authority of the *protomedicato* was strengthened after 1646 in that only qualified applicants with university degrees were allowed to practice legally, especially outside the larger urban areas; this prompted the development of an extensive illicit practice of medicine by empirics and *curanderos*,[15] especially in rural areas.

Among those in New Spain who filled the vacuum created by the small number of physicians and surgeons were clerics, especially those belonging to the mendicant orders that labored in hospices and hospitals. Mine operators often took care of their Indian work force, and a large number of native healers, relying on the predominantly magico-religious Aztec medicine, ministered to Indians, blacks, and mestizos.[16] Such *curanderismo* or folk healing, officially ridiculed by the Spaniards, and later persecuted by the Inquisition, assumed an importance beyond furnishing health care to the vast majority of rural poor. In fact, by preserving religious and social values, the *curandero* became an essential figure in the survival of the traditional native culture. Use of magical procedures in healing helped native populations to maintain their identity and distinctiveness. Thus *curanderismo* became the most effective defense mechanism against Spanish acculturation, especially after 1620.

Medical education

In 1570 Philip II[17] justified the mission of Francisco Hernández[18] to the New World by declaring: 'Wishing that our subjects should enjoy a long life and preserve perfect health, we take care in providing them with physicians and teachers who will direct, teach, and cure their illnesses. With this goal in mind, we have established chairs of medicine and philosophy at the most important universities of the Indies'. The Royal and Pontifical University of Mexico had already been founded in 1551 by order of Charles V. A quarter of a century later, in 1575, the Rector of the University . . . proposed the establishment of a medical chair. His recommendation, however, was rejected. . . .

After assurances of funding from the king, however, the Mexican *audiencia*[19] finally created a *prima* chair of medicine in 1578, follow-

---

[15] Native healers.

[16] Spanish-American Indian.

[17] Philip II, king of Spain (1556–98).

[18] Francisco Hernández (1517–87) was appointed court physician to Philip II in 1567. Three years later he was made *protomédico*, or chief medical officer, in New Spain; see also below extract 12.5.

[19] The viceroy's governing body which possessed judicial powers.

ing the regulations and curriculum then in use at the University of Salamanca. . . .

[. . .]

It is significant that almost three decades passed between the foundation of the university and the creation of a medical chair. At the very
least it suggests that colonial authorities did not consider such studies
to be an effective remedy for the chronic shortage of physicians and the
proliferation of irregular healers and quacks. The relatively small
number of physicians trained by the university during its early years
indicates that the authorities were wise to look elsewhere for a solution
of their problem.

Given the constant trickle of Spanish graduates arriving in the colony
to treat the Spanish urban elite, the university probably saw little
reason to endow a new chair of medicine. . . . Not surprisingly, the medical profession in the capital seems to have been equally reluctant to
support formal medical training; at least there is no indication that any
of its members pressured the academic authorities into creating a chair.
Because of the shortage of competent healers, these physicians were in
great demand and were able to exact high fees for their services; they
had little interest in fostering more competition. . . .

Medical education in both Spain and the colonies stressed a rational
orientation to matters of health and disease that appealed primarily to
gente de razón – people of reason. For the vast majority of New Spain's
residents, whether Indian, black, or mestizo, sickness continued to
have a supernatural significance that no logical exposition of humors,
temperaments, and qualities could fully explain or justify. For these
people, eloquence and debating skills, philosophical argumentations
and flawless quotations of texts sharpened through numerous examinations and *oposiciones*,[20] meant little. Hippocrates had indeed come to
the colonies, but he was known only among the educated elite.

Hospitals

Hospitals in New Spain also followed Spanish models. As early as 1502,
Isabel of Castile instructed Nicolás de Ovando, Columbus' successor
as governor of the island of Hispaniola, 'to build hospitals where the
poor can be housed and cured, whether Christians or Indians'. The
royal order instituted a social welfare system called *beneficencia* developed by the Spanish rulers and the Church to insure the wellbeing of

[20] Disputations.

colonial inhabitants and to facilitate evangelization of the indigenous population.

[...]

There were two types of hospitals in New Spain: general and specialized. In cities, general hospitals, which took care of sick Spaniards and Indians of both sexes, were usually located near the central plaza and the church. No doubt prompted by the repeated epidemics and the conviction that miasma, or bad air, caused disease, a royal decree in 1573 required that 'when a city, village or place be founded, the hospitals for the non-contagious sick are to be placed next to the church, and for the contagious sick, erected in an elevated place where no ill winds passing through the hospitals are going to hurt the population'.

In 1521 the conquistador Hernando Cortés founded the first general hospital in New Spain, in the City of Mexico. . . . [T]his institution was designed specifically to care for the sick poor, both Spaniards and Indians; however, it excluded patients suffering from leprosy, syphilis, madness, and St. Anthony's fire. Cortés financed the establishment from his own personal fortune as a gesture of thanksgiving and penance, and he made elaborate arrangements in his will for a permanent endowment. . . .

Special hospitals existed for patients believed to be suffering from leprosy. Traditionally dedicated in Europe to Saint Lazarus, these establishments or lazarettos were generally located outside of towns to insure the isolation of their inmates. In the early 1520s, Cortés built the Hospital de San Lázaro in Tlaxpana, outside the City of Mexico. In 1539, Bishop Juan de Zumárraga[21] founded the Hospital del Amor de Dios exclusively for patients suffering from syphilis, since they were excluded from Cortés' general hospital. In 1567 Bernardino Alvarez, an affluent former conquistador, erected the Hospital de San Hipólito on the outskirts of Mexico City and dedicated it to convalescents and mental patients.

In 1555 the colonial authorities in Mexico City discussed in earnest the establishment of hospitals exclusively devoted to Indians, who composed about 80 percent of the city's inhabitants. If the natives could be congregated in one place during the epidemics, it would be easier for clergy to administer last rites. Aided by new instructions from Philip II a year later, local authorities expanded and rebuilt the Hospital San José de los Naturales, originally established in the early 1530s . . . for

---

[21] Zumárraga (1468–1548) was the first bishop of Mexico.

the care of the Indians. With eight wards, this establishment could accommodate more than 200 sick and destitute Indians.

The reorganized hospital was supported by Indian tribute, the *medio real de hospital*. Each Indian village in New Spain was enjoined to pay the institution one Spanish bushel of corn out of every hundred collected. Additional income came from items willed by patients to the hospital. The new building, completed in 1556, housed one ward for contagious cases and another for persons suffering from rabies. An ambulatory department treated emergency cases. The staff consisted of five chaplains, two physicians, two surgeons, and various apprentices. As in certain Spanish hospitals of the period, autopsies of patients dying in the institutions were permitted in order to ascertain cause of death.

Although the health care of natives in the City of Mexico and its environs remained in the hands of the Crown, elsewhere Franciscans and Augustinians ran hospitals exclusively for Indians. Most of these institutions were erected without specific donations and were maintained by the contribution of religious *cofradías*.[22] The sick usually resided in a small building adjacent to the church or convent. . . .

The Hospital de Santa Cruz, established in 1569 at Huaxtepec by Bernardino Alvarez, well known for his charitable works, merits special attention. This hospital was located about fifty miles from the City of Mexico, on a beautiful site previously used as a retreat by Aztec rulers. Many plants, including a large number of medicinals . . . grew in Montezuma's gardens, a popular spa, which, according to the natives, possessed healing powers. Alvarez' establishment was designed to care for convalescents and patients suffering from chronic ailments, who were shuttled from Mexico's St. Hippolytus Hospital by members of the Brotherhood of Charity dedicated to this saint. The physicians at the Hospital de Santa Cruz used native herbs to treat a variety of medical problems, including syphilis.

When the *protomédico* Francisco Hernández visited the hospital, perhaps in 1574, he learned a great deal about medicinal plants and returned to the capital with a rich harvest of information. Gregorio López (*ca.* 1542–*ca.* 1596), a hermit and medical author, had a similar experience during his stay as a patient. His unpublished 'Tesoro de la Medicinas' ['Treasure of Medicines'] contains observations concerning medical treatments with botanical remedies. The excellent reputation of the Hospital de Santa Cruz as a spa with innovative therapeutics attracted patients from all over New Spain and from as far away as Guatemala and Peru.

---

[22] Confraternities.

Among the most distinctive of New Spain's private hospitals were the so-called pueblo-hospitals established by Vasco de Quiroga (1477–1565), a judge of the second Mexican *audiencia*. Like other Spanish officials and clerics in the colony, Quiroga desired to educate and convert the Indians as well as ameliorate the abuses they were suffering at the hands of their new lords. Influenced by Thomas More's *Utopia*,[23] Quiroga advocated the creation of pueblos composed of 6,000 extended families, each consisting of ten to sixteen married couples from the same lineage. A central feature of each settlement was a hospital containing separate facilities for patients with contagious diseases. A *mayordomo* (superintendent) and a *dispensero* (literally a dispenser of first aid) administered the hospital, which was also served by a physician, surgeon, and apothecary.

[. . .]

As an experiment in converting and educating Indians, Quiroga's scheme proved successful. In providing health care, however, it seems to have been less efficacious, especially after the establishment of hospitals for natives in the City of Mexico and in the province of Michoacán.

[. . .]

In many respects the hospitals of New Spain served a social function similar to those in the mother country. Even the effort to use them to convert the Indians had been anticipated in Spain, on a much smaller scale, when the Spanish kings employed hospitals to help Christianize the reconquered Moors.[24] The novel feature of hospitals in New Spain was their role in reversing the dispersal of the indigenous population, frightened by ruthless *encomenderos*[25] and threatened by disease. Hospitals attracted Indians not only temporarily, such as during epidemics, but permanently, for example in the pueblos. With their large patient populations and *cofradías*, they functioned as centers for Spanish acculturation. Both religious celebrations and medical routines allowed the natives not only to learn Christian dogma and values, but a new language and a sense of community.

---

[23] First published in Latin in 1516 by the English humanist, diplomat and statesman, Thomas More (1478–1535), *Utopia* described a perfect society in which the traditional rules of early sixteenth-century society no longer applied. It contains a description of a hospital for contagious diseases.

[24] The Arab inhabitants of Spain. The *reconquista* of Moorish Spain was completed in 1492 following the fall of Granada.

[25] Spaniards who were given the use of land and the labour of all those who lived on the land, while ownership remained in the hands of the Spanish crown. Many became very rich.

[. . .]

Medical theory and practice

In his instructions to Francisco Hernández in 1570, Philip II not only stressed the potential benefits that would accrue from a knowledge of New World medicinal plants, but spelled out the methods to acquire the desired data. The king directed the *protomédico* to gather information 'from all physicians, surgeons, Spanish and Indian herbalists, and other curious persons with such abilities who evidently could understand and know something, and obtain in general an account of all medicinal herbs, trees, plants, and seeds that exist in a given province'. Furthermore, he ordered Hernández to ask informants about the faculties, temperaments, and dosages of these medicines and, if possible, to perform clinical tests or at least secure affidavits from experts certifying all therapeutic claims.

These royal instructions reflected the great interest of both the Crown and Spanish medical circles in American drugs. Their concern was more than scientific; it stemmed as well from economic considerations related to trade in spices and drugs, an issue of paramount importance. . . . [G]uaiacum, the holy wood from the Caribbean islands, was already being employed in Spain by 1516 to treat syphilis, and its use spread rapidly to other European countries. The profits made by those who imported this wood from the New World suggested that fortunes awaited the discovery of new remedies.

Since the time of Columbus, accounts of miraculous cures with New World plants had flooded Spain. . . . [In the 1550s], the Crown received a manuscript titled 'Libellus de Medicinalibus Indorum Herbis' ['A Book of Herbal Medicines of the Indies'] from the Franciscan Colegio de Santa Cruz in Tlatelolco, an institution devoted to the education of young Indians and to the preservation of Aztec culture. This document, a Latin translation of an Aztec work written by a native healer, Martín de la Cruz, summarized traditional medical knowledge. It also included hundreds of drawings depicting a great variety of medicinal plants. Although it was never published, this work proved to the royal court that herbal riches awaited the colonists.

Hernández closely followed the methodology suggested by Philip II for gathering medical information. As revealed in his letters and reports, he viewed Aztec medicine within the context of his own humoral pathology and therapeutics and constantly sought to explain favorable effects in those terms. He often tasted medicinal products in order to classify them and assign them fundamental Galenic qualities, a method that more than once made him gravely ill. Stripped of their magico-religious context, native practices made little sense to a foreign practitioner who adhered to a naturalistic system of medicine, and Hernández often expressed doubts about claims made by Indians if he could not readily find humoral explanations.

Hernández summarized his criticisms of Aztec medicine in a manuscript entitled 'De Antiquitatibus Novae Hispaniae' ['On the Antiquities of New Spain'], which discussed Indian customs, ceremonies, and laws. Written during the early 1570s, Hernández' comments typify the reactions of learned Spanish physicians who had occasion to observe native healing. His foremost complaint was that Aztec healers or *ticitl* did not study the nature of individual diseases or differentiate between individual ailments. In his view, their histories and examinations of the sick were too superficial to facilitate differential diagnoses. He was also dismayed by what he felt was insufficient dietary recommendations for the sick, a fundamental part of his therapeutic regimen. The Indians, moreover, did not perform phlebotomies, so common in European practice, but restricted their bloodletting to occasional scarifications. Above all, Hernández thought that native remedies were prescribed irrationally and without enough flexibility to deal with changing clinical situations. Hence he concluded that Aztec healers were merely empirics, rigidly using their materia medica according to traditions passed on from generation to generation.

[. . .]

Hernández' reservations about indigenous medicine must be kept in mind when analyzing the early medical literature of New Spain, our best source of information about medical theory and practice in the colonies. All of those who wrote on this subject were Spanish physicians and surgeons motivated by a desire to correct the same deficiencies Hernández had perceived and thereby recast Aztec medicine according to classical Hippocratic and Galenic models. In their opinion, a theoretical knowledge of humors and qualities was needed in order to understand the nature of disease, to distinguish between clinical pictures, and to render a correct prognosis. Likewise, they thought that humoralism could transcend blind Aztec empiricism and enable the establishment of rational therapeutics, flexible enough to incorporate many valuable elements from the native pharmacopoeia.

12.5
The Europeanisation of native American remedies

*The Mexican Treasury. The Writings of Dr. Francisco
Hernández,* ed. Simon Varey and trans. R. Chabrán,
C. L. Chamberlin and S. Varey (Stanford, Stanford University
Press, 2000), pp. 138, 139, 140.

Francisco Hernández (1517–87) was appointed court physician to
Philip II in 1567. Three years later he was made *protomédico* in New
Spain. He translated and commented on Pliny's *Natural history* (not
published until the twentieth century), and wrote his own *Natural history of New Spain,* which was only published in parts in the seventeenth century. The excerpts here, taken from this work, first appeared
in a selection of Hernández' writings in the *Quatro libros de la naturaleza* (1615). They were the fruits of his seven years' travels in New
Spain, where he spent much of his time identifying plants and gathering
information about them from Spaniards and native American Indians.

Tzocuilpátli

The herb called tzocuilpátli has leaves resembling those of the basil,
only much smaller and serrate, but profoundly rough. On one side they
[are] whitish and not very different from those that the [herb] called
cihuapatli produces. The stalks [are] round, hirsute, and whitish, yellow
on their upper parts. The flowers [are] round and pilose.[26] The root [is]
full of fibers. It grows in the wooded hills of a hot land, such as the
province of Pánuco. The root is odoriferous, resinous, and hot and dry
in the fourth degree. When a decoction has been made of the root, and
reduced by one third and [it is] drunk, once only, in a moderate amount,
they say that it restores lost mobility. Instilled into the nostrils, it cures
migraine by evacuating phlegm from the head by this route.

Hemionitic Cihuapatli

Because this herb cures the indispositions of women, and resembles
the hemionitidis – for it is a species of satinwood [to judge by] the shape

---

[26] Covered with hair.

of its leaves – they call it the hemionitic cihuapatli; but the Spanish women of New Spain call it 'mother's herb'. It produces many slender, round, straight, villous[27] stalks from its one fibrous root. The leaves [are] long and soft, and in a certain way resemble those of the hemion-itidis, whence comes its name. The flowers are white and in calyxes. It grows in all areas, both temperate and hot. It is dry in the third degree. For this reason three or four ounces of its decoction are generally pre-scribed for women who are giving birth, so that they may deliver [their babies] more easily with a good outcome. The decoction or juice is very useful for the breast. When a handful of the leaves has been crushed and given to be drunk in water or some appropriate liquid, they relieve stomach cramps, cure dropsy, and provoke menstruation. They plant it from root cuttings and from seed. They usually cultivate it as a pleasing and nice-looking thing, not only in gardens and orchards, but also in flowerpots and clay receptacles. Ladies and gentlewomen are in the habit of beautifying their halls and windows with it, and [also] their pri-vate pleasure gardens.

Tepetlachichicxíhuitl, or Bitter Herb That Grows in Wooded Hills

The tepetlachichicxíhuitl, which other people call chichixíhuitl, is an herb with fragrant, serrate, rough, whitish leaves like a wall german-der's. The slender, dark, round, smooth stalks grow three spans in length;[28] on the ends of the stalks are hirsute white blossoms with yellow [in them], shaped like little stars, from which grows an oblong small fruit. The root is white and fibrous. It grows in hot hills. The root is fragrant, hot and dry in the third degree, with subtle parts that have a certain bitterness, from which it takes its name. It is an herb of great importance, whose juice greatly alleviates indigestion and afflictions of the chest when it is administered every day in the morning, since it purges phlegmatic and bilious humors by means of the upper channel as well as the lower.

---

[27] Soft and hairy.
[28] About two feet three inches.

12.6
The reception of American drugs in early modern Europe

Andrew Wear, 'The Early Modern Debate about Foreign Drugs:
Localism versus Universalism in Medicine', *Lancet* 354 (1999),
pp. 149–51.

In this extract, Andrew Wear discusses the controversy surrounding
the introduction of foreign remedies to Europe in the sixteenth century, including the use of medical and religious arguments to support
the view that local diseases were best cured by local remedies, which
were also more readily affordable by the poor. However, Wear also
points out that exotic foreign remedies were popular. Commercially
profitable, Galenic physicians had few problems incorporating them
into traditional practice. At the same time, the medical knowledge of
the indigenous peoples who used them was jettisoned. Wear makes
the analogy with the globalising tendencies of present-day scientific
medicine.

In the 16th and 17th centuries the intense search for new drugs in the
new-found world of America and in the rediscovered one of the East
aroused controversy, which, as today, centred around issues of univer-
sality and localism. However, the focus of the arguments was on the
appropriateness of foreign remedies for Europeans, rather than on the
economic and cultural consequences for indigenous peoples of the
drug trade and of the spread of European medicine across the globe.

Part of the commercial imperative for the voyages of European discovery was the search for spices and remedies. . . . The association of
the new remedies with large-scale commercial opportunities helped to
give them universal appeal; remedies that were believed to work only
within a geographical area were worth less than those that were marketed as being effective across geographical, cultural, and national
boundaries. It was also to some extent important to note how indigenous people used remedies because prospective settlers might benefit
from local drugs for local diseases. . . .

However, a form of intellectual and mercantilist appropriation took
place when foreign drugs came into Europe. Exotic remedies remained
exotic. It was part of their commercial appeal; it was what made them
expensive and, therefore, big money-earners for merchants and apothe-

caries. But the original cultural associations of the remedies and how they were understood in terms of the medical systems of their places of origin were of no interest and ignored. Instead, the remedies from the East Indies and America were quickly integrated into the orthodox qualitative-humoral system of medicine taught in the universities. 16th-century writers such as Garcia d'Orta . . . and Nicolas Monardes,[29] . . . described the therapeutic powers of the new remedies and assigned them qualitative characteristics. This meant that they became part of the allopathic medical system derived from Galen. . . . Tobacco, for instance, was famously described by Monardes as being able to cure, by means of its hot and dry qualities, toothaches, bad breath, chilblains, ulcers, old sores, worms, pains in the joints, poisonous bites, poisoned wounds, kidney stones, carbuncles, and weariness.

However, there was resistance to the use of foreign remedies. Some of it was pragmatic. Foreign remedies were especially prone to be counterfeited, adulterated, and substituted since the profits to be made from [them] were generally greater than those from drugs produced with local ingredients. . . .

Foreign remedies, even unadulterated, also provoked strong opposition on other grounds – nationalistic, religious, economic, and medical. The message of die-hard opponents of the new exotic drugs was that because these substances were foreign they would not suit European bodies. Their argument was one based on locality: a place and especially its climate . . . shaped the constitution or qualitative-humoral balance of people and plants . . . so local plants were most suitable for local people and their diseases. . . .

Within medicine, the argument that local drugs were best was used mainly by the Paracelsian opponents of the establishment medicine. . . . Just as modern scientific medicine makes claims that it can be applied globally, so the practitioners of Galenic medicine claimed that the scope of its theory and of its therapeutics was universal, even though both had originated in the Mediterranean and Asia Minor. . . . It was in this context that Paracelsus . . . used the argument from local remedies to contest the global remit of Galenic medicine. The dispute about foreign and local remedies thus got caught up in the fight between two competing medical systems. . . .

Religion, the dominant ideology of the 16th century, was also brought into the argument by the opponents of foreign drugs. They cited *Eccle-*

---

[29] Garcia d'Orta (b. c. 1490) was a Portuguese merchant and physician based in Goa, in India, and the author of an Indian herbal, first published in Spanish in Goa in 1563. For Monardes, see above note 13.

siasticus ch 38 v 4, 'The Lord hath created medicines out of the earth' to bolster their case. In England, Timothie Bright[30] . . . wrote an extensive critique of foreign remedies partly based on the passage from *Ecclesiasticus*. He argued that just as God had provided food and clothing so also had he placed medicines nearby, since the preservation of human beings was part of the providential goodness of the creator. He added that it detracted from God's providence to depend on the 'adventures of Merchants' for health, and 'the disease being in the one part of the world, to have the medicine in the other . . .' Bright also argued for a local rather than a global materia medica on the grounds that there was a fit between the qualitative . . . constitution of a place, its inhabitants, its diseases, and the remedies growing there. . . . The belief that climate and place shaped a people's nature and its health and illness had its roots in Hippocratic medicine and it dovetailed easily with the Christian view that God created through his providence a particular environment that affected each person for good and ill.

Opponents of foreign remedies also pointed to their cost and consequent effect for the treatment of the poor. Paracelsians presented themselves as especially concerned with providing cheap or charitable care for the poor in contrast to the Galenists, who had a reputation for being expensive and uncharitable.

[. . .]

In contrast to remedies, foreign medical theories were not imported into Europe at this time. European knowledge was generally regarded as being superior. Historians might interpret this attitude as an early example of western medical imperialism. . . . James Primrose,[31] a staunch English defender of orthodox Galenic medicine, noted approvingly that 'it was wisely ordered by the Spaniards and Portugals, that in India where they bear rule, physic should be practised after the self same manner that it is in Europe according to the doctrine of Galen and Hippocrates'. He claimed that because Galenic medicine was founded on 'universal' principles, it could be applied to different places and climates. . . .

. . . Even a writer like Bright, who argued for local remedies, did not argue for local knowledge whether of English wise-women or of indigenous people. The wish among Galenists and Paracelsians for a medi-

---

[30] Bright (1550–1615) was physician to St Bartholomew's Hospital in London and a moderate Paracelsian, who later became a clergyman. He was the author of *A treatise: wherein is declared the sufficiencie of English medicines* (London, 1580).

[31] For Primrose, see extract 2.3 above.

cine that was based on expert rather than on popular or folk knowledge meant that rival sources of knowledge were not recognised, though their remedies might have been.

12.7

Medicine and slavery

Richard B. Sheridan, *Doctors and Slaves: A Medical and Demographic History of Slavery in the British West Indies, 1680–1834* (Cambridge, Cambridge University Press, 1985), pp. 329–31, 335–6.

In this work, Sheridan analyses the interaction between slave owners, slaves and doctors in the context of the working and living conditions experienced by slaves. He is concerned to trace the biomedical and demographic outcomes of slavery. In the process, his book combines historical analysis with present-day biological and medical knowledge.

European doctors in the Sugar Colonies were at their best when they urged planters to enhance the life chances of their slaves by providing better diets, clothing, housing, and sanitation; tempering work loads and punishment; and taking care of pregnant women, mothers and children. They were at their best when they made an effort to understand their black patients in a clinical sense and also the intimate union of medicine and magic in the minds of Afro-Caribbean slaves, the culture shock they suffered, and their suspicion and fear of white doctors and their medicines. They were at their best when they made an effort to learn the folk wisdom of the blacks, study their herbal remedies, and search out indigenous plants that have medicinal value. They were at their best when they combined the practice of medicine and surgery with scientific investigation and the publication of books concerned with tropical medicine and natural history. They were at their best when they were skeptical of fashionable theories of disease causation and sought to advance rational conceptual schemes adapted to the disease environment in the West Indies. They were at their best when they were alert to the baneful influence of certain medicines and limited their prescriptions to therapeutically effective drugs.

Very few, if any, medical men conformed to this ideal. One important source of error and malpractice was the humoral-climatic and miasmatic theory of medicine. . . .

[. . .]

Extreme bleeding, vomiting, and purging, or heroic medicine, appear to have been widely practiced in the West Indies. Advocates of venesection or bloodletting claimed that it relieved pain, prompted relaxation and sleep, subdued fever and the force of the circulation, checked vomiting, and prevented hemorrhage. . . .

Bloodletting reached its peak of popularity in Europe and America in the early nineteenth century, although it met with a mixed response by certain doctors in the British Sugar Colonies. In treating cases of pneumonia, Dr. James Thomson[32] noted that in several instances within a sixty-hour period he had 'taken away eighty ounces of blood from a robust negro and saved his life'. Immediately after the first copious bleeding he administered a strong purge consisting of neutral salts with James's or antimonial powders. He warned, however, that after the second or third day bleeding became very dangerous and by many doctors was altogether interdicted. . . .

Practitioners in the West Indies were not unlike their counterparts in North America and Europe in overdosing their patients with drugs. There is reason to believe that overdosing was carried to even greater lengths owing to both the belief that tropical diseases needed to be arrested quickly with strong remedies and the racist myth that blacks were less sensitive than whites to strong medicine. Dr. Collins[33] voiced the latter belief in pungent language, pointing out that:

the most nauseous drugs, unless of the emetic tribe, seldom ruffle the stomachs of negroes, or dispose them to vomit. Bark they retain in almost any quantity, and their bowels resist the most drastic purges, without suffering much inconvenience. I have given, for the tape-worm, ten grains of calomel, and twenty-five of gamboge,[34] to a constitution, which I had

---

[32] James Thomson, M.D. (d. 1822) was the author of *A treatise on the diseases of Negroes, as they occur in the island of Jamaica: with observations on the country remedies* (Jamaica, 1820).

[33] David Collins was both a doctor and a successful planter on the island of St Vincent. His *Practical rules for the management and medical treatment of Negro slaves in the sugar colonies*, first published in 1803, is concerned with the management and discipline of slaves, and with the need to keep them healthy as well as treating those diseases most prevalent among them.

[34] A purgative made from the resin of the tree of the same name.

before found to be almost immoveable, without their occasioning one puke, or more than four or five motions of the belly.

[. . .]

. . . [I]t is perhaps true that the European practitioners as a group had little positive impact on the health of their black patients. They lacked the authority and resources to alleviate the major medical problems of poverty, ignorance, poor nourishment, hard labor, and ill-regulated conditions of life. The white doctor often lacked authority to keep a slave in the hospital for treatment when the master or manager was convinced that the slave was feigning illness to avoid labor. The white doctor was both a technician and a colonizer who confronted a colonized and enslaved patient who was reluctant to entrust his life to a stranger. Slaves were generally alienated from colonial society and tended to fear and mistrust the white doctors who treated their illnesses. Lacking the ability to communicate and establish rapport with his patients, the white doctor could only practice plantation medicine as if he were a veterinarian. Slaves might be expected to resist the poisonous potions and pills that constituted the pharmacopoeia of European-trained doctors. . . .

Black slave medics – whether attached to plantation hospitals or in informal practice – were often more effective in their cures than their white counterparts. . . . Afro-West Indian slaves depended on their own medical knowledge and art without much help from white professionals during the seventeenth and most of the eighteenth centuries. Rather than routinely purging, puking, and bleeding their patients, the black doctors administered herbs and roots that frequently contained curative properties. Even if their remedies did not cure, they did not kill as did opium, mercury, antimony, and venesection. Black medics were able to communicate with their patients in their native tongue, to make them feel better and thus speed recovery by caring for the whole patient.

The role of black medics on the plantations of the Sugar Colonies is difficult to reconstruct from written records. What we know is largely what has survived from accounts of slave hospitals and their black attendants. We do not know the nature and extent of black medical treatment of blacks outside the hospitals and of black self-care, which was hidden from white view. Indirect evidence that the African medical culture survived the Middle Passage is the substantial number of medicinal plants that are common to both African and Caribbean countries today.

Because women played a key role in the day-to-day medical practice of Africa in the era of the Atlantic slave-trade, it is reasonable to assume

341

that they continued to minister to the sick and wounded as plantation slaves. Sick nurses often combined supervisory, professional, and menial duties as they labored long hours in the slave hospitals. Whereas the white doctors and overseers visited the hospitals intermittently, black nurses provided sustained care of the sick and injured. They were more likely to be familiar with black-related diseases and cures than their white counterparts. They treated 'their own kind', which probably gave them a more personal interest in effecting a cure. Although handicapped by age and frail health, black nurses often exhibited qualities of competence, patience, gentleness, and self-devotion that more than compensated for their physical limitations. Outside the hospitals women no doubt cared for the sick and injured family members and friends, but this aspect of plantation health care has gone unrecorded. More than any other contribution, the black medics comforted the sorrowing and invoked supernatural vengeance against oppressors, and thus strengthened their brothers' and sisters' defenses against the psychological assaults of slavery. In this way, their contribution to survival against racial oppression outweighed the health services provided by white doctors.

12.8

The survival of African medicine in the American colonies

Sharla M. Fett, *Working Cures: Healing, Health, and Power on Southern Slave Plantations* (Chapel Hill and London, University of North Carolina Press, 2002), pp. 62–9.

Sharla Fett's work is concerned with health, illness and healing from the point of view of the slaves who lived on the plantations in the American South. She seeks to show how the power relations between owners and slaves made health a contested area, as well as demonstrating that conflict between slaves lay at the heart of conjuring medicine. In this extract she discusses another characteristic feature of black, slave medicine – its debt to herbalism. Here the situation was more porous with the movement of plants across continents and a much greater interchange of knowledge between black slaves and their white owners.

Southern herbal medicine was characterized by a high degree of exchange across lines of race, ethnicity, class, and region. . . .

The eclectic character of antebellum[35] remedies had its roots in the colonial period, when European newcomers, African natives, and indigenous Americans avidly sought medicines to survive in their changing worlds. Indeed, the colonization of the Americas initiated a global movement of plants as well as of peoples and diseases. Early European colonists set out to document and collect new plant species from the Americas, hoping to find new commodities and make their American colonies less dependent on European medicines. The Enlightenment project of European botanical classification emerged in part from the collection of exotic plants that accompanied colonization of native American lands and the forced transportation of Africans to plantation labor. At the same time colonists transplanted European flora such as apple, dandelion, and mullein that became quickly natu ralized to the North American landscape. In South America as well, where sugar planters and Jesuits brought pennyroyal, basil, and English plantain, the 'frenetic' rate of 'floristic exchange' led to an astonishing revision of the indigenous biotic inventory.

The Atlantic slave trade also fostered an exchange of Old World and New World plants. Some West African captives undergoing the terror of the transatlantic crossing may have worn strings of red and black wild licorice seeds and thus brought the licorice plant to the Caribbean. The roots of the licorice plant served as a common medicine aboard slaving vessels, and West African descendants in the Caribbean continued to use wild licorice medicinally for coughs and fevers. African grasses crossed the Atlantic with slavers who discarded on American shores the straw used to line the putrid holds of slave ships. In addition, benne (sesame), yams, okra, and black-eyed peas originated in Africa and were later grown by enslaved Africans for food. Some of these culti-vated foods served medicinal purposes in the New World as well. Africans in the Americas employed okra leaves as poultices, Jamaican senna as a laxative, 'Surinam poison' as a cure for chronic sores, and kola seeds for belly pains. By the eighteenth century the herbal medi-cines of enslaved Africans included not only native African plants but also indigenous American plants, such as Jerusalem oak and capsicum (red pepper), which had circulated in the Atlantic world for over a cen-tury. This colonial exchange of plants across the Atlantic reorganized the pharmacopoeia that both European and African descendants drew on for medicines in North America.

[35] That is, before the American civil war (1861–65) and the formal abolition of slavery in the United States of America.

[. . .]

Enslaved black practitioners also carefully guarded their herbal recipes, occasionally exchanging a cure for precious freedom. Significantly, this avenue to manumission was offered only to enslaved men. In 1729 Virginia authorities freed the aging Papan in return for a venereal disease remedy that he had kept 'as a most Profound secrett' until that time. The Virginia burgesses judged the exchange a good bargain. They hoped that Papan's recipe of 'Roots and Barks' would save 'the lives of a great number of Slaves' afflicted with yaws and other venereal diseases. In 1749 the South Carolina Assembly manumitted Caesar in exchange for snakebite and poison cures that would become popular in antebellum recipe books. Six years later the South Carolina Assembly made a similar proposal to Sampson, a healer known for his fearless handling of rattlesnakes. He received his freedom and a fifty-pound annuity as payment for his rattlesnake bite medicine made from heart snakeroot, polypody, avens root, and rum. English colonists clearly saw something of value in eighteenth-century slave herbalism and did not hesitate to appropriate African cures.

[. . .]

Daily interactions among plantation women, however, produced the most fertile ground for exchange between planter and slave herbal medicine. Slaveholding women who viewed the oversight of children's health as part of their domestic duties frequently dosed slave children with herbal remedies. . . .

[. . .]

Though the herbal repertoires of slaves and slaveholders were by no means identical, the remedies themselves sometimes circulated with surprising fluidity. Despite a widespread assumption of black intellectual inferiority, the planter class willingly absorbed reputed cures from African American practitioners. In their turn, despite distrust of white medical interference as a whole, African Americans also borrowed from the stock of planter remedies. White and black herbalism on antebellum plantations thus formed two related but distinct spheres of knowledge; necessity and circumstance led to some overlap, while class and race divisions created important differences.

Several historical developments contributed to the differences between the herbalism of elite white planters and of enslaved blacks. Literacy, direct access to white physicians, and participation in distant markets marked the herbal practices of southern white elites in ways not seen among slaves (or poorer whites, for that matter). In turn, enslaved African Americans, by virtue of their labor and subsistence patterns, maintained an intimate knowledge of the surrounding landscape. The herbal repertoire of the slave quarters as a result drew heavily from African American local botanical expertise.

[. . .]

Household remedy books . . . revealed southern planters' participation in expanding commercial markets. Throughout the eighteenth century, wealthy southern whites had routinely employed medicines imported from Europe through the seaport cities or produced domestically in the North. The market revolution of the antebellum period further increased slaveholders' access to imported botanical products. Plantation medicine chests were filled with ipepac from South America, jalap from Mexico, opium from the Far East, quinine from the Andes, and chamomile from Europe. Consumption of internationally marketed botanicals reflected the increase in medical consumerism in middling to wealthy white households. Though they did not abandon homegrown medicines, many slaveholders grew less knowledgeable about local medicinal plants even as they expanded their purchase of commercially marketed medicines. . . .

In contrast . . . the slave quarters of southern plantations harbored many botanical experts. . . . [E]nslaved African Americans who worked in the fields developed a 'keen awareness and precise knowledge of the environment'[36] not available to planter families. . . . Agricultural labor, subsistence hunting and gardening, and the domestic economy all oriented enslaved African Americans toward a working knowledge of the local flora. The complex repertoire of North American black herbalism grew out of this particular relationship to the natural environment.

---

[36] The quotation is taken from Mart Stewart.

Part thirteen

Medical organisation, training and the medical marketplace in eighteenth-century Europe

---

13.1
Challenging the physicians' monopoly in London: the Rose Case (1704)

Sir George Clark, *A History of the Royal College of Physicians of London* (2 vols, Oxford, Clarendon Press, 1964–66), vol. 2, pp. 476–9.

The House of Lords' judgement in the Rose Case permanently destroyed the Royal College of Physicians' legal monopoly over medical practice in London. The extract is taken from the official history of the College. The balanced narrative, devoid of analysis, reflects the character of most institutional histories of medicine before the present.

The Rose Case is extremely complex. The apothecary was initially denounced to the College for practising medicine illegally by an irate patient who felt he had been overcharged. The College then prosecuted Rose before the Court of King's Bench, where its monopoly was upheld and the apothecary fined for misbehaviour. It seems, however, that both the judge and the jury were unhappy with the privileged position of the College, even if it did have the law on its side, and the jury brought in an ambiguous verdict. Rose, it was found, had merely received payment for making up medicines, not for giving advice. For this reason, Rose was able to argue that the sentence was unjust and obtain a writ of error from the crown, which allowed the case to be retried in the highest court of the land, the House of Lords. There the original judgement was overturned. Henceforth, the position under common law was that the College could not pursue

unlicensed practitioners of physic in the capital who did not charge
for their services.

In the winter of 1699–1700 John Seale, a butcher in Hungerford Market,
fell ill and was given physic by William Rose, apothecary, of St. Nicholas
Lane, with the result that he was never the better but much worse. He
paid a vast deal of money, and more than a year after his original attack
the apothecary sent in another large bill. With this in his hand John
Seale came to the *comitia minora*.[1] It is not stated that the apothecary
was heard in his own defence or even that he was summoned; the College did not intend to try his case but to send him before a judge and
jury. The Annals[2] merely give their decision: 'that Mr. Swift, the attorney
of the College prosecute the said William Rose forthwith'. Mr. Seale
came again to report that Mr. Rose had come to see him, had railed
against the College and had been very troublesome. Mr. Swift and the
court of king's bench did their duty. The jury found a special verdict that
Rose, without any fee for advice, did make up and compound several
medicines, and sold and delivered them to Seale, to be drunk and taken
as proper to his distemper. By the judgment of Sir John Holt,[3] which followed, Rose, as might have been foreseen, was fined, £5 for one proved
month of practice.

The common law made no provision for an appeal against this decision, but it was possible to obtain a writ of error if the Crown ordered
the attorney-general to issue his *fiat* for such a writ. A writ of error
alleged that there was an error in the record of the case, whether truly
or not had then to be decided judicially. None of the apothecaries who
had been convicted in the past 200 years had ever resorted to this
expensive and chancy procedure; but at least twice in the king's bench
hearings things had been said which encouraged the Society of Apothecaries[4] to go on with the fight. . . .

William Rose brought his writ of error to the [H]ouse of [L]ords, the
supreme judicial tribunal, which had never yet adjudicated on any business of the College. Each side had to present its case in print. The College case was the regular water-tight recital of the charters and the Acts
of Parliament, with an account of . . . the facts of Rose's case. The

---

[1] The governing body of the College of Physicians.

[2] The minute book of the College's proceedings.

[3] Sir John Holt (1642–1710) was a leading Whig judge who was appointed Lord Chief Justice on 17 April 1689 shortly after the Glorious Revolution and the accession of William III and
Mary.

[4] Rose was a member of the Society, which supported him throughout the legal proceedings.

apothecaries took their stand on usage against obsolete law. They represented the physicians as monopolists and themselves as rendering indispensable services by practising among the poor and often among patients of all classes. The committee summoned all the members of the College of Physicians to be present at the trial. The hearing was on 15 March 1703/4. Sir Thomas Powys, led off for the apothecaries . . . contending that the charter was never intended to restrain any man – any apothecary, that is – in his trade. Mr. Dodd on the same side spoke boldly: 'I am not only for the apothecaries but for all the poor people of England'. Mr. Cooper, for the physicians, said that the apothecaries of London pretended to greater privileges than any others; the question was . . . the practice of physic; if the judgement were reversed there was no pretender to physic but he would practise on the same account as Rose. Sir Thomas Powys in reply denied this, and he fell upon the record of the trial. This showed, he said, that the physicians did not find what Seale was sick of, and admitted that his sickness was trivial. The record did not prove that Rose gave advice or even that he sold his medicines, only that he made them up. For that single act, done without reward, he was prosecuted.

When the lawyers had done, a doctor proposed to speak, but their lordships would not hear him. After debate the question was put. The judgement was reversed.

13.2

The Académie Royale de Chirurgie and medicine in *ancien régime* France

Laurence Brockliss and Colin Jones, *The Medical World of Early Modern France* (Oxford, Clarendon Press, 1997), pp. 578–81.

Set up in 1731, the French Académie de Chirurgie (Academy of Surgery) was one of a number of medical and surgical academies that were established in eighteenth-century Europe to foster medical progress. In the course of the seventeenth century, the French crown had established a number of academies to promote and police the arts and the sciences, starting with the Académie Française in 1635, which was set up to standardise and embellish the French language. At this date, the promotion of medicine had not been considered a national priority, although a number of physicians were members of the Académie des Sciences, founded in 1666, which included anatomy in its remit. The creation of academies of surgery (1731) and medicine (1776) emphasised the new importance attached to medical knowledge in the age of the Enlightenment, even if the seventeen-year gap between the foundation of the former and its receipt of a specific royal warrant suggests that many around the king had still to be convinced. Like other learned *ancien régime* institutions, it carefully guarded its privileges and membership was restricted to a select few. Its impact on French surgery was probably limited, however, and it was finally abolished, along with other royal institiutions and academies, in the Revolution in 1793.

The Academy of Surgery was established by royal letters patent in November 1731 through the efforts of the two leading promoters of the surgical art at court, Mareschal and La Peyronie.[5] The initial aim of its founders was that the new institution would be from the start under royal protection, like the other academies in the capital, such as the Academy of Sciences. The king, however, did not confer this privilege immediately, insisting that royal status would only be granted the Academy once 'experience has revealed the benefits that the public will draw from it'. As a result, the Academy was first established as a *société académique*, no different in status from the majority of provincial academies which, though receiving state authorization, equally did not enjoy specific royal patronage. It was only in 1748, after successful lobbying by La Martinière,[6] La Peyronie's successor as the king's premier surgeon, that the surgical society became officially known as the Académie Royale de Chirurgie, a title it thereafter retained until it was abolished, along with all the French academies, by the Convention[7] in August 1793.

In contrast to the other Parisian academies founded in the reign of Louis XIV,[8] the Academy of Surgery was always closely associated with an existing institution: the Paris community of surgeons. Not only did the Academy meet in the community's headquarters but every member of the corporation was *de jure* a member of the Academy. From the outset, however, a distinction was drawn between a hard core of élite members of the Academy and the majority of Paris surgeons from whose midst they were drawn. All Paris surgeons could attend meet-

[5] Georges Mareschal (d. 1733) and François Gigot de La Peyronie (d. 1747) were premier surgeons to Louis XV. La Peyronie succeeded Mareschal on the latter's death in 1733.

[6] Germain Pichaut de La Martinière.

[7] The governing body set up by the revolutionaries after 1789.

[8] Louis XIV (1643–1715), popularly known as 'the Sun King'.

ings of the Academy and present papers but only the hard core could enjoy the dignity and emoluments (never great) of an academician. Initially in 1731 this hard core consisted of sixty ordinary academicians and ten associates (out of a Paris surgical community of some 250). Twenty years later, after various distributional changes in the interim, the number of ordinary academicians, henceforth called *conseillers du comité*, was finalized at forty and the number of *adjoints* or resident associate members at twenty. At the same time, the method of appointing academicians changed. From 1739 two-thirds of the élite hard core had been elected annually by the Paris community of surgeons; the other third had been directly nominated by the king's premier surgeon. The aim, according to the *règlement* drawn up by La Peyronie, was to excite a spirit of competition among the Paris surgeons. In 1751 the crown changed the rules and the method of recruitment became less open. Academicians still had to be drawn from the Paris community of surgeons, but their appointment was now for life and their selection was controlled by the hard-core élite, who on a vacancy presented the king with a list of three nominees. The Paris surgeons attempted to fight the new arrangements, but in vain. From 1751 to 1793 the Academy of Surgery was a typical Ancien-Régime academy: corporatist, self-perpetuating, and élitist. It was also closely tied to the court for the king's premier surgeon was always its president.

The overt purpose of the Academy was to foster surgical progress by collecting, vetting, and publicizing observations and discoveries with the ultimate intention of composing a sort of surgical equivalent to Justinian's law code.[9] According to the 1751 *réglement*:

> The Academy will busy itself in perfecting the theory and practice of surgery through [promoting] research into and discoveries about the physical structure [*la physique*] of the human body and the causes, effects, and indications of surgical diseases. It will especially be involved with determining with precision the cases in which an operation is or is not necessary, when and how operations should be performed, and what [treatment] should precede and follow them. It will indicate the surgical remedies which are appropriate for each disease and the reasons which determine their employment.

In addition, the Academy was required to collect extraordinary observations about particular remedies and new operations, and compile histories of surgical practices, highlighting where new methods had been substituted for traditional ones and explaining the change.

---

[9] The Byzantine Emperor, Justinian (527–65), was responsible for issuing a massive codification of Roman Law based on a digest of all known classical authorities on the subject.

The Academy performed its statutory function as a creative policeman with a large degree of success, if unsurprisingly, it never produced a definitive statement about the surgical art. From the beginning academicians . . . accepted the authority of the institution and duly reported their observations and discoveries at the Academy's weekly meetings; indeed, from 1751 members were threatened with dismissal if they failed to produce at least one or two papers per year. Provincial researchers, however, had to be enticed to send their findings to a completely Parisian institution, especially before the Academy was granted a royal warranty. This was achieved by adopting strategies already deployed by other Parisian academies anxious to establish an authoritative voice over their disciplinary field. The primary carrot was the annual prize competition. Each year from 1732 the academicians presented a gold medallion, designed by the Académie des Inscriptions[10] and eventually worth 500 *livres*,[11] to the author of the best essay on a surgical subject previously specified. Academicians themselves were not allowed to apply. Even in the early years the competition attracted numerous candidates: twenty-five papers were received in its second year, when the prize was won by Claude-Nicolas Lecat (1700–68), chief surgeon at the Rouen Hôtel Dieu.[12]

But the annual prize by itself could not ensure that the Academy was kept supplied with a flood of observations from the provinces, so other carrots were gradually introduced to maintain provincial interest and enthusiasm. One was to award assiduous and valued provincial and foreign reporters the title of associate membership. This status was granted from at least 1740 when Lecat and the Marseilles oculist Daviel[13] were admitted but the number of surgeons thus honoured was never great, presumably from fear lest the title be devalued. By 1750 there were only fourteen foreign and nineteen provincial associates and the figure, though not determined by statute, hovered around this level thereafter. In the second half of the eighteenth century, however, associate membership was not the only honorific carrot the Academy had at its disposal. In 1752 a new category of corresponding member was invented, and from 1759, if not before, five French surgeons a year who were not academicians and had presented the Academy with a detailed

---

[10] The French Society of Antiquarians.

[11] £20.

[12] The city's poor house.

[13] Jacques Daviel (1693–1762) was a Marseilles surgeon who came to national prominence following his development of innovatory techniques for dealing with cataracts in the 1730s and 1740s.

paper or at least three interesting observations in the previous twelve months were awarded a gold medal worth 100 *livres*.[14]

As a result of these manoeuvres the Academy was able to attract a fairly constant supply of books, papers, and observations from all over France. On their receipt, they were placed in the hands of the *commissaire pour les extraits*, whose job was to prepare an accurate and neutral account of their contents. In due course, this account would be read to the assembled members, who would either decide there and then on the value of the submission or would pass it to a special committee for detailed evaluation. Once the Academy had reached a decision, the task of communicating the verdict to the author was given to the *commissaire pour les correspondances*. The latter would draw up a letter containing the Academy's views, which would be read to the assembled company before it was dispatched, thereby ensuring that its message had been officially approved by the academicians.

By successfully soliciting information about new surgical observations and techniques from surgeons all over the country and sitting in judgement on their importance, the Academy throughout its existence fulfilled, albeit imperfectly, its role as the guardian and arbiter of surgical progress. However, as the academicians met in secret . . . and the correspondence with provincial and foreign surgeons was private, its activities as thus far described hardly belonged to the public domain. In order to fulfil its wider brief, to publicize as well as evaluate new surgical findings and eventually to create an authoritative code of surgical practice, the Academy had to imitate further its sister institutions in the capital and publish the observations and discoveries it felt worthy of becoming part of surgical lore. In this regard, however, it was less successful. While the Academy of Sciences published annual transactions throughout the eighteenth century, the Academy of Surgery was only able to make public and permanent its contribution to surgical progress on five occasions: 1743, 1752, 1757, 1768, and 1774.

[14] §4.

13.3

Medicine and the state in eighteenth-century Germany: the plight of the *physicus* or state-physician

'Letter of Georg Spangenberg to the Collegium Medicum of Braunschweig (May 1747)' in Mary Lindemann, *Health and Healing in Eighteenth-Century Germany* (Baltimore and London, Johns Hopkins University Press, 1996), pp. 3–6.

Medical practise in the states of northern Germany in the eighteenth century was policed at local level by government representatives, who had to report periodically to a central committee. The document here is an English translation of a report sent in to the Braunschweig-Wolfenbüttel Medical Board, or Collegium Medicum, in 1746 and offers a good idea of the frustrations felt by a *physicus* or state-physician employed to work in the countryside. Spangenberg was an obscure physician eking out a living in a district of Brunswick (Braunschweig) covering four villages and inhabited by some 5,000 people. He also practised in two neighbouring areas, one belonging to the king of Prussia (a reminder that Germany was a hotchpotch of interlocking states at this period).

An apothecary once lived in Walkenried [but no longer does]; about half an hour from here, in the town of Ellrich, are two apothecaries; there are two more in the town of Bleichrode, about three hours distant; and one [living] about two miles away in Nordhausen. The apothecary shops in Bleichrode and Nordhausen are in good condition; the shop in Ellrich is, however, [only] just adequately maintained. The drugs I use routinely I order from the New Apothecary in Nordhausen. Those medicines that require no special apparatus [to make], I concoct myself; prescriptions, however, I write sometimes for one, sometimes for another apothecary, depending on which is closer to my patients. . . .

At present, only one surgeon, Siegfried Nezel by name, lives in the Walkenried district, in the village of Zorge. He was examined by Physicus Blumen in Blankenburg, and sworn in . . . [and] since that time everyone has seemed quite satisfied with his performance. He visits his patients diligently and willingly, his fees are very moderate, he attempts no treatments without asking for further information and instruction, and, in difficult cases, when [for example] an operation becomes necessary . . . he always consults another, [more] experienced surgeon in Nordhausen or elsewhere, [calling him in] to perform such operations, while he pays close attention in order to learn what he does not know.

As to midwifery, the situation is very unsatisfactory. The three villages [in my district] – Zorge, Wiede, and Hohegeiss – are large and populous. Each village holds about two hundred families, yet each has only a single midwife. When she is ill, or when, as often happens, two women go into labor simultaneously, then the mothers must turn to other women . . . to assist them [in childbed]. According to local custom, each [lying-in] woman may choose any matron as her midwife; the authorities only insist that she pay the regular midwife the [normal] fee of six groschen. No one is ever denied the right to select any woman she pleases as midwife. This principle is sound insofar as it provides the [regular] midwife with an adequate income, but the public [as a whole] suffers. Previously, I supervised the midwives in Walkenried . . . yet am no longer asked to do so. Frau Neuhofer has acted as midwife for several years now [in Zorge?], without being either examined or sworn in; [and] I can do nothing to remedy such [disorders] because Amtmann[15] Heiland completely shuts me out [of affairs and does not allow me] to busy myself with the tasks generally incumbent on a physicus. [Thus] for some years now I have had to let everything take its own course. [At first] I believed that Heiland would eventually see the light and put the common good above all other considerations . . . [but this has not happened].

I took the liberty, then, to denounce the midwife in Zorge officially for her brutal treatment of a birthing woman; she sought to force her into labor too soon and even tried to pull [the child] out of her. For my 'audacity', the ecclesiastical court reprimanded me harshly, fully without cause and quite contrary to any sense of justice.

Because I am allowed knowledge of nothing going on around here and am permitted to attend to nothing, the entire medical situation in Walkenried, since Heiland has become Amtmann, has fallen into the worst possible disarray. Twenty years ago, I received a gracious concession [from the privy council] . . . to practice medicine here, and from the very beginning [of my residence] and until the previous Amtmann Mattenberg died, I executed all the official duties of a physicus, conducted the *visa reperta*[16] [on corpses] and [inspected] all severely wounded persons, tested the abilities of *operateurs* before they . . . cut

---

[15] Magistrate.
[16] A visual inspection; i.e. a coroner's report.

for the stone, or repaired hernias, or couched cataracts, and I super-vised all such operations personally. Whenever workers at one of the ducal ... mines or foundries fell ill or suffered injury, I treated them without charge, even journeying to them at my own expense. When dysentery, or *febres maligna, purpure et petectia* raged,[17] as often hap-pens here, I went in person to visit all patients without distinction, and assisted many of the needy among them, and even gave them medica-tions free of all charge. For all these and [many] similar services, I have never received a penny's worth of salary or in *accidentzen*,[18] except for an annual grant of six cords of firewood and nine shocks of grain, and [as a result] performed these tasks completely without recompense and merely in hope of future preferment. I do not even enjoy the freedom [from taxes] granted to the surgeon [here] ... but rather must pay all contributions and levies, [provide] all services, and [even] hire some-one to do corvée[19] for me. For eighteen years I was allowed to pasture my few animals [on communal meadows] without fee. [But] in the past two years, through the instigation of a certain someone [Heiland], I have been sharply warned that if I wish to enjoy this right in the future, I must request special authorization ... from the ducal treasury. In the Geröder districts, about three hours' journey from here, I have held the office of physicus for eighteen years. In 1743, His Royal Highness the king of Prussia named me as adjunct-physicus for the County of Hohen-stein. ... [A] dispensation granted me by the king of Prussia has per-mitted me to reside in Walkenried, almost in the middle [of the various areas entrusted to me], only one hour away from the city of Sachsa, and scarcely one-half hour distant from Ellrich. Thus I can attend to my duties in Hohenstein ... and there as well as in Geröder ... every aspect of public health is in perfect order. In Walkenried, however, ... every-thing is going to the dogs because I have not been appointed physicus and Heiland opposes me. All kinds of people have settled here, who were not tolerated in Hohenstein and were driven from there. [These], however, wander freely around in Walkenried, cajoling the inhabitants into unnecessary treatments and depriving them of both their money and their health. A tanner's apprentice named Prümann, who was ban-ished from Hohenstein because of his medicating, dwells in the village of Wiede without fear; he has cheated many people out of their money and their health. A baptised Jew, who calls himself Christian Fridrich

---

[17] Three types of fever: malignant, puerperal and petectal. The first type was considered highly contagious; the other two were characterised by the appearance of purple and reddish spots on the skin.

[18] An unexpected or one-off payment.

[19] A feudal due of unpaid work owed by a vassal to a lord.

and was born in Dessau, was found out in Hohenstein and was sentenced to the workhouse in Halberstadt because he violated the Royal [Prussian] Medical Ordinance. Now he practices unhindered in Walkenried. Eight days ago, he treated the mining clerk Fischer, who was consumptive, and in all probability caused his death. [But] last year Amtmann Heiland himself asked Fridrich's help [for an illness], [an action] that prejudices and affronts all [proper] physicians, and engenders feelings of trust in persons [like Fridrich] throughout the population. [Such consultation] clearly transgresses ... the ducal Medical Ordinance. A vagrant, who pretends to be an *operateur*, and goes by the name of Winsil, attempted to couch the cataract of Gürze Kylingen in Hohegeiss. With Heiland's permission, and in the presence of the local pastor Schlegel and the village headman Grimme, he so badly botched the operation that the vitreous humor of both eyeballs welled forth to about the size of a pea. Kylingen, whom a skilled oculist could probably have helped, now stumbles about stone blind. ...

In January of this year, a journeyman blacksmith and Catholic convert from Quedlinburg took up lodgings in Hohegeiss and Zorge and, posing as a priest, sought to cure many people with all sorts of superstitious nonsense, by blessings and by the laying on of consecrated vestments; he also promised to exorcise evil spirits. ... Pastor Colditz in Zorge wrote to Heiland about one of the parish paupers who had taken ill, requesting that Heiland instruct me – according to the provisions of the ducal regulations on poor relief – to assist the man with essential medicines. Heiland responded that such [aid] had to be requested, not from me, but from the district physicus in Blankenburg, who lives five miles [from Zorge], and the medicines must be procured from him. About three years ago, a man from Hohegeiss ... was discovered dead on the road to Zorge. [The body] was only perfunctorily viewed by the military surgeon [Feldsher] who, finding no wounds [on it], allowed the body to be buried without any further investigation. Similar deeds that contravene the Medical Ordinance occur daily, and the public has to suffer under them, [and] I must hold my tongue, no matter what, because I am not a regularly appointed physicus and must fear the fierce enmity [Heiland bears] against me. ...

Over sixty years ago, Nicolaus Kästner was physicus here; almost forty years ago [c. 1707], Dr. Meder [became physicus]. Although he enjoyed a handsome salary, [Meder] found himself unable to make a go of it [and] left. ... From then on, and until I arrived in 1727 ... there was no physician here. The reason why Meder could not remain – the great poverty of the inhabitants – still exists. In Walkenried, there are approximately 700 to 750 large families ... who have no farmland, and who are also not artisans. [They] work either as day laborers, wood choppers, sharecroppers, miners, stokers, smiths, or the like. [And for] all of these, on the day they do not work, they also do not eat, and [they] often are not able to come up with four groschen to save their lives. Among these poor people, many are chronically ill. For every one [of them] that can afford medicines, there are two or three that I must treat for free. . . . This makes it impossible for a physician to earn his bread here or for an apothecary to make a living. What I obtain from my practice outside [of Walkenried] in the Brandenburg jurisdictions and in Geröder and then only [by undertaking] long and wearying journeys, I am forced to spend and throw away again [here] in Walkenried.

13.4

Reforming the medical curriculum: Toulouse (1773)

J. Barbot, *Les Chroniques de la Faculté de Médecine de Toulouse du XVIIIe au XIXe Siècle* (2 vols, Toulouse, Dirion, 1905), vol. 1, pp. 270–2. Translated by Elizabeth Rabone.

The medical Faculty of Toulouse was never one of Europe's most progressive in the eighteenth century, but this extract from the revised statutes of the University, dating from 1773, shows it embraced the new emphasis on teaching medical students anatomy, surgery, chemistry, botany and pharmacy as much as more celebrated institutions. Given that new statutes were only promulgated once the old were obsolete, it can be assumed that the Faculty had expanded its curriculum some time before this date.

Article I

Those who are to study in the Faculty of Medicine at the University of Toulouse in order to take a degree will be required to register in their own hand, on the Faculty registers intended for that purpose and kept with the Secretary of the Faculty, four times a year, in the first month after the schools open and in January, April and July. Each time they register, students are to write the names of the professors whose lectures they will take.

Article II

During the first year, students shall take physiology and hygiene; they shall attend demonstrations of anatomy, chemistry and botany. They shall enrol with the following professors. The first two courses shall be taken by the professors of physiology and anatomy and the last two by the aforementioned professor of physiology and the professor of chemistry and botany.

Article III

In the second year, the students shall follow the lessons of the professor of medicine until Easter, and from Easter until the end of the year, they shall take the lecture dictated by the professor of surgery. These first two courses will be taken by the professors of pathology and medicine and the last two by the aforementioned professor of pathology and the professor of surgery. Students will be required to attend lessons and demonstrations of anatomy, chemistry and botany, without it being necessary for them to enrol under the professors of these various subjects.

Article IV

In the third year, students shall take the lecture taught by the professor of practical medicine; until Easter, they shall continue to follow the lectures of the professor of surgery. The first two courses shall be taken by the professors of practical medicine and of medicine and the last two by the aforementioned professor of practical medicine and the professor of surgery. Students shall also attend lectures and demonstrations in anatomy, chemistry and botany.

Article V

All those who want to take a degree shall be required to take, at the end of three years' study, an examination of two hours' duration on at least those branches of medicine that they have been taught in the preceding year and in the third examination, they will be examined on all the lessons they have taken throughout their medical studies. To this end the candidates for a degree shall submit their applications to the Secretary of the Faculty at the beginning of July. In the application they shall write the names of the professors whose lectures they have attended. The Secretary shall then present the aforementioned applications to the Faculty assembly, which will regularly take place on the first Thursday in July, and in this assembly examiners will be assigned to each of the candidates and the candidates will be given the date of their examination.

[. . .]

The Dean then told those present that it was the custom that one or several of the students was employed in looking after the lecture theatre during anatomy lessons, likewise the chemistry laboratory and other small details relating to the Schools. The students were chosen and nominated by the professors. The Dean said that the distribution of these jobs should be formalised.

On this subject it was decided that three students (one from each of the three years of study) would be chosen to perform these tasks and would be given the name 'monitors' and that in future those who are to perform these tasks will present six students to the professors on Saint Catherine's Day (25 November), two from each of the three years, from amongst whom the professors shall choose three to take over from the previous monitors. So it is concluded.

13.5

The clinical education of the physician in late eighteenth-century France: Philippe Pinel (1793)

Philippe Pinel, *The Clinical Training of Doctors. An Essay of 1793*, ed. and trans. Dora B. Weiner (Baltimore and London, Johns Hopkins University Press, 1980), pp. 77–9, 85–93.

The eighteenth century saw the slow introduction of official hospital-based courses in clinical medicine for the first time, although even on the eve of the French Revolution they were not commonplace. This extract, taken from an essay by the French physician, Philippe Pinel (1745–1826), in 1793, discusses the importance of such courses and how they should be organised. In the 1780s, a number of reform-minded French physicians had called for the establishment of faculty courses in clinical medicine, aware that France was lagging behind other countries in this regard. It was only with the Revolution and the establishment of the National Assembly, however, that clinical medicine became a political issue. In 1790, the Health Committee of the Assembly asked for proposals on the reorganisation of health care in France. Félix Vicq d'Azyr (1748–94), on behalf of the Société Royale de Médecine, produced a hefty report, calling, among other things, for the establishment of medical teaching in hospitals. Initially, nothing came of this initiative, but the Société continued to lobby for reform, and in 1793 (no longer a royal institution) set an essay question on the best method of teaching practical medicine in a hospital. The physician, Philippe Pinel, was one of several respondents.

Pinel took his medical degree at Toulouse in 1773, then moved to Paris where he gained a living before the Revolution as a medical journalist and translator. In 1792 he became a hospital physician and quickly established a reputation as a private teacher of clinical medicine and an expert in mental disorders who promoted a more humane treatment of the mad.

Urgent need for teaching hospitals in France

We hope that the French nation, having just reconquered its most inalienable rights, will create a clinical school promptly. Such an establishment is an urgent and indispensable priority since one of the worst ills that can afflict humanity is ignorance and lack of principles on the part of physicians. We must therefore profit from the experience of other nations and also put the progress made in the other sciences to use in our new establishment. Good judgment and precision will render medical observations useful and conclusive.

Should teaching wards be located in a large or small hospital?

A fundamental question is whether teaching wards should be located in a large or small hospital. This question is solved for surgery: experience indicates that this part of medicine has flourished and progressed only in large hospitals like the Hôtels-Dieu of Paris and Lyon or St. Thomas' Hospital in London. Indeed, small or medium-sized hospitals cannot provide a sufficiently large number of clearly characterized surgical cases such as serious and compound fractures, numerous varieties of hernia operations, kidney stones, aneurysms, lachrymal fistulas, etc. Students [at a small hospital] therefore cannot survey the total subject matter during their academic studies nor can they progress in surgery. Therefore I believe that a surgical teaching ward must be part of a large hospital in order to be an effective center of instruction.

But for medicine a medium-sized hospital like the Charité[20] can be sufficient since it can always provide twenty or thirty well-defined illnesses. Also, the acute illnesses characteristic of each season are available there in sufficient variety to offer students correct and precise data. It is worth mentioning that the basic goal of a teaching hospital is to give students a good grasp of what is already known in medicine. The description of illnesses and all that concerns diagnosis and prognosis offers little medical ground for new research, but relies on repetitious references to the medical literature.

In contrast, there is a part of medicine susceptible of great simplification or rather of complete renewal in contrast to present practice, namely the whole field of materia medica and dietetics. Physicians must totally discard the monstrous hotchpotch of medications, use only simple plants and their derivatives, and designate them by their specific characteristics, as botanists do. As for chemical substances, physicians should use only the simplest and least complicated materials and specify them according to the new nomenclature.

Lastly, dietetics offers endless resources if it is skillfully used and strictly delimits medication. Dietetics can make enormous progress owing to new knowledge in natural history, the analysis of plants, and the cultivation of a large number that have been successfully adapted to our climate. It is from these various points of view that medicine is very liable to improvements and that a medium-sized hospital can provide enough illnesses, enough subject matter for fruitful new research on teaching wards. Simple medication can assist the healing powers of nature and provide a solid base for the art of medicine.

Number of patients on teaching wards

On a teaching ward, painstaking care must be expended on each disease: therefore their number must not exceed the time-limit of medical rounds nor the physician's attention span. The teaching ward at Vienna holds only twelve patients; that at Edinburgh, thirty-two. This last number seems large to me, if one aims at rigorous observation. It is very demanding to see fifteen or twenty patients consecutively. And we wish to banish the disgraceful ease with which the most mediocre doctor seems to run for the door when he makes rounds. The clinical physician must fulfill the double role of exact and faithful observer and of skillful professor who must teach young students the art of observation. He must proceed with wise deliberation, going from one patient to the

[20] Another Paris hospital.

next. His zeal, I would even say his enthusiasm, for the art he practices will often make him prolong the time allotted to certain patients. In the practice of medicine, as in the other arts and sciences, progress results from hard work and rigorous self-criticism, even when others judge you with much indulgence.

Grouping of patients on teaching wards

However one might group and distribute illnesses, one cannot avoid being somewhat arbitrary. The Society of Medicine[21] has proposed several schemes in its *New Plan for the Reform of Medicine in France* [1790]. I believe that nature suggests a distribution according to age and sex. Every age has, so to speak, its own way of life and sickness, and demands fundamentally different therapy for the same disease. This holds equally true for the two sexes. One should first establish two general divisions, one for men, the other for women. The first would be sub-divided into 1) boys up to puberty; 2) adults to about fifty years of age; 3) men from the climacteric to senescence. The women's section would be sub-divided in a similar way and would comprise 1) childhood up to menstruation; 2) the whole period of fertility, that is, from onset to the end of menstruation; 3) from menopause to what is called *femina effeta*. Each of these subdivisions might hold three or four patients, a total of eighteen to twenty-four, a maximum, if one wishes to avoid hasty judgment caused by an excess of work.

[. . .]

Only well-defined diseases admissible to teaching ward

. . . Still another factor one must heed in a teaching hospital is to admit only cases with well-defined symptoms. These diseases will be used to teach students who must confront clear and logical ideas. Therefore it is essential that the total disease picture be as coherent and typical as possible. The students must be shown case histories where a sequence of clearly defined symptoms leads to a favorable or fatal outcome, so that one can classify the illness by simple comparisons and relate it to cases in the literature or in medical practice. I feel I should illustrate this assertion with an example taken from one of the most famous clinical hospitals. The best way of indicating what needs to be done is often to show what was not done.

---

[21] Founded in 1778.

De Haen[22] speaks in his journals . . . of a woman tormented by inveterate and intolerable headaches. When she was young, she had fallen on her head and developed an abscess that had suppurated through the ears. At the age of six she developed smallpox with malignant complications and lost all her hair owing to suppuration. The mother was unable to tell whether this cephalalgia was due to the fall or to some dessicating remedy used after the smallpox to stop the oozing from the head. The sickness lingered, with frequent vomiting, hemorrhaging from the nose, spasms, etc., and finally a dry cough and palpitations. M. De Haen says that this patient provided him with the opportunity of a lengthy disquisition to his students in which he discussed the causes, symptoms, diagnosis, and prognosis of this illness from the beginning of medicine to our day and deduced the required therapy. I beg the pardon of M. De Haen and the whole Vienna School: agreed, one may discuss this sickness for years in learned and vague discourse. But I defy the most acute mind to say anything exact and precise about such an illness or to base treatment on any solid data. M. De Haen's procedure confirms my opinion: he hesitates between placing a seton[23] on the neck, prescribing hydragogous purgatives,[24] sublimate of mercury, leeches and cupping, etc., and ends with childish nonsense, the wearing of verbena[25] around the neck as an amulet. He then submits this sickness to the medical students as a topic for their weekly discussion. I would have acted with more wisdom, had I been professor: I would have forbidden any speeches about a problem with insufficient data and would have directed the students' attention to some other complicated case with well-defined characteristics.

[. . .]

First year of academic studies

The first year of academic studies should be used chiefly for anatomy in the amphitheatres and for the study of some elementary works on physiology and hygiene. . . .

---

[22] Anton de Haen (1704–76) was one of the most celebrated pupils of Boerhaave and a leading proponent of his clinical methods which he taught at Vienna.

[23] A thread inserted in a fold of the skin in order to maintain a channel for the discharge of superfluous matter.

[24] Medicines which remove water or serum from the body.

[25] Vervain.

[. . .]

Main studies in the second year

I think that second-year students should not be admitted to clinical lessons right away. They have not yet mastered the general principles of practical medicine nor acquired the habit of grasping pathologic symptoms. They have not yet reached the level that diagnosis and prognosis require. I would therefore propose that these students spend a great deal of time during their second year attending medical rounds on the general hospital wards. At the same time they should concentrate on studying the best elementary text of practical medicine, for example that of Cullen.[26] One should also try to rid them as much as possible from the habit of seeing through someone else's eyes and trusting someone else's judgment. In order to train them to see for themselves, one might encourage them to follow three or four patients closely. They could write a history of these illnesses while profiting from the remarks of the physician on rounds or from those of some more advanced student. Thus they would learn to recognize external and manifest signs that indicate the nature and severity of illnesses. They would carefully record their observations. In order to stimulate rivalry in a sort of competition, one might encourage two or three students to write the history of the same case, individually and without comparing notes, as soon as their competence permits.

The reading of these case reports would take up part of the professor's class in practical medicine. This course is essential in a teaching hospital. The professor's presentation of the subject matter should be as brief as possible since the students can consult the required textbooks. The other, longer part of the class should be used for the reading and critique of the students' individual work. This would encourage strict habits and teach them to master difficulties. Such classes, or rather, such informal groups, could meet without the paraphernalia of pedantry and give burgeoning talent free play. The professor could enjoy the moving experience of watching passionate and well-motivated young men make rapid progress, unrestricted by sterile efforts at memorization.

[. . .]

Third year studies: structure of sickbed lessons

Students who have mastered the first two years of medical school will have the maturity needed for clinical lessons. They are worthy of learn-

---

[26] William Cullen, Professor of Medicine at Edinburgh. For Cullen, see extract 6.7 above.

ing from the clinical professor according to their ability and knowledge. He will be able to identify the particularly talented students who can assist him in the strict supervision and care of patients. For, of course, each patient shall have his student supervisor, like at the Vienna clinical school, or his assistant supervisor, like at Pavia. It is here especially that an important principle must be applied: always confront the student with difficulties that make him practice under the watchful eye of the professor who will rectify mistakes, fill the lacunae, and preside without fail over the prescription of remedies.

[. . .]

Means of training the students' judgment rather than their memory

The physician's visit to the clinical ward thus essentially consists of listening to the student in charge report on the illness of each patient. In the third year of medical school especially, the progress of the students' knowledge and the acquired habit of observation relieves the professor from going into a host of details. He can be content to remedy omissions, rectify errors, and offer new thoughts on difficult cases. Thus patient care can be prompt, attentive, and enlightened, and at the same time the students can gain experience, a solid foundation for further progress. Every case they observe will be fresh in their minds because it is grounded in concrete observations. It adds to their knowledge and illustrates nature's resources for the cure of diseases and, in certain cases, her errors and impotence. The students' attention is livelier and deeper when concentrated on one object at a time or at least only on similar cases found in the literature or elsewhere in the hospital.

The several patients whom they successively supervise in the same room would thus allow students to investigate and master several diseases in the course of one year. After successful completion of this task, they might continue to pursue it for several more years and even advise other students on the wards. It is obvious that such dedication for two or three years would result in greater expertise in theory and practice. It would also serve to identify the men who are worthiest of public confidence since they will have had the experience of observing several diseases closely and studying their several forms and variations. They could broaden their knowledge to include the influence of the seasons on diseases by an awareness of the acute illnesses prevalent on the general hospital wards. Sydenham[27] developed these principles expertly in his writings.

[27] Thomas Sydenham (1624–89). For the English clinician, Sydenham, and his observations on the seasonal nature of many distempers, see above extract 11.5.

13.6
Surgical instruction in early eighteenth-century Paris

Johannes Gessner's, Pariser Tagebuch 1727,
ed. and trans. U. Boschung (Bern, Hans Huber, 1985), pp. 352–3.
Translation by Rod Boroughs.

Throughout the eighteenth century, medical students who wanted hands-on instruction in the ancillary medical arts had to seek a private tutor. In the second quarter of the eighteenth century, students flocked to Paris to study anatomy and surgery with Europe's acknowledged masters. One of these, the Swiss Johann Gessner (1709–90), kept a diary of his six-month stay in the French capital in the autumn and winter of 1727.

Gessner and his brother came to Paris from Leiden in August 1727 after sitting at the feet of the great Boerhaave. For about a month they attended several courses of lectures on osteology, given by François Le Dran (1685–1770) and others, and enrolled in Le Dran's practical anatomy class at the Charité, which was due to begin in early October and where they would have the opportunity to dissect. Unfortunately, however, the dissection class was put back to November on royal orders, perhaps because the autumn was too warm to make autopsies a practical possibility. In the meantime, Le Dran gave the two Gessners a body illegally and allowed them to learn the basics of dissection in their own lodgings helped by his assistant. The anatomy course in the Charité finally began on 4 November and lasted until Christmas, when the diary ends. The extract describes how the two brothers spent a day in mid-December.

15 December, 7 a.m.
We observed a leg amputation carried out below the knee.[28] The amputation was performed on the right side where the surgeon also stood. A double ligature was applied higher up, together with a second tourniquet a little lower to draw the skin together. He performed the amputation quickly as he only had to saw through one bone. He bound the arteries with two sutures which was enormously painful for the

---

[28] The diarist is in error here; as becomes clear later, the amputation must have been carried out above the knee.

patient. Afterwards the patient was full of praise for the operation. Some of those present were appointed to take care of his truncated limb. The bone was rotten in places; the muscles were all without colour; there was stiffening of the knee joint; and there was water, yellow in colour, instead of blood.

In the afternoon Dr Le Dran bandaged a multiple fracture of the tibia, administered a digestive,[29] and cut away the callused surface skin on the sole of the foot.

He operated on a phimosis.[30] The man who had been afflicted by nature with this condition three times previously was about twenty years old. The cellulous covering membrane of his prepuce would become so inflated that his penis became as thick as a fist. The condition had previously been relieved by means of dispersing poultices, but this fourth time the swelling was so great that it could not be stopped by these remedies and it was feared that gangrene would set in, and so a slot for an operation was granted. He inserted a pointed, ridged instrument into the glans and the penis as far as the crown of the glans. Then he opened up the contracted prepuce with a remarkable knife which was long but exceptionally fine. Due to the patient's violent movements, he was unable to make an incision above the crown. So then he repeatedly opened up the prepuce above the crown of the glans with a scissors. It was incredible how much pain this operation caused the wretched patient, and how much he groaned. Finally, part of the prepuce was also cut away with the scissors.

Today, we received a cadaver afflicted with haemorrhoids, causing the whole body to emit a foul smell. I started dissecting the muscles of the femur while my brother dissected those of the forearm.

During supper, the cook came in. He had almost completely severed the upper part of his thumb so that it was only attached by the skin. A lint dressing containing balsam de copayba was immediately applied, and the thumb was bound with a bandage. As he was being bandaged, the cook fainted, and he was brought round by having cold water sprinkled on his face and by drinking cold water.

---

[29] An application or ointment promoting suppuration.
[30] A contraction of the orifice of the prepuce, so that it cannot be retracted.

13.7
Popular criticism of the medical profession: Tobias Smollett's *Humphry Clinker* (1771)

Tobias Smollett, *The Expedition of Humphry Clinker*
(1st edn 1771; Harmondsworth, Penguin, 1985), pp. 51–3.

English novels, plays and correspondence from the eighteenth century abound in accounts of illness from the perspective of the patient. In this extract, taken from the highly popular picaresque novel, *Humphry Clinker* (1771), we are introduced, in a letter to his confidante, Dr Lewis, to the ailments of Matthew Bramble, a Gloucestershire squire, and his view of the medical profession. Bramble is a curmudgeonly but kind old gentleman, much concerned about the state of his health, whose first ports of call are understandably the Hot Wells at Bristol and the Pump Room at Bath. The author, Tobias Smollett (1722–71), was himself a practising London surgeon, though not a very successful one.

To Dr LEWIS

HOT WELL, April 20.

I understand your hint. There are mysteries in physic, as well as in religion; which we of the profane have no right to investigate – A man must not presume to use his reason, unless he has studied the categories, and can chop logic by mode and figure – Between friends, I think every man of tolerable parts ought, at my time of day, to be both physician and lawyer, as far as his own constitution and property are concerned. For my own part, I have had an hospital these fourteen years within myself, and studied my own case with the most painful attention; consequently may be supposed to know something of the matter, although I have not taken regular courses of physiology *et cetera et cetera*. – In short, I have for some time been of opinion (no offence, dear Doctor) that the sum of all your medical discoveries amounts to this, that the more you study the less you know. – I have read all that has been written on the Hot Wells, and what I can collect from the whole, is, that the water contains nothing but a little salt, and calcarious earth, mixed in such inconsiderable proportion, as can have very little, if any, effect on the animal economy. This being the case, I think the man deserves to be fitted with a cap and bells, who for such a paultry advantage as this spring affords, sacrifices his precious time, which might be employed in taking more effectual remedies, and exposes himself to the dirt, the stench, the chilling blasts, and perpetual rains, that render this place to me intolerable. If these waters, from a small degree of astringency, are of some service in the *diabetes, diarrhœa*, and *night sweats*, when the secretions are too much increased, must not they do harm in the same proportion, where the humours are obstructed, as in the *asthma, scurvy, gout* and *dropsy*? – Now we talk of the *dropsy*, here is a strange fantastical oddity, one of your brethren, who harangues every day in the Pump-room, as if he was hired to give lectures on all subjects whatsoever – I know not what to make of him – Sometimes he makes shrewd remarks; at other times he talks like the greatest simpleton in nature – He has read a great deal; but without method or judgment, and digested nothing. He believes every thing he has read; especially if it has any thing of the marvellous in it; and his conversation is a surprizing hotch-potch of erudition and extravagance. – He told me t'other day, with great confidence, that my case was dropsical; or, as he called it, *leucophlegmatic*: A sure sign, that his want of experience is equal to his presumption; for, you know, there is nothing analogous to the dropsy in my disorder – I wish those impertinent fellows, with their ricketty understandings, would keep their advice for those that ask it – *Dropsy*, indeed! Sure I have not lived to the age of fifty-five, and had such experience of my own disorder, and consulted you and other eminent physicians, so often, and so long, to be undeceived by such a – But, without all doubt, the man is mad; and, therefore, what he says is of no consequence. . . . Let me know what you think of this half-witted Doctor's impertinent, ridiculous, and absurd notion of my disorder – So far from being dropsical, I am as lank in the belly as a grey-hound; and, by measuring my ancle with a pack-thread, I find the swelling subsides every day – From such doctors, good Lord deliver us! – I have not yet taken any lodgings in Bath; because there we can be accommodated at a minute's warning, and I shall choose for myself – I need not say your directions for drinking and bathing will be agreeable to,

Dear Lewis,

Yours ever,

MAT. BRAMBLE

P.S. I forgot to tell you, that my right ancle pits, a symptom, as I take it, of its being *œdematous*,[31] not *leucophlegmatic*.

---

[31] Typical of a localised form of dropsy.

13.8

Alternative therapies in Georgian England: James Graham's Celestial Bed

Roy Porter, *Health for Sale: Quackery in England, 1660–1850*
(Manchester and New York, Manchester University Press, 1989),
pp. 161–2.

James Graham (1745–94) was one of the most outrageous but earnest entrepreneurs and sex therapists to strut the medical stage of late-Georgian England. In this extract the late Roy Porter allows Graham to describe in his own words his apparatus for rejuvenating the barren marriage. Porter's work contains the only modern analysis of the life of Graham. A great self-publicist and author, who produced lengthy accounts of his therapeutic methods, the description here of his Grand Celestial bed is taken from his *A sketch or short description of Dr Graham's medical apparatus* (London, 1780).

Graham resists being categorised solely as an impresario, or as a fanatic; he was both, and it is through this double vision that we must approach the object which won him his notoriety, contemporary and present: in the most private part of the Temple,[32] there stood the Celestial Bed. Graham apostrophised it thus:

> The Grand Celestial Bed, whose magical influences are now celebrated from pole to pole and from the rising to the setting of the sun, is 12 ft. long by 9 ft. wide, supported by forty pillars of brilliant glass of the most exquisite workmanship, in richly variegated colours. The super-celestial dome of the bed, which contains the odoriferous, balmy and ethereal spices, odours and essences, which is the grand reservoir of those reviving invigorating influences which are exhaled by the breath of the music and by the exhilarating force of electrical fire, is covered on the other side with brilliant panes of looking-glass.
>
> On the utmost summit of the dome are placed two exquisite figures of Cupid and Psyche,[33] with a figure of Hymen[34] behind, with his torch flaming with electrical fire in one hand and with the other, supporting a celes-

[32] Graham's Temple of Health was located in the Adelphi, and later in Pall Mall, in London.

[33] Cupid was the Roman god of love, the son of Mercury and Venus. In Greek mythology, Psyche was the butterfly-winged attendant of Eros (Cupid).

[34] In Greek and Roman mythology, Hymen was the god of marriage, usually represented carrying a torch and a veil.

tial crown, sparkling over a pair of living turtle doves, on a little bed of roses.

The other elegant group of figures which sport on the top of the dome, having each of them musical instruments in their hands, which by the most expensive mechanism, breathe forth sound corresponding to their instruments, flutes, guitars[,] violins, clarinets, trumpets, horns, oboes, kettle drums, etc.

At the head of the bed appears sparkling with electrical fire a great first commandment: 'BE FRUITFUL, MULTIPLY AND REPLENISH THE EARTH'.[35] Under that is an elegant sweet-toned organ in front of which is a fine landscape of moving figures, priest and bride's procession entering the Temple of Hymen.

The chief principle of my Celestial Bed is produced by artificial load-stones. About 15 cwt. of compound magnets are continually pouring forth in an everflowing circle. The bed is constructed with a double frame, which moves on an axis or pivot and can be converted into an inclined plane.

The bed was presented to the late-Georgian fashionable world as a fertility shrine, available to couples on a nightly basis:

Should pregnancy at any time not happily ensue [i.e., that is from the regular course of conjugal love] I have the most astonishing method to recommend which will infallibly produce a genial and happy issue, I mean my Celestial or Magnetico-electrico bed, which is the first and only ever in the world: it is placed in a spacious room to the right of my orchestra which produces the Celestial fire and the vivifying influence: this brilliant Celestial Bed is supported by six massive brass pillars with Saxon blue and purple satin, perfumed with Arabian spices in the style of those in the Seraglio[36] of a Grand Turk. Any gentleman and his lady desirous of progeny, and wishing to spend an evening in the Celestial apartment, which coition may, on compliment of a £50 bank note, be permitted to partake of the heavenly joys it affords by causing immediate conception, accompanied by the soft music. Superior ecstasy which the parties enjoy in the Celestial Bed is really astonishing and never before thought of in this world: the barren must certainly become fruitful when they are powerfully agitated in the delights of love.

The Celestial Bed was Graham's much-bruited *chef d'oeuvre*. He clearly intended it as a source of income, since he charged £50 a night for its use. It provided him with vast publicity, and was the subject of smutty lampoons such as *The Celestial Beds* (1781), and *Il Convito Amoroso*

[35] Genesis 1:22.
[36] Harem.

(1782) – this latter probably a self-satire by Graham himself, trading on the assumption that all publicity is good publicity – which depicted jaded couples flocking in, as if to a new ark, to repopulate the species.

Was the bed used, as contemporaries smirked, for debauch and prostitution? There is no evidence for this. Graham himself insisted that the bed was not for voluptuaries but for couples desiring children . . . being designed to overcome flaccidity or barrenness by 'an electrical stroke or two'; and, he hoped, it would work towards the 'propagating of Beings rational, and far stronger and more beautiful in mental as well as in bodily endowments, than the present puny, feeble, and nonsensical race of probationary mortals, which crawl, and fret, and politely play at cutting one another's throats for nothing at all, on most parts of this terraqueous globe'. There was already a plethora of resorts to which the smart set could repair for amorous adventure . . . and bagnios and classy brothels aplenty where attractive bed-mates were to be had (Casanova found one paid up to six guineas). Hence it is unlikely that Graham's high-minded sentiments about sexual rejuvenation served merely as a façade for libertinism or commercial sex. In fact, we have no direct knowledge of what went on between the sheets of the Bed.

Index